Clinical
Obstetrics
AND
Gynecology

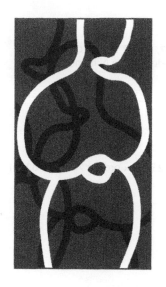

Clinical
Obstetrics
AND
Gynecology

A PROBLEM-BASED APPROACH

Alexander F. Burnett, MD

Assistant Professor
Division of Gynecologic Oncology
University of Southern California
Los Angeles, California

b

**Blackwell
Science**

© 2001 By Alexander F. Burnett

EDITORIAL OFFICES:

Commerce Place, 350 Main Street, Malden, Massachusetts 02148, USA
Osney Mead, Oxford OX2 0EL, England
25 John Street, London WC1N 2BL, England
23 Ainslie Place, Edinburgh EH3 6AJ, Scotland
54 University Street, Carlton, Victoria 3053, Australia

OTHER EDITORIAL OFFICES:

Blackwell Wissenschafts-Verlag GmbH, Kurfürstendamm 57, 10707 Berlin, Germany
Blackwell Science KK, MG Kodenmacho Building, 7-10 Kodenmacho Nihombashi,
Chuo-ku, Tokyo 104, Japan

DISTRIBUTORS:

USA Blackwell Science, Inc.
Commerce Place
350 Main Street
Malden, Massachusetts 02148
(Telephone orders: 800-215-1000 or 781-388-8250; fax orders: 781-388-8270)

Canada Login Brothers Book Company
324 Saulteaux Crescent
Winnipeg, Manitoba, R3J 3T2
(Telephone orders: 204-837-2987)

Australia Blackwell Science Pty, Ltd.
54 University Street
Carlton, Victoria 3053
(Telephone orders: 03-9347-0300;
fax orders: 03-9349-3016)

Outside North America and Australia
Blackwell Science, Ltd.
c/o Marston Book Services, Ltd.
P.O. Box 269
Abingdon
Oxon OX14 4YN
England
(Telephone orders: 44-01235-465500; fax orders: 44-01235-465555)

Acquisitions: Laura Berendson
Development: Jessica Carlisle
Production: Irene Herlihy
Manufacturing: Lisa Flanagan
Marketing Manager: Toni Fournier

Director of Marketing: Lisa Larsen
Cover design by Meral Dabcovich, VisPer
Interior design by Leslie Haimes
Typeset by Northeastern Graphic Services, Inc.

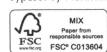

00 01 02 03 5 4 3 2 1

The Blackwell Science logo is a trade mark of Blackwell Science Ltd., registered at the United Kingdom Trade Marks Registry

Library of Congress Cataloging-in-Publication Data

Clinical obstetrics and gynecology : a problem-based approach / edited by Alexander F. Burnett.
 p. ; cm.
ISBN 0-632-04353-9
 1. Obstetrics—Problems, exercises, etc. 2. Gynecology—Problems, exercises, etc. I. Burnett, Alexander F.
 DNLM: 1. Obstetrics—Problems and Exercises. 2. Genital Diseases, Female—Problems and Exercises. 3. Women's Health—Problems and Exercises. WQ 18.2 C641 2001]
RG111.C655 2001
618—dc21
                  00-039760

To Martha,
for her love and encouragement
each step of the way

CONTENTS

IV. REPRODUCTIVE ENDOCRINOLOGY AND INFERTILITY 229

CONTRIBUTORS

Brian D. Acacio, MD
Fellow, Division of Reproductive
 Endocrinology
USC Keck School of Medicine
Los Angeles, California

Raquel D. Arias, MD
Associate Professor, Obstetrics and Gynecology
Associate Dean of Women
USC Keck School of Medicine
Los Angeles, California

Kevin R. Brader, MD
Assistant Professor, Gynecologic Oncology
Vanderbilt University
Nashville, Tennessee

Megan E. Breen, MD
Assistant Professor, Obstetrics and Gynecology
Georgetown University Medical Center
Washington, DC

Brendan F. Burke, MD
Assistant Professor, Obstetrics and Gynecology
Georgetown University Medical Center
Washington, DC

Alexander M. Burnett, MD
Clinical Professor, Obstetrics and Gynecology,
 Retired
Georgetown University Medical Center
Washington, DC

D. A. Dessouky, MD, PhD
Professor, Obstetrics and Gynecology
Georgetown University Medical Center
Washington, DC

Gary D. Helmbrecht, MD
Assistant Professor, Obstetrics and Gynecology
University of Nebraska, Omaha Campus
Director, Maternal Fetal Medicine
Avera Health System
Sioux Fall, South Dakota

William H. Hindle, MD
Professor, Obstetrics and Gynecology
USC Keck School of Medicine
Los Angeles, California

Jeffrey F. Hines, MD
Staff Gynecologic Oncologist
Brooke Army Medical Center
Fort Sam Houston, Texas

Mark H. Incerpi, MD
Assistant Professor, Maternal–Fetal Medicine
USC Keck School of Medicine
Los Angeles, California

John K. Jain, MD
Assistant Professor, Reproductive Endocrinology
 and Infertility
USC Keck School of Medicine
Los Angeles, California

John J. Klutke, MD
Assistant Professor, Gynecologic Urology
USC Keck School of Medicine
Los Angeles, California

Shaun G. Lencki, MD
Division of Perinatology
Western Pennsylvania Hospital
Pittsburgh, Pennsylvania

Michele E. Martin, MS, CGC
Genetics Counselor
Columbia Hospital for Women
Washington, DC

James L. Moore, MD
Gynecologic Oncology
Women's Specialty Center
Jackson, Mississippi

Eva A. Olah, MD
Vice-Chairman, Department of Obstetrics
 and Gynecology
Washington County Hospital
Hagerstown, Maryland

Thomas Pinkert, MD
Director of the Center for Maternal Fetal
 Medicine and Reproductive Genetics
Adventist Health Care
Rockville, Maryland

Ronald K. Potkul, MD
Professor, Chief Division of Gynecologic
 Oncology
Loyola University
Maywood, Illinois

Michele B. Prince, MS, CGC
Division of Genetics, Department of Obstetrics
 and Gynecology
Georgetown University Medical Center
Washington, DC

Tina Raine, MD
Assistant Professor, Obstetrics and Gynecology
University of California, San Francisco
San Francisco General Hospital
San Francisco, California

Preston C. Sacks, MD
Reproductive Endocrinology and Infertility
Columbia Fertility Associates
Washington, DC

Luis E. Sanz, MD
Professor, Chief of Division of Gynecology
  and Obstetrics
Director, Urogynecology and Vaginal
  Reconstruction Clinic
Georgetown University Medical Center
Washington, DC

Young K. Shin, MD
Professor, Anesthesiology
Georgetown University Medical Center
Washington, DC

Cathy Spong, MD
Instructor, Division of Maternal Fetal Medicine
Georgetown University Medical Center
Washington, DC

Jean-Gilles Tchabo, MD
Professor, Obstetrics and Gynecology
Georgetown University Medical Center
Washington, DC

Melvin H. Thornton, MD
Clinical Assistant Professor, Obstetrics
  and Gynecology
USC Keck School of Medicine
Los Angeles, California

do not necessarily have the approval by the Food and Drug Administration for use in the doses and dosages for which they are recommended. The recommendation for each drug should be given only as guidance to the ... ...

With the vast amount of knowledge available today to medical students, prioritization becomes critical in studying clinical subjects. This text presents the core curriculum in obstetrics and gynecology in a new way—utilizing problem-based learning. The data are presented in concert with clinical scenarios that illustrate the key points. This method of teaching facilitates better retention of the material, as concepts are immediately reinforced with clinical correlations. The cases presented are representative of typical patient problems seen in obstetrics and gynecology; in fact, they are modifications of the authors' own clinical experiences. These cases are not trivial detail situations—they are "nuts and bolts" of this field and are typical of what a student may expect to see during his or her third- and fourth-year rotations.

The text utilizes the learning objectives of the Association of Professors of Gynecology and Obstetrics (APGO) and surpasses the student objectives for each area of the specialty. The text is divided into six sections: introduction with the obstetrical/gynecological history and physical and basic procedures; primary care medicine as it relates to obstetrics and gynecology; obstetrics with prenatal, gestational, and post-partum care and complications of obstetrics; reproductive endocrinology and infertility; gynecology and gynecologic oncology; and ethical and legal aspects of care in obstetrics and gynecology.

Each chapter has review questions appearing at the end of the book, which are formatted as board-type questions. These questions allow students to quickly determine whether they have retained the salient points of each chapter. More than 150 figures and photographs illustrate the material and more than 130 charts and tables provide quick access to it. This compact, yet thorough book offers students a unique means of retaining the information presented with the clinical problems and will prove to be a valuable reference during their third- and fourth-year clerkships and beyond.

I would like to acknowledge Joy Denomme, Kathleen Broderick, and Elisabeth Garofalo for their editorial assistance and encouragement in bringing this manuscript to fruition.

A. F. B.

PART I

History and Procedures

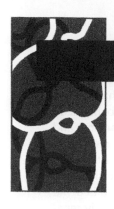

CHAPTER 1

History of Obstetrics and Gynecology

Alexander F. Burnett

The history of obstetrics and gynecology is the history of humanity itself. Only in the last 200 years, however, have practitioners in these fields had any effect on morbidity and mortality from childbirth and infirmities of the female reproductive system. Previously, interventions were undertaken mostly for the purpose of dissecting dead fetuses in utero in an effort to save the mother's life. Sometimes, however, the mother's life was not the primary consideration.

ANCIENT HISTORY

Superstition surrounding conception and childbirth characterizes the ancients' view toward obstetrics. There was clear understanding that the act of intercourse was responsible for conception, but the exact mechanics of the mixture of sperm and egg were rife with unfounded notions. Soranus, the great Roman physician, described contraceptive methods that included utilization of a sponge-like device placed into the vagina to absorb sperm.

Historically, a number of plants were known to act as abortifacients. Included in this group was a plant called *Silphium*, which was used for centuries by the Greeks and Romans. A member of the fennel family, it grew on the coast of what is now Libya. So efficacious and in demand was this agent that the over-harvesting of the plant led to its extinction by the first century A.D. Other, less potent agents survive until today. Reportedly, women in the Appalachian Mountain regions of North Caro-

lina and Tennessee continue to use seeds from Queen Anne's lace for contraceptive purposes. These seeds were heralded by Hippocrates for their contraceptive and abortive properties. Research in 1986 identified compounds within Queen Anne's lace that block the production of progesterone, the hormone necessary for the maintenance of the endometrial lining early in pregnancy.

Post-coital douching was employed in ancient Egypt as early as 1500 B.C., often using concoctions containing such additives as garlic, wine, fennel, and tar. Barrier methods of contraception have been described in ancient China and Japan using oiled silk paper placed against the cervix as a diaphragm. In Europe, Casanova (the well-known lover) described using the rind of a half-lemon placed against the cervix to prevent pregnancy. The oldest known condoms came from ancient Rome, where animal bladders were fitted over the penis, mostly to prevent sexually transmitted diseases. In the 1700s, a resurgence in the condom made from sheep cecum was seen in Europe. By the 1880s, vulcanization of rubber allowed mass production of condoms, which became easily available for the first time.

Contraceptives introduced in the twentieth century include the intrauterine device, the oral contraceptive pill, implantable steroid contraceptives, and the female condom. Newer forms of contraception, such as RU-486, will undoubtedly affect future choices of birth control methods.

Childbirth assistance historically was relegated to midwives, as it was often considered beneath the dignity of physicians. In the past, intervention in delivery most often consisted of perfecting methods of destruction of dead fetuses to attempt to save the mother's life. The Romans had scalpels, dilators, vaginal speculums, decapitators, and cranioclasts available (Figure 1.1). The purpose of the cranioclast, for example, was to decompress the head in cephalo-pelvic disproportion to permit delivery of the dead fetus.

Little advancement in childbirth assistance occurred over the next two millennia. It is clear to see why the obstetrician in these times was held with suspicion, given that his only tools were those of destruction. Consider the way in which William Smellie (1697–1763), the great Scottish obstetrician, described his attendance at the delivery of a dead fetus from a transverse lie in 1754:

"One of the arms had descended, and been so pulled by the midwife, that the shoulder was down to the Os Externum.

I tried to raise the shoulder by passing up along the arm which was excessively swelled and livid, it having been down in that position above four and twenty hours; but I could not introduce my hand. Considering that the child was probably dead from its being so long in that situation, and its not being felt to move by the mother for many hours, I thought it was most expedient to separate the arm from the shoulder. This last being low down, I guided the points of the scissors to it, and easily separated the arm; partly by cutting the skin and ligaments, and partly by pulling and twisting."

Smellie continued to dismember the fetus in an effort to deliver it. He eventually was able to deliver the breach, but had difficulty in delivering the aftercoming head:

". . . I wrapped a cloth round the shoulders, and pulled at them with so great force, as almost to separate the head. By these means, the head was brought a little lower; yet not daring to exert again such violence at the body, I pulled by the crotchet, which brought the head down to the Os Exter-

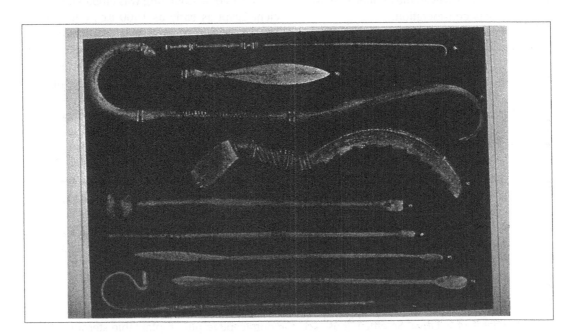

Figure 1.1   Obstetric and gynecologic instruments. First or second century BC. On the top, curettes, uterine sounds, and a catheter; in the center, half of a cranioclast for crushing the skull; on the bottom, a blunt hook, embryotome for incising or dismembering the fetus, and a membrane hook.

Source: Speert H. Obstetrics and gynecology: a history and iconography, 2nd ed. San Francisco: Normal Publishing, 1994:270.

num; and in raising the body and pulling it upwards, it at last separated.

The head however being brought low, I took hold of the under jaw, and pulling at that, while I exerted more force at the crotchet, the head was also delivered."

Forceps (Figure 1.2) were developed around 1600 by Peter Chamberlen of England, but remained a closely held family secret for at least 100 years. The first published description of forceps was made in 1733. Since then, these instruments have undergone many modifications to provide different axises of traction and rotation of the head. In addition, Edmund Piper in 1924 developed forceps for application to the aftercoming head in a breach delivery to provide flexion of the head, rather than traction.

PUERPERAL FEVER

As obstetrics became a more recognized study, an increasing number of women were assisted in delivery by physicians. This care was not always fortuitous, however, as the lying-in hospitals became places of high maternal mortality from puerperal sepsis. As early as 1795, it was proposed that post-partum septic fever may have been caused by an infectious agent that was spread by the hands of the birth attendants. When Oliver Wendell Holmes did a review of the subject for the *New England Quarterly Journal of Medicine and Surgery* in 1843, he concluded that the etiology of this fever was related to an infectious agent spread by the physician or midwife. For his pains, Holmes was roundly denounced by the prominent Boston obstetricians of the day.

Ignaz Semmelweis (1818–1865) sought to study puerperal fever on the wards of the lying-in hospital in Vienna, Austria. In his day, separate wards existed for those patients delivered by physicians and those patients delivered by midwives. The physician ward had a 10-fold increase in puerperal sepsis relative to the midwife ward. When one of Semmelweis's associates at the hospital performed an autopsy on a woman who died of puerperal sepsis, he was cut during the procedure and subsequently developed sepsis and died. Semmelweis concluded that the high incidence of puerperal fever on the physician ward was due

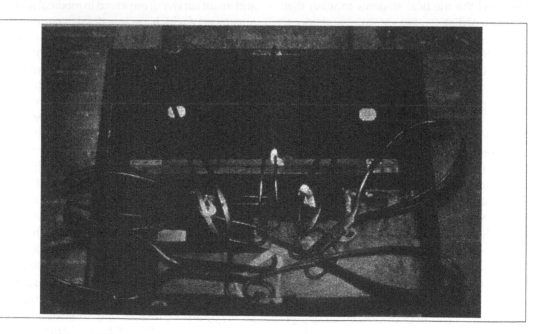

Figure 1.2 The Chamberlen forceps. The original instruments and their attic repository in the home of Dr. Peter Chamberlen.

Source: Speert H. Obstetrics and gynecology: a history and iconography, 2nd ed. San Francisco: Normal Publishing, 1994:281.

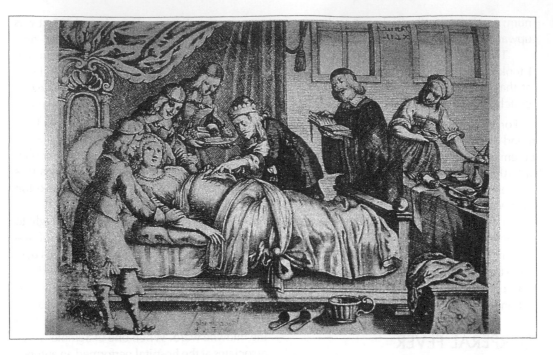

Figure 1.3 Cesarean section. From Scultetus' *Auctarium ad armanentarium chirurgicum,* published posthumously in Leyden, 1653.

to an infectious agent being passed from the autopsy suite to the birthing suites. In 1846, he instructed the medical students to wash their hands immediately after autopsies and prior to deliveries. In four months, the ward had a reduction in post-partum mortality from 45% to 4%, the lowest in Europe.

CESAREAN DELIVERY

Probably no area of obstetrics and gynecology is the source of as much unfounded folklore as the abdominal delivery. Even the name of the procedure is the subject of historical controversy. Julius Caesar was certainly not born by this method, in that his mother was still alive during his early adulthood. In Roman times, this method of delivery was reserved for pregnant women who were dying or dead. Under Pompilius's rule (715–672 B.C.), a decree was issued stating that all women who died late in pregnancy should undergo incisional delivery of the child. This decree became a Lex Regia (royal law), which under the era of Caesar became known as Lex Caesarea. Alternatively, the origin of "cesarean" delivery may be from the Latin *caedere,* to cut.

Numerous reports of successful cesarean deliveries (that is, those in which both mother and infant survived) are found in medical literature, most of which are anecdotal in nature and reported quite distant from the time of the event. The majority of women died from the surgery due to blood loss or, if they survived the initial procedure, peritonitis in the post-partum period. One questionable cesarean delivery involved Lady Jane Seymour, who went into spontaneous labor on October 10, 1537 (Figure 1.4). Lady Jane was the third wife of Henry VIII of England. At one point in her long difficult labor, King Henry is reported to have said to the court physicians, "Save the life of the child, for another wife can easily be found." It is unclear whether the method of delivery, which took place two days later, was cesarean or vaginal. Lady Jane did attend the baptism on a stretcher on October 16, but succumbed to presumed peritonitis on October 24. The son born to Lady Jane, Edward VI, reigned only six years.

In the late 1800s, Edward Porro (1842–1902) established what became know as the Porro operation, in which the cesarean delivery was followed by a supra-cervical hysterectomy. The theory was that the retained uterus

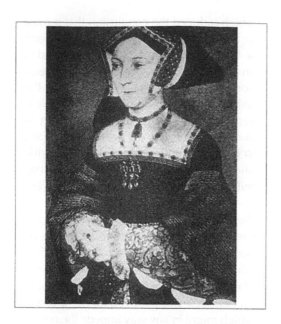

Figure 1.4　Jane Seymour, third wife of Henry VIII (1536). From the painting by Holbein in the Belvedere Gallery, Vienna.

Source: Hellman LM. Three deliveries that changed the history of the world. Maryland State Medical Journal, November 1972:41–48.

after delivery was the chief culprit of postpartum infection. A dramatic account, complete with photographs, of the delivery of Julia Cavallini (a ricketic dwarf; see Figure 1.5) on May 21, 1876, is provided by Porro:

"I did not press the matter until 4 p.m. By now the pains were quite strong, and these alone sufficed to persuade the patient to accept our advice . . . At 4:40 p.m. she was taken to the obstetric amphitheater . . . At 4:42 p.m. the chloroform anesthesia was begun . . . At 4:51 p.m. we began to cut through the abdominal wall . . . After the peritoneal cavity was opened . . . the uterus was immediately incised in the same direction and to the same extent as the abdominal incision . . . We extracted a large [3300-gm] female infant, alive, healthy, well formed, and crying spontaneously . . . we proceeded to extract the placenta, which was removed intact.

The uterus bled from its cut edges. We brought the organ out through the abdominal incision . . . but adequate hemostasis could not be obtained . . . Holding the uterus up out of the abdominal wound . . .

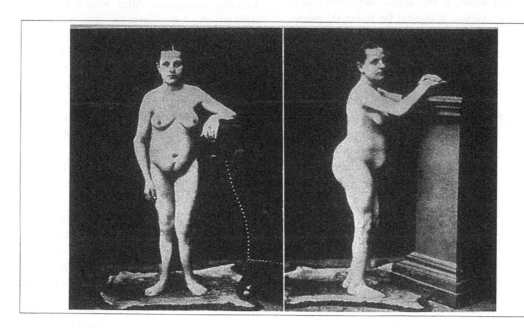

Figure 1.5　Julia Cavallini: a ricketic dwarf on whom Eduardo Porro performed a successful cesarean hysterectomy in 1876.

Source: Porro E. Dell'amputazione utero-ovarica come complemento di taglio cesareo. Ann Univ Med e Chir 1876;237:289.

we placed the strong wire snare of Cintrat at the level of the internal os and drew it very tight . . . After we ascertained that the blood flow was completely shut off, we excised the uterus above the ligature."

GYNECOLOGIC SURGERY

The history of gynecologic surgery is shorter, but no less dramatic than that of obstetrics. Surgery in ancient times consisted mainly of excision of necrotic lesions. The Romans listed four manners of treating uterine prolapse:

1. Suspend a woman upside down on a ladder for 24 hours, then put her to bed and restrict her to cool drinks.

2. Introduce a piece of beef into the vagina.

3. Distend the vagina with bellows, replace the prolapsed uterus, and keep it in place by introducing into the vagina a pomegranate that has been peeled and hardened with vinegar.

4. Prescribe bedrest to reduce the prolapse, then place a tampon soaked in astringents into the vagina to keep the uterus in place for three days, followed by sitz-baths in warm wine. If the organ becomes black (gangrenous), it should be removed surgically, which is generally done without danger to the patient.

The history of gynecologic procedures after this time consisted of mostly anecdotal reports with little verification. In 1809, the first reported successful oophorectomy in the United States occurred in Danville, Kentucky, by Ephraim McDowell with the assistance of his nephew. He describes the case of Jane Crawford:

"In December, 1809, I was called to see a Mrs. Crawford, who had for several months thought herself pregnant. So strong was the presumption of her being in the last stage of pregnancy, that two physicians, who were consulted on her case, requested my aid in delivering her. The abdomen was considerably enlarged, and had the appearance of pregnancy, though the inclination of the tumor was to one side, admitting of an easy removal to the other. Upon examination, per vaginam, I found nothing in the uterus; which induced the conclusion that it must be an enlarged ovarium. Having never seen so large a substance extracted, nor heard of an attempt, or success attending any operation, such as this required, I gave to the unhappy woman information of her dangerous situation. She appeared willing to undergo an experiment, which I promised to perform if she would come to Danville (the town where I live), a distance of sixty miles from her place of residence. This appeared almost impracticable by any, even the most favourable conveyance, though she performed the journey in a few days on horseback. I commenced the operation, which was concluded as follows: Having placed her on a table of the ordinary height, on her back and removed all her dressing which might in any way impede the operation, I made an incision about three inches from the musculus rectus abdominis, on the left side . . . the tumor then appeared full in view, but was so large that we could not take it away entire. We put a strong ligature around the fallopian tube near to the uterus; we then cut open the tumor . . . [and] took out fifteen pounds of a dirty, gelatinous looking substance. After which we cut through the fallopian tube, and extracted the sack, which weighed seven pounds and one half. We then turned her upon her left side, so as to permit the blood to escape; after which we closed the external opening with the interrupted suture, leaving out, at the lower end of the incision, the ligature which surrounded the fallopian tube. Between every two stitches we put a strip of adhesive plaster, which, by keeping the parts in contact, hastened the healing of the incision. In five days I visited her, and much to my astonishment found her engaged in making up her bed. I gave her particular caution for the future; and in twenty-five days; she returned home as she came, in good health, which she continues to enjoy."

Keep in mind that these procedures were performed in an era prior to antibiotics, sterilization, or anesthesia. On January 19, 1847, James Young Simpson (1811–1870), the famous Scottish obstetrician, first administered ether to a woman in labor. He was greatly criticized as being unnatural, and even heretical, in trying to eliminate the pain of labor. He and his associates experimented with various concoctions after dinner each evening in an attempt to find better anesthetic agents. On November 4, 1847, Simpson came upon chloroform, with which he subsequently had great success in alleviating labor and delivery discomfort. His critics were finally silenced after chloroform was given to Queen Victoria during a delivery, after which she made Simpson a baron in appreciation of his discovery.

James Marion Sims (1813–1883) is considered the father of modern gynecologic surgery. Sims, who was raised and educated in South Carolina, set up practice in Alabama after the unfortunate deaths of his first two patients in South Carolina. In the era of slavery, the issue of vesico-vaginal fistulae became one of economics and convenience for slave owners. If a house slave developed a fistula (generally from protracted childbirth), she would constantly leak urine and be quite odorous. Therefore, she would be relegated to the fields—an inconvenience to the slave owner. Sims performed more than 40 vaginal procedures on three slave women (Anarcha, Betsy, and Lucy) before discovering appropriate suture materials and techniques to affect a cure. He became an extremely influential gynecologist in his day, eventually practicing in Europe and in New York. Sims is credited with founding the forerunner of the Memorial Sloan Cancer Institute, and his legacy persists in the form of the Sims retractor, which he developed, and the Sims position, which he utilized in repair of vesico-vaginal fistulae. Sims was also a strong proponent of hand-washing prior to any surgical procedure.

The late 1800s saw major advances in gynecologic surgery, with the Johns Hopkins Hospital leading the way in this regard. Howard Kelly was one of the first professors at Johns Hopkins. He is credited with developing the cystoscope, developing techniques for uterine suspension, and improving vesico-vaginal fistula repair. In addition, he was the first to advocate treatment of gynecologic cancers with X rays and radium. Further improvement in gynecologic cancer care was achieved by another Johns Hopkins surgeon, John Clark, who is credited with performing the first radical hysterectomy for removal of cervical carcinoma.

With improvement in anesthetics, antibiotics, blood products, surgical equipment and techniques, such procedures are now considered commonplace and suffering from gynecologic problems has been greatly reduced. For instance, George Papanicolaou (1883–1962) developed a screening technique for detecting invasive and preinvasive cancers of the cervix that has diminished the incidence and mortality from this disease in the United States. The development of ultrasound imaging during the last 30 years has revolutionized the care of high-risk pregnancies, and more recent techniques have allowed procedures to be performed on fetuses in utero. These two examples represent the types of developments that can be predicted in the coming century for obstetrics and gynecology, when we can expect further improvements in screening and prevention of disease, as well as improvements in techniques to treat existing maladies.

SUMMARY

The history of obstetrics and gynecology reflects the history of humankind. It is a fascinating story entwined with much myth and legend. Superstition continues to play a dominant role in issues surrounding childbirth, even among the educated population. Advances in science have improved obstetrics from a service of dismembering dead fetuses in an effort to save the mother's life to commonplace close management and surgical delivery of gestations who may be in danger. Refinement in preconceptual screening, improved reproductive techniques, better identification and management of high-risk pregnancies, and better medical care of mothers with systemic illnesses will be explored in detail in this book, where we will emphasize the advances made in the field of obstetrics. In gynecology, improved knowledge of the disease processes, surgical and medical advances, and increased screening for diseases in earlier stages will continue to diminish the suffering in women with genitally related illnesses.

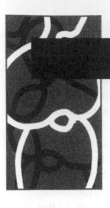

CHAPTER 2

Clinical Anatomy of the Pelvis

Alexander F. Burnett

Gynecology is a surgical specialty; therefore, a thorough understanding of the anatomy of the pelvis is crucial before exploration or treatment of the female genital tract can begin. One must become familiar with the internal and external organs in the reproductive system, as well as adjacent tissues that may produce symptomatology in the same region. Critical to the anatomy of these organs is their blood supply, lymphatic drainage, and enervation. This chapter will present the basics of gynecologic anatomy, with clinical correlations.

EXTERNAL GENITALIA

The external genitalia of the female reproductive tract are presented in the reproductive state (Figure 2.1)—that is, in a woman who has gone through puberty and has not yet reached menopause. These genitalia consist of the vulva, the mons, the introitus with the urethral and vaginal openings, and the perineum between the vulva and the perirectal area. The vulva contains the outer labia majora, the smaller inner labia minora, and the clitoris. The labia are analogs of the male scrotum. The clitoris contains two corpora and a glans, similar to the penis; it does not, however, contain the urethra. The majority of the blood supply to the external genitalia comes from branches of the internal pudendal artery, which is itself a branch of the anterior hypo-

gastric artery. The lymphatic drainage of the external genitalia flows to the lymph nodes in the groin region.

CLINICAL CORRELATION

B. T. is a 72-year-old woman with an exophytic cancerous growth on her right labia majorum. The tumor measures 4 cm, and a biopsy reveals a squamous cell carcinoma. Where is she at risk for lymphatic metastases?

In vulvar cancer, the groin nodes are the most likely area of initial lymphatic metastases. If the lesion is limited to one side of the vulva, the most likely region to be involved is the ipsilateral groin. Treatment of this tumor consists of radical resection of the tumor with dissection of the ipsilateral groin nodes. If any of the nodes are grossly positive, the contralateral nodes should be dissected as well.

The nerve supply to the female perineum is from the pudendal nerve, which arises from S2–S4. This nerve branches further to provide the inferior rectal nerve, the superficial and deep branches of the perineal nerve, and the dorsal nerve of the clitoris.

The vagina is a tubular structure that is approximately 10 cm in depth, and capable of expanding with sexual intercourse or childbirth. The vascular supply comes from branches of the internal pudendal artery as well as direct

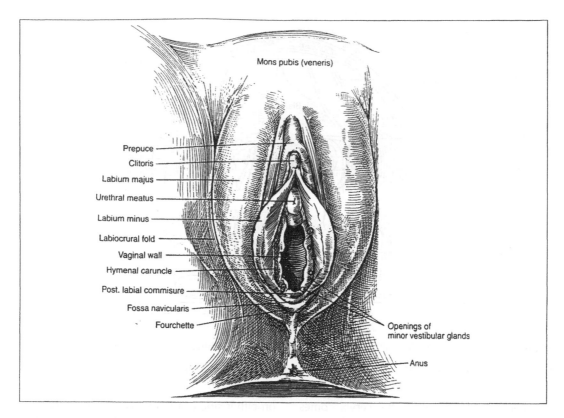

Mons pubis (veneris)

Prepuce
Clitoris
Labium majus
Urethral meatus
Labium minus
Labiocrural fold
Vaginal wall
Hymenal caruncle
Post. labial commisure
Fossa navicularis
Fourchette

Openings of
minor vestibular glands

Anus

Figure 2.1 External female genitalia

Source: Copland textbook of gynecology. Philadelphia: W. B. Saunders, 1993:50.

branches from the hypogastric artery and branches from the uterine artery. The lymphatic drainage from the lower one-third of the vagina flows to the groin nodes, and the upper two-thirds of the vagina drains to the pelvic lymph nodes. During sexual excitement, lubrication is released from the vaginal walls as a transudate. Under normal circumstances, there are no glands within the mucosa of the vagina. Instead, the vagina is covered with squamous epithelium that responds to estrogen by cornification (thickening of squamous cells). If a woman lacks estrogen, as might occur with menopause, the skin of the vagina may become atrophic, and the patient may have difficulty with sexual lubrication and may easily bleed.

The innervation of the vagina and the upper genital tract occurs mainly from the hypogastric plexus. The lowest portion of the vagina is also innervated by the pudendal nerve. Pain fibers from the vagina travel with the sacral parasympathetics and enter the cord via nerves S2, S3, and S4.

UPPER GENITAL TRACT

The uterus consists of the body (corpus) and the cervix (Figure 2.2). The cervix is that part extending into the vagina; it measures approximately 5 cm in length. The central canal of the cervix—the endocervical canal—functions as a conduit between the uterus and vagina. Through this canal will travel sperm to fertilize the egg at the time of ovulation; in addition, menstrual blood will pass out the same route to the vagina at the time of menstruation. The canal of the cervix is lined with glandular epithelium, which undergoes metaplasia to squamous epithelium at the transformation zone on the exocervix. The majority of cervical dysplasias and carcinomas develop within the transformation zone. The glandular elements of the cervical canal extrude a thick mucus for the majority of the woman's ovulatory cycle. At the midcycle when ovulation occurs, however, estrogen causes the mucus to become watery, which is more favorable to sperm penetration.

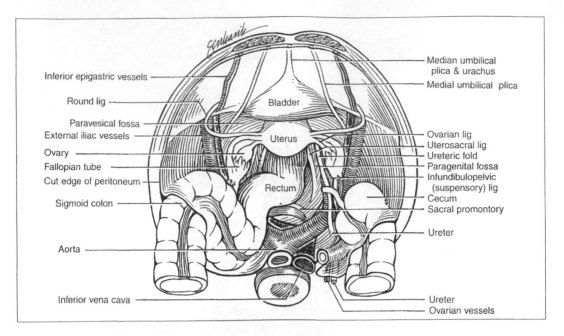

Figure 2.2   The upper female genital tract demonstrating the relationship of the uterus, bladder, and rectum

Source: Morrow CP, Curtin JP, eds. Gynecologic cancer surgery. New York: Livingstone, 1996.

The vascular supply to the cervix comes from vessels from the hypogastric and uterine arteries. The major vessels run along the lateral portion of the cervix, which corresponds to the 3 o'clock and 9 o'clock positions if one is viewing the cervix through a speculum with the round exocervix being analogous to a clock face. Sutures may be placed in these regions to diminish bleeding from the cervix for minor procedures such as a cervical conization. During labor and delivery, the cervix becomes progressively thinner as the presenting part of the baby pushes downward through the birth canal. In a primiparous woman, the cervix typically thins completely before beginning to dilate. Progressive dilation of the cervix must occur to allow passage of the baby. In multiparous women, the cervix may dilate a significant amount without thinning as it has previously been stretched from childbirth.

The uterine corpus (body) contains the endometrial cavity and connects with the fallopian tubes. The uterus is maintained in position by several ligamentous attachments to the pelvis. Along the superior aspect of the uterus on either side is the round ligament, which traverses to the pelvic sidewall, then through the inguinal canal to attach to the labia majora. The broad ligaments are folds of peritoneum on either side of the uterus that cover the lateral aspects of the uterus to the sidewall. Also covered by the broad ligaments are the parametria, the uterine vessels, the ureters, the round ligaments, and the para-ovarian regions. The posterior aspect of the uterus is connected to the sacrum via the utero-sacral ligaments. The anterior aspect of the uterus is connected to the bladder by the vesico-uterine ligaments, or bladder pillars.

The lower aspect of the uterus, the cervix, and the upper vagina connect to the lateral pelvis by the Cardinal ligaments (parametria). These ligaments are important for supporting the uterus and preventing descensus (relaxation) of the uterus into the vagina. In addition, they carry the lymphatic channels from these areas to their regional lymph nodes. During surgery for cervical carcinoma, the Cardinal ligaments are resected to remove the lymphatics from the cervix. Other critical structures that are contained in the Cardinal ligaments include the ureters and the uterine vessels.

The wall of the uterus consists of a thin serosal covering in the peritoneal cavity, an inner endometrial layer that changes with the ovulatory cycle, and a thick middle layer—the myometrium—that is composed of smooth muscle. The muscular portion is responsible for uterine contractions with childbirth and with menstruation. These contractions function to expel the fetus and to constrict the vascular channels within this organ. The endometrium is a dynamic layer that responds to the sex steroids by initially increasing in thickness under the influence of estrogen, then stabilizing in thickness under the influence of progesterone, and finally becoming ischemic and sloughing with the withdrawal of both hormones. If implantation of a fertilized zygote occurs during the cycle, then the corpus luteum of the ovary continues to secrete progesterone, which allows maintenance of the endometrium to nourish the zygote.

The major blood supply to the uterus is the uterine artery, which is a branch of the hypogastric (internal iliac) artery. On occasion, with severe uterine hemorrhage, the hypogastric artery must be ligated to diminish the blood supply to the uterus. The venous return takes place parallel to the arterial supply of the uterus. The lymphatic drainage from the uterus consists of the pelvic lymph nodes and the lymph nodes in the region of the aortic bifurcation (the para-aortic lymph nodes).

On either lateral side of the uterus lay the ovaries and fallopian tubes. The ovaries connect to the uterus via the utero-ovarian ligaments. The vascular supply to the ovaries occurs via the infundibulopelvic ligament. The ovarian arterial supply originates from the aorta. The venous return takes place through the vena cava on the right and the renal vein on the left. The lymphatics from the ovary follow the vascular supply. The ovaries' primary functions include the recruitment and ovulation of an egg each cycle and production of the female sex steroids. A delicate balance occurs between the hypothalamus, the pituitary, and the ovary for the production of gonadotropin-releasing hormone, gonadotropins, and the two sex steroids, estrogen and progesterone. The ovary is also capable of producing androgens, the majority of which are eventually aromatized within the ovary to estrogens.

The fallopian tubes (oviducts) are adjacent to the ovaries. The distal ends of these tubes contain the fimbria—finger-like projections that assist in the capture of the ovum after ovulation. The tubes, which are approximately 10 cm in length, are divided into four segments (Figure 2.3). Going medially from the fimbriae is the ampulla, which progressively narrows, then the isthmic portion, then the interstitial portion, which traverses the myometrium and terminates in the uterine ostia. Lining the fallopian tubes are ciliated cells that assist in moving the ovum through the tube to the uterus. After ovulation, the ovum is picked up by the fimbria and brought into the ampullary portion of the tube.

Normally, fertilization takes places within the ampulla. The fertilized zygote will reach the endometrial cavity in approximately four to five days and become implanted in the endometrium in another one to two days. Women who have severe damage of the cilia secondary to scarring or infection, or women who have congenital absence of the cilia in the fallopian tubes, are generally infertile. Lesser damage to the fallopian tubes may allow fertilization to occur with inadequate transport of the pregnancy, leading to an ectopic gestation. The most common site for an ectopic pregnancy is the fallopian tube—most frequently in the ampulla (55%), followed by the isthmic region (20% to 25%), the fimbria (17%), and the interstitial segment (2% to 4%).

The vascular supply to the fallopian tube is mostly from the ovarian vessels, and the lymphatic drainage parallels that of the ovaries.

THE URETER

While not considered a part of the female genitalia, the ureter (Figure 2.4) has an intimate relationship with the female pelvic anatomy. It runs from the hilum of the kidney to the bladder. It begins in a position lateral to the pelvic vessels, then crosses over the bifurcation of the external and internal iliac arteries to continue medially to these vessels. The ureter is adherent to the medial leaflet of the peritoneum in the pelvis. It comes proximal to the uterus at Wertheim's canal (the ureteral tunnel), which begins where the uterine vessels come medially over the ureter. The ureter travels then along the cervix until it enters the bladder at the trigone.

The areas where the ureters may be in-

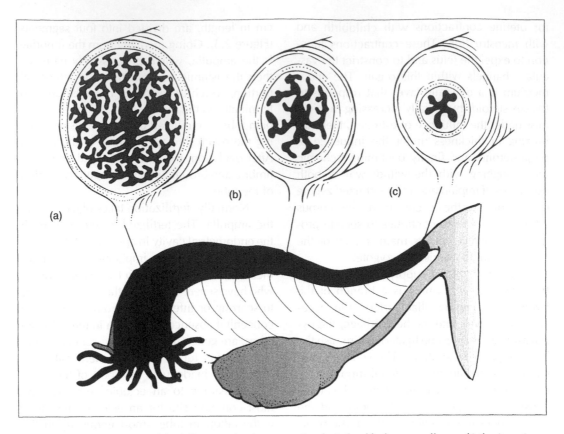

Figure 2.3   Cross sections of the fallopian tube demonstrating the infundibular, ampullar, and isthmic regions
Source: Droegemueller.

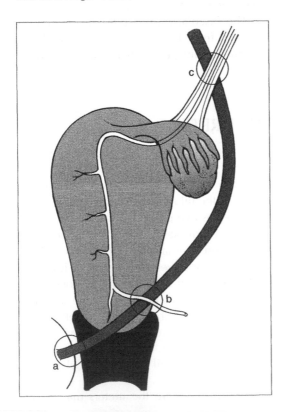

jured during gynecologic procedures are as follows (Figure 2.4):

a.   Proximal to the utero-vesical junction near the trigone

b.   Proximal to the uterine vessels at the tunnel

c.   Proximal to the infundibulo-pelvic ligament at the pelvic brim

Visualization of the ureter and use of proper surgical technique will diminish injury to these structures.

THE AVASCULAR SPACES

The female pelvis contains eight avascular spaces that may be utilized during surgical approach to the pelvic organs (Figure 2.5). These spaces provide convenient regions for manip-

Figure 2.4   Common sites of ureteral injury associated with hysterectomy

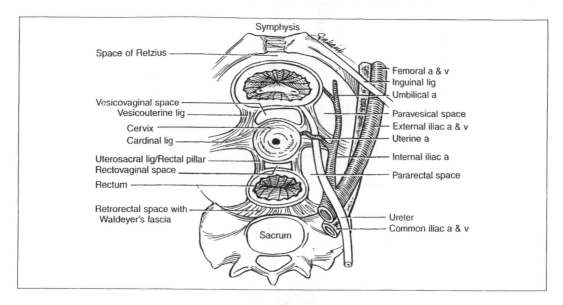

Figure 2.5 Female anatomy at the level of the bladder, cervix, and rectum, demonstrating the avascular spaces of the retroperitoneum

Source: Morrow CP, Curtin JP, eds. Gynecologic cancer surgery. New York: Livingstone, 1996.

ulation of the pelvic organs so that surgery can be accomplished safely. All of these spaces are outside the peritoneal cavity.

Beginning anteriorly, the area anterior to the bladder is called the prevesical space or space of Retzius. This area is important when suspending the bladder neck to correct anatomical urinary incontinence. The next avascular space in the midline is the vesico-vaginal space, which separates the bladder from the cervix and vagina. This space must be developed to safely remove the uterus and cervix when performing a total hysterectomy. Next is the rectovaginal space between the rectum and vagina. This space, like all of the avascular spaces, can be developed down to the pelvic floor. It is most critical to develop it when undertaking radical cancer procedures or during a hysterectomy when the rectum is adherent to the posterior cervix and vagina secondary to scarring. Most posteriorly is the rectorectal space, which is utilized only during surgery to remove the distal colon.

Laterally, two spaces appear on either side, called the pararectal and paravesical spaces. Surgical exploration of the pararectal space involves identifying the ureter medially, the hypogastric artery laterally, and the Cardinal ligament inferiorly. This space also goes down

to the pelvic floor. The benefit of opening it comes in displacing the ureter away from the pelvic vessels so as to gain access to the uterine vessels from a lateral approach. The paravesical space is found between the external iliac artery lateral and the superior vesical artery medial. Utilization of these avascular spaces will allow better access to the genital organs and will decrease injury to adjacent pelvic organs.

PELVIC FLOOR

The pelvic floor is an interconnecting sling of muscles that includes openings for the vagina, the urethra, and the rectum and, at the same time, provides support for the pelvic viscera. When weakening of the pelvic floor occurs because of prolonged labor or multiple childbirths, hernias can occur that affect the continence of stool and urine. Chapter 43 deals specifically with the consequences of pelvic relaxation.

The floor consists of the coccygeus muscles and the levator ani, which is a composite of three muscles: the puborectalis muscle, the iliococcygeus muscle, and the pubococcygeus muscle (Figure 2.6). The puborectalis and pubococcygeus muscles are critical for the external sphincter mechanism of the rectum. Re-

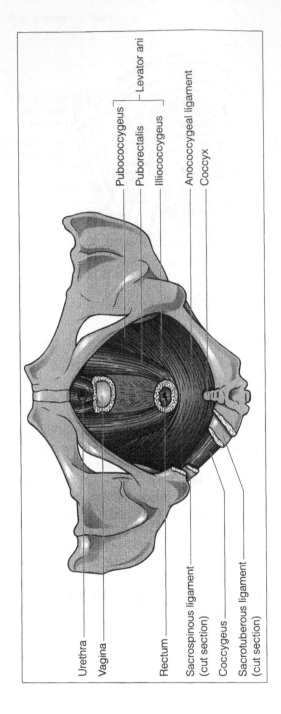

Figure 2.6 Structural support of the pelvis demonstrating the levator ani muscles

Source: Callahan TL, Caughey AB, Heffner LJ. Blueprints in obstetrics and gynecology. Malden, MA: Blackwell Science, 1998:114.

Table 2.1 Blood Supply, Lymphatics, and Nerves of the Female Genitalia

	VULVA	VAGINA	CERVIX	UTERUS	TUBES AND OVARIES
Artery	Internal pudendal External pudendal Clitoral	Descending branch of uterine Internal pudendal Inferior rectal	Uterine artery	Uterine (from hypogastric)	Gonadal artery from aorta
Venous (if different from artery)					Right ovarian vein drains into inferior vena cava Left ovarian vein drains into left renal vein
Lymphatics	Inguinal nodes	Upper: pelvic nodes Lower: inguinal nodes	Pelvic nodes	Pelvic and para-aortic nodes	Predominantly para-aortic aortic nodes
Nerves	Pudendal (S2–S4) Ilionguinal (L1) Genito-femoral (L1–L2)	Sensory: Pudendal Autonomic: vaginal plexus	Sensory accompanies parasympa-thetics to S2, S3, and S4	Sensory accompanies sympathetics (T11, T12) Parasympa-thetics to S2, S3, and S4	Sensory to T11, T12, and L1 Autonomics to uterine and ovarian plexus

pair of anatomical causes of stool or urinary incontinence requires a surgical restoration of the pelvic floor.

SUMMARY

A thorough understanding of the blood supply, innervation, and lymphatic drainage of the pelvic organs is necessary to diagnose and treat maladies of the female genital tract. This information is critical in the surgical approach to gynecology, obstetrics, and gynecologic oncology. Table 2.1 summarizes these key elements for each structure of the female genitalia.

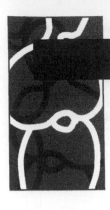

CHAPTER 3

History and Physical Examination

Megan Breen

The gynecologic history and physical examination should be incorporated into every woman's general medical history and examination. Many of the topics covered are of a sensitive nature dealing with women's sexuality. It is essential that the physician maintain a nonjudgmental, professional attitude, regardless of personal opinion. It is preferable to interview the patient initially in a room separate from the examination room, with the patient fully clothed. At the completion of the examination, findings and future management should be discussed in a similar manner in the office, rather than the examination room.

A thorough obstetric and gynecologic history and physical examination will include the following components.

HISTORY

A general history is required in addition to the specifics for obstetrics and gynecology. For many women in the reproductive age group, the gynecologist will serve as the primary physician.

CHIEF COMPLAINT

This statement summarizes the primary reason for the patient's visit, preferably in her own words.

HISTORY OF PRESENT ILLNESS

This history consists of a thorough review of the associated symptoms, duration, and aggra-

vating or alleviating factors of the chief complaint. Portions of the history are reviewed if relevant. For instance, for a woman presenting with a suspicious pelvic mass, her family history for breast, ovarian, endometrial, and colon cancer is pertinent. The information in this section is used to describe the chief complaint in detail. The introduction of the patient should include her gravity and parity (discussed later in this chapter) and the date of the onset of her last normal menstrual period, if relevant.

OBSTETRICAL HISTORY

Record all prior pregnancies and their outcomes, including complications, molar gestations, ectopic gestations, and spontaneous and elective abortions. For deliveries, state whether normal spontaneous vaginal delivery occurred or whether a cesarean delivery was required, and the reasons for such intervention. Also include the number of weeks at which delivery occurred. In addition, operative vaginal delivery should be documented (forceps or vacuum). For a woman presenting for prenatal care, documentation of prior deliveries in terms of weight, sex, length of labor, anesthesia, and congenital malformations should be described.

Two commonly used abbreviations in describing obstetrical history are G for "gravida" (total number of pregnancies) and P for "parity" (results of the pregnancies). Parity is further subclassified into full-term deliveries, premature deliveries, deliveries prior to 20 weeks (abortions, either spontaneous, induced, or ectopic), and number of living children. For example, a woman who had two miscarriages at eight weeks gestation and then delivered three term infants who are all currently living would be G5P3023 (five pregnancies, three full-term, no preterm, two abortions, and three living children).

GYNECOLOGIC HISTORY

The menstrual history should include the age of menarche, the frequency and regularity of menstrual cycles, and the duration of menses. This history may be expressed in an abbreviated form, such as 12 y.o. × 28 d. × 5–6 d. (onset at age 12, menses every 28 days, and menstrual flow lasting 5 to 6 days). The amount of flow and any pain associated with the menses (dysmenorrhea) should be discussed. The woman should be questioned about bleeding between her periods, even if it is slight, and post-coital bleeding (bleeding after intercourse). Any post-menopausal bleeding requires a thorough evaluation.

The basic gynecologic history should include the time of last Pap smear and the regularity of Pap smears, if the patient has any history of an abnormal Pap smear and if any therapy was required for that abnormality. Also, the patient should be questioned about any history of ovarian masses or pelvic abnormalities, and any history of recurrent vaginal yeast infections or discharge.

The sexual history is also an integral part of the gynecologic history. The age at first intercourse (coitarche) and total number of lifetime sexual partners are relevant to the development of cervical dysplasia. The patient should be asked if she has any pain during intercourse (dyspareunia) and, if so, the complaint should be characterized. Many women will not volunteer this information unless directly questioned. A history of contraception, including types used, failures, and reasons for discontinuation, should be discussed.

As the patient ages, urologic issues become more important. Many post-menopausal women develop symptoms of urinary incontinence, but may not mention it unless directly questioned. All women should be questioned about urinary tract infections, as well as history of kidney stones or other urinary tract problems.

PAST MEDICAL HISTORY

Record any major illnesses, hospitalizations, or conditions. This area should include any known drug allergies with specific reactions. In addition, specify any current medications, including dosages. For pregnant women, vaccination history and exposure to communicable diseases should be recorded.

PAST SURGICAL HISTORY

List operations with types of anesthesia and any reactions to anesthesia.

SOCIAL HISTORY

Note the patient's living situation and occupation, citing any particular stresses or problems. Detail use of alcohol, tobacco, or drugs.

FAMILY HISTORY

Ask the patient if there is any history of cancer in her family, especially cancer of the breast, ovary, colon, or endometrium. Other conditions that may have a familial predisposition include diabetes, autoimmune disorders, cardiac disease, and depression.

REVIEW OF SYSTEMS

For the gynecologist, particular attention to women's problems should be addressed. These issues include discussing any symptoms of eating disorders (particularly among young women), and inquiring about domestic or sexual abuse. Abused women have an increased number of visits to doctor's offices for nonspecific complaints, and domestic abuse exists in all social stratas.

CLINICAL CORRELATION

T. B. is a 38-year-old Caucasian female, G5P2032, who presents to the office complaining of a "fishy smelling vaginal discharge."

HPI: She has noted this malodorous discharge for several weeks. The discharge is watery and yellow. It causes a great deal of itching and burning at the introitus. She denies any dyspareunia. She is sexually active and has a new partner. She uses oral contraceptives for birth control.

OB Hx: She delivered two full-term children without complications. The largest was 7 lb, 10 oz. She had two miscarriages and one ectopic pregnancy that was removed via laparoscopy.

Gyn Hx: 12 × 28 × 3 days. Her menses are regular on oral contraceptive pills. She notices heavier flow and increased cramps when she is not taking the pills. She has yearly Pap smears and reports all of them to have been normal. Coitarche was at age 20 years and she has had seven lifetime partners. She denies any other gynecologic or urologic complaints.

PMH: She is healthy and has no known drug allergies. She does not take any medications other than oral contraceptive pills.

PSH: In 1986, she underwent a laparoscopy-salpingostomy for ectopic pregnancy without complications.

Soc Hx: She denies tobacco or illicit drug use. She averages two alcohol drinks per week. She is recently divorced and works as a journalist.

Fam Hx: Both parents are alive and well. There is no family history of cardiac disease, diabetes, or cancer.

ROS: Noncontributory. She denies any history of violence or abuse.

THE PHYSICAL EXAMINATION

A comprehensive examination should be undertaken. The following basics should be included:

- *Vital signs:* Including height, weight, blood pressure, pulse, respirations, and temperature.
- *HEENT:* Routine examination.
- *Neck:* Thyroid enlargement may effect menstrual cycles.
- *Lungs:* Routine examination.
- *Cardiac:* Routine examination.
- *Breasts:* Any masses or irregularities should be thoroughly evaluated. Galactorrhea may represent either breast disease, pituitary abnormalities, or side effects of medications (for example, antipsychotics). Patients should be questioned about a self breast examination and should be in-

structed at this time as to how to conduct one. This examination is described in detail in Chapter 48.

- *Abdomen:* Pelvic masses become abdominal masses if they are large enough. Myomatous uterus, ovarian tumors, pregnancy, or bladder distention may all present with an abdominal mass. A routine abdominal examination should include palpation of the liver edge, identification of any masses, and localization of any abdominal discomfort.
- *Back:* Pyelonephritis frequently has costovertebral angle tenderness. Curvature of the spine should be noted and signs of osteoporosis documented.
- *Extremities:* Routine examination.
- *Neurological:* Urogenital complaints, such as incontinence, may be a presenting symptom of a neurologic process such as multiple sclerosis.
- *Skin:* Acne and abnormal hair distribution are often the result of elevated androgens, which may be produced by the ovaries or adrenal glands. Hair distribution in a normal female follows a characteristic pattern of development during puberty and alterations in the female hair pattern may be an indicator of pubertal abnormalities (discussed in Chapter 40).
- *Lymphatic:* These glands are important in assessing either infection or cancer.

THE PELVIC EXAMINATION

This step is generally the last part of the physical examination. A chaperone should be present to assist, irrespective of the sex of the practitioner. This practice protects both the patient and the examiner, and the assistant will aid in collection of specimens. The patient's privacy should be respected as much as possible throughout the examination.

Prior to the examination, have the patient empty her bladder. Ideally, the rectum as well should be emptied for an optimum pelvic exam.

- *External genitalia:* Note hair distribution and any skin irritation or signs of infection.

The inguinal lymph nodes should be palpated for enlargement. The skin of the labia majora should be smooth. Any lesions need inspection and require biopsy if a concern arises regarding dysplasia or carcinoma. The urethra should also be examined. Palpation of the labia may note any nodularity or enlargement, with particular attention to enlargement of the Bartholin's glands and Skene's glands.

- *Vagina:* The vaginal mucosa should be assessed for atrophy. Lesions of the vagina should also be noted, including any nodular lesions felt on bimanual exam.

- *Speculum examination:* The speculum should be warmed if possible, and a small amount of water or lubricant may aid in ease of insertion (Figure 3.1). The cervix position may be distorted by changes in uterine anatomy or pelvic masses. The cervix is inspected for friability (easy bleeding), lesions, or discharge. The Pap smear is performed, generally using a cytobrush for the endocervical portion of the smear. If the patient has undergone a hysterectomy, a Pap smear should continue to be performed on the vaginal cuff. If appropriate, cultures of the cervix should be done after the Pap smear. A wet mount examining a vaginal discharge with the addition of saline or potassium hydroxide will often determine the offending organism in a vaginal infection.

- *Bimanual examination:* This examination is performed with one or two lubricated fingers of the gloved hand gently placed into the vagina. Personal style will dictate preferences, but generally the dominant hand is placed on the abdomen, with the vaginal hand supporting the genital structures being palpated. The virginal patient may not permit vaginal examination, in which case the entire pelvic examination is performed via the rectum. The bimanual examination should note any cervical motion tenderness, which may be an indication of pelvic inflammatory disease. For the obstetric examination, a description of the cervical length, position, thickness, and any dilation should be noted, as early dilation may indicate a risk for cervical incompetence. A more thorough description of the obstetric cervix (the Bishop's score) is detailed in Chapter 26. The contour and

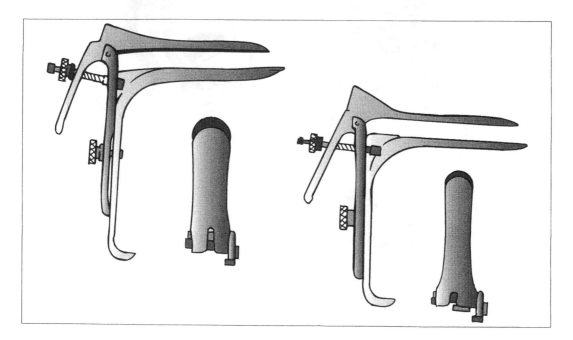

Figure 3.1   Graves (left) and Peterson (right) specula

size of the uterus should be assessed as well as the position and mobility. Two-thirds of women have anteverted uteri (uteri that tip anteriorly); the remaining one-third have either midline uteri or retroverted uteri (Figure 3.2). The ovaries are palpated on either side by sweeping inferiorly and medially from approximately the anterior superior iliac spine to the lower lateral aspect of the uterus. The ovaries are normally 2 to 4 cm in length, but may be enlarged with functional cysts, follicles, or neoplasms.

- *Recto-vaginal examination:* This examination is a critical component to the pelvic examination. Pathology of the posterior cul-de-sac is generally palpable only by recto-vaginal examination (Figure 3.3). Likewise, the parametria are best assessed by recto-vaginal exam. This step is particularly important in assessing a patient for cancer. Anal sphincter tone can be assessed as well. Stool occult blood testing should be performed on all patients older than age 40, or on younger patients if there is any symptomatology of colon cancer. Palpation of a bulge from the lower rectum into the posterior vagina would identify a rectocele.

CLINICAL CORRELATION
Physical Examination

T. B. is a well-appearing, somewhat anxious female
VS: 5 ft 3 in, 135 lb
BP: 114/70
P: 80
R: 16/min
HEENT: Normal
Neck: No thyromegaly or nodules
Lungs: Bilaterally clear to auscultation
CV: Regular rate and rhythm, no murmurs
Breasts: No masses, discharge, or tenderness; axillae negative for nodules
Abdomen: Soft, flat, nontender; well-healed laparoscopy scars; no masses palpable

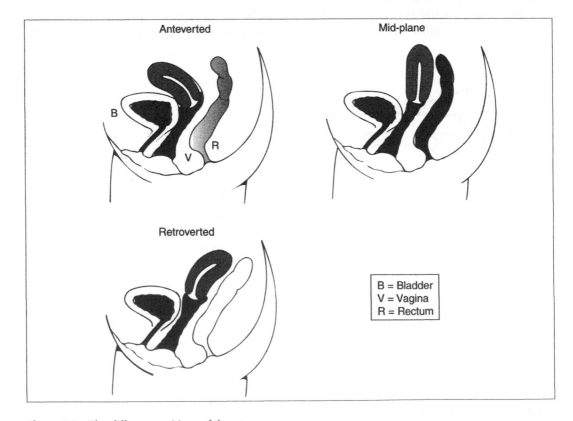

Figure 3.2   The different positions of the uterus

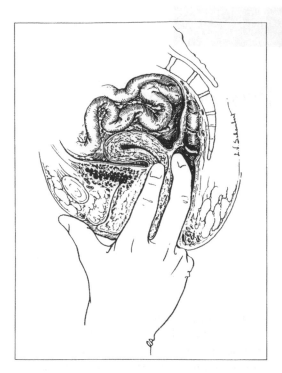

Figure 3.3 The recto-vaginal examination

Source: Callahan TL, Caughey AB, Heffner LJ. Blueprints in obstetrics and gynecology. Malden, MA: Blackwell Science, 1998.

Back: Straight, no costo-vertebral angle tenderness
Extremities: No clubbing, cyanosis, or edema
Neuro: Grossly intact
Skin: No lesions or nodules
Peripheral lymph nodes: Nonpalpable

Pelvic Examination

External genitalia: Some erythema noted in the posterior forschette; no lesions apparent; Bartholin's and Skene's glands normal; urethra normal
Vagina: Copious yellow discharge, no lesions, normal mucosa
Cervix: Somewhat friable; cultures and wet mount specimens taken; no lesions noted
Bimanual: Normal-size anteverted uterus, nontender, no cervical motion tenderness; normal-size bilateral ovaries, mobile and nontender
Rectovaginal: Confirmatory with no masses in the posterior cul-de-sac
Wet mount: Numerous white blood cells and mobile trichomonads

Assessment/Plan

A 38-year-old with *Trichomonas* infection. She will be treated with metronidazole and instructed to have her partner treated as well before resuming sexual relations. She is counseled regarding other sexually transmitted diseases. Her gonorrhea and Chlamydia cultures subsequently return negative.

SUMMARY

Once the exam is concluded, the patient should be given the opportunity to dress and discuss the results and management. Future visits will build on the foundations of the initial visit and require substantially less time.

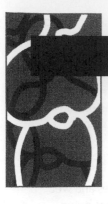

CHAPTER 4

Gynecologic Procedures

The evaluation of the gynecologic patient frequently involves the use of diagnostic and therapeutic surgical procedures. The practitioner needs to fully understand the indications and contraindications for these procedures so that adequate counseling is provided for the patient on the potential risks and benefits. The patient should be educated in language which she understands, allowing her to make informed choices from the options available. The practitioner should also be aware of the financial cost of various procedures, as cost containment is an important issue in health care today.

OFFICE PROCEDURES

CLINICAL CORRELATION

E. K. is a 23-year-old white female, gravida 0, who presented to the community clinic for a routine gynecologic exam. She has regular menses every 29 days. Her last Pap smear was one year ago and reported as normal. She is sexually active, using condoms occasionally. Her review of systems, past medical, surgical, and family histories are negative. Social history revealed that she smokes one pack of cigarettes per day, but does not drink or use illicit drugs. She lives with her parents and has a good relationship with her siblings.

The physical examination reveals a healthy-appearing female with no obvious abnormalities. The pelvic examination was normal. Two weeks later, however the Pap smear returns as abnormal and the patient returns to the office for evaluation.

COLPOSCOPY

Colposcopy is a procedure that is indicated in the work-up of an abnormal Pap smear (Figure 4.1). The colposcope is a binocular instrument that magnifies images by approximately 10 to 16 times. To perform a colposcopy, a solution of 3% to 5% acetic acid (dilute vinegar) is first applied to the cervix and vagina, and then careful examination with the colposcope, usually with a green filter, is carried out, noting any abnormalities. The dilute acetic acid causes cytoplasmic changes in the nonkeratinized cervical epithelium. Normal surface cells show no change after application of acetic acid, whereas dysplastic cells become a white color. These patches of dysplasia are referred to as "aceto-white," and they indicate an area of concern that should be closely inspected.

A satisfactory examination requires the following: (1) the entire transformation zone (the junction of the squamous and columnar epithelium of the cervix) be visualized; and (2) that if an abnormality is noted, the entire extent of the lesion is seen (Figure 4.2). Abnormal areas, such as those that turn white with the application of acetic acid (aceto-white

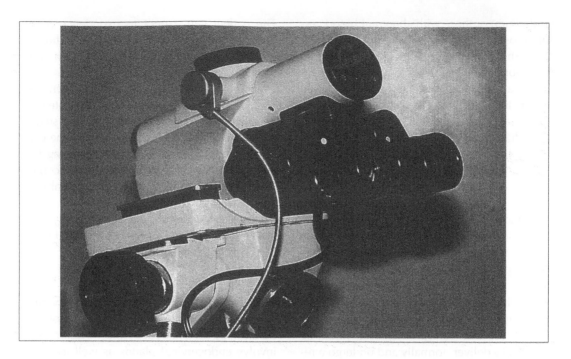

Figure 4.1 Colposcope

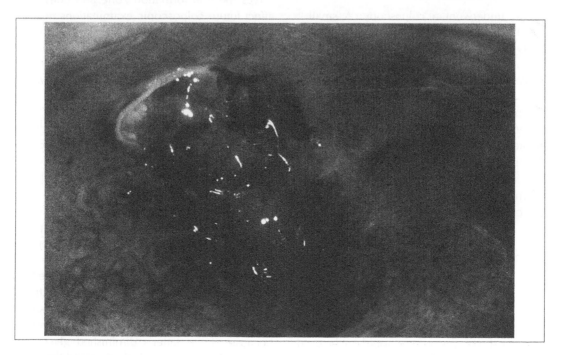

Figure 4.2 Colposcopic view of the cervix. The abnormalities on this cervix are consistent with micro-invasive cancer.

epithelium) or those with abnormal blood vessels (mosaicism or punctation), should be biopsied. An endocervical curettage (ECC) should be performed unless the patient is pregnant. An ECC is a scraping of the endocervical canal to sample the tissue lining the canal. In contrast to a cervical biopsy, an ECC is essentially a blind procedure. The risks of the procedure include minor discomfort and minor bleeding related to biopsy. Bleeding can usually be controlled with silver nitrate or Monsel's solution.

The pregnant patient with an abnormal Pap smear should be evaluated colposcopically. Generally, biopsy is reserved for those women with lesions with vascular abnormalities suspicious for microinvasive or invasive cancer. Cervical biopsy is safe during pregnancy, but may be accompanied by greater bleeding than biopsy in the nonpregnant patient. Those women with dysplasia should be allowed to deliver normally and undergo a repeat colposcopy six weeks after delivery. A more thorough explanation of dysplasia of the lower genital tract is provided in Chapters 49 and 50.

CLINICAL CORRELATION

E. K. underwent a colposcopy. A small area of white epithelium was noted on the cervix, and a biopsy and ECC were subsequently performed. A small lesion was also noted on the upper aspect of the vagina; this area was biopsied as well. The vaginal biopsy and ECC were negative, but the cervical biopsy was consistent with moderate dysplasia (cervical intraepithelial neoplasia II or CIN II). Treatment options discussed with the patient included cryotherapy, laser vaporization, and the loop electrosurgical excision procedure.

CRYOTHERAPY

Cryotherapy uses nitrous oxide or carbon dioxide to freeze the dysplastic lesion of the cervix. It can be used only if the entire lesion can be visualized and does not extend into the cervical canal. This procedure should not be used during pregnancy. The lesion is frozen for three to five minutes, with an ice ball extending approximately 5 mm beyond the lesion.

The patient can expect to experience some mild cramping during the procedure, although this discomfort is usually alleviated with nonsteroidal anti-inflammatory agents.

A vaginal discharge may be present for several weeks after the procedure. Potential long-term side effects include cervical stenosis, infertility related to destruction of the cervical glands, and difficulty in visualizing the transformation zone on future colposcopies should the patient again experience an abnormal Pap smear. For this last reason most particularly, a physician should not routinely perform cryotherapy if some other modality of treatment is available.

LASER VAPORIZATION

An alternative to cryosurgery is carbon dioxide laser vaporization of the cervix. This procedure can be used to treat dysplastic lesions that involve endocervical glands as well as those that remain confined to the exocervix. With laser therapy, intracellular water absorbs the energy of the laser beam, resulting in vaporization of the tissue. This procedure may be performed under local or general anesthesia.

Unlike cryosurgery, laser surgery preserves the transformation zone and does not affect future colposcopic examinations nearly as much. It is ideal for treating external genitalia for condylomata (warts) or dysplasia (vulvar intraepithelial neoplasia—VIN), as the cosmetic results from appropriate treatment with laser are excellent.

LOOP ELECTROSURGICAL EXCISION PROCEDURE

Loop electrosurgical excision procedure (LEEP; see Figure 4.3) uses a thin wire loop to excise the transformation zone with the cervical lesion. Unlike laser vaporization, which destroys tissue, LEEP provides a specimen for pathological examination. This procedure is usually performed in the office after infiltrating the cervix with a local anesthetic. The cervix may be painted with Lugol's solution to identify the lesion. Lugol's solution is a strong iodine solution that stains glycogen in normal cervical tissue dark brown, but does not stain dysplastic tissue because of the latter's diminished glycogen content. The wire loop is then passed through the cervix, thereby excising the lesion and cauterizing the base simultaneously. After the le-

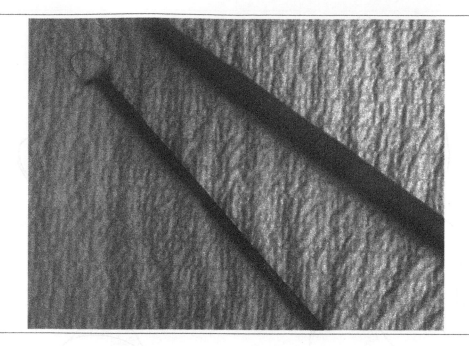

Figure 4.3   Wire electrode for performing the LEEP (loop electrosurgical excision procedure)

sion has been excised, cauterization may be obtained with a ball probe that works via the LEEP electrocautery current. The patient may experience some cramping, discharge, or bleeding during LEEP.

CONE BIOPSY

Cone biopsy involves removal of a cone shaped portion of the cervix encompassing the cervical os, which is then submitted for pathologic evaluation. Conization of the cervix is indicated in several instances:

- If the endocervical curettings are positive for dysplasia

- If the transformation zone cannot be adequately visualized and evaluated

- If the cervical biopsy obtained contains carcinoma in situ or microinvasive carcinoma

- If the cytological findings on Pap smear cannot be adequately explained by the colposcopic findings

The amount of tissue removed from the exocervix can be determined by doing the procedure under colposcopic guidance or by staining the cervix with Lugol's solution to outline abnormal areas. The apex of the cone bi-

opsy should be above the lesions in question but below the internal os to prevent cervical incompetence. The cone specimen may be excised with a scalpel (cold knife cone), a laser, or a loop electrode (Figure 4.4). Endocervical curettage should be performed after the cone is removed to document complete excision of the lesion. The base of the cone may be cauterized or sutured to achieve hemostasis.

Potential complications of cone biopsy may include bleeding, cervical stenosis, infertility due to removal of the cervical glands, and cervical incompetence if the cone reaches the internal os. As with cryosurgery, laser, or LEEP of the exocervix, a follow-up Pap smear should be performed three to four months after the procedure.

ENDOMETRIAL BIOPSY

CLINICAL CORRELATION

E. F. is a 45-year-old female, gravida 2, para 2, who presented to her gynecologist complaining of increasingly heavy menstrual cycles (menorrhagia) along with episodes of heavy intramenstrual bleeding (menometrorrhagia), which have progressively

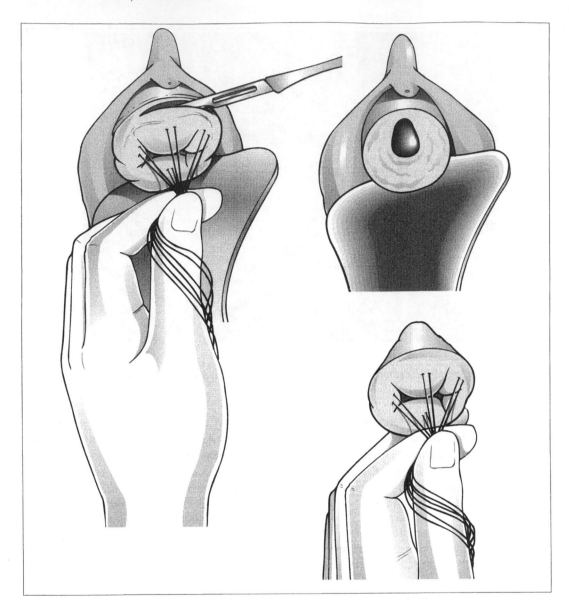

Figure 4.4   Method of cold-knife conization of the cervix

Source: Callahan TL, Caughey AB, Heffner LJ. Blueprints in obstetrics and gynecology. Malden, MA: Blackwell Science, 1998:181.

worsened over the last six months. Her cycles still occur every 28 days, but the flow is heavier, lasting about 8 to 10 days, and it can be incapacitating. She frequently will bleed for an additional 3 days at midcycle. Her review of systems is remarkable only for fatigue. No bowel or bladder changes have occurred, nor has the patient suffered any recent illnesses. Her last Pap smear was normal six months ago. She is sexually active and uses condoms for birth control. Past medical and surgical histories are negative. A complete physical examination was performed and was negative except for an enlarged midline uterus consistent with 10- to 12-week gestational size. No adnexal masses were palpable. Rectal exam and stool guaiac were negative.

Endometrial biopsy samples the uterine lining. Indications for endometrial biopsy include the following: (1) abnormal uterine bleeding; (2) dating of the endometrium in an infertility work-up; and (3) evaluation of a chronic endometrial infection. Contraindications include pregnancy and active acute pelvic infection. Endometrial biopsies do not require anesthesia and are typically performed in the office.

After a negative pregnancy test is obtained, a bimanual examination is conducted to ascertain the position of the uterus. Various instruments may be used to obtain the sample, including a plastic pipelle or a sharp metal curette to which a syringe is attached for aspiration. The curette is introduced through the cervical os into the endometrial cavity and the sample is aspirated. In menopausal women, the cervical os may be stenotic, and a paracervical block may be helpful to allow passage of the curette. The most serious complication of endometrial biopsy is uterine perforation, which occurs in 1 in 1000 cases. In addition, infection is possible but occurs only rarely if sterile procedure is followed.

DILATION AND CURETTAGE

Dilation and curettage (D&C) is an alternative to endometrial biopsy for uterine sampling, although it is used for other indications as well. In patients who are hypovolemic due to severe bleeding from a miscarriage or dysfunctional uterine bleeding, D&C is the treatment of choice for the acute situation. If endometrial biopsy fails to obtain a specimen due to cervical stenosis or patient discomfort, a D&C should be performed. If an office biopsy reveals atypical adenomatous hyperplasia of the endometrium, D&C should be done to rule out a more serious lesion prior to medically treating the patient (see Chapter 51 on uterine disorders). Pregnancy status should be determined prior to going to the operating room.

In the operating room, the patient may be administered either local or general anesthesia. She is placed in a lithotomy position with the ankles elevated. An examination under anesthesia is performed to determine the uterine size and position. Using a speculum, the ante-

rior lip of the cervix is visualized and then grasped with a teneculum. An endocervical curettage is performed first to prevent contamination by the endometrial sampling. Serial dilators are employed to enlarge the cervical opening sufficiently to allow passage of the uterine curette. Next, the uterus is sounded to determine the size of the endometrial cavity. Endometrial curettage is then performed.

Potential complications include perforation of the uterus, bleeding, infection, and anesthetic risks. Contraindications are the presence of a viable pregnancy (unless D&C is performed for the purpose of termination) and active pelvic infection. The major disadvantage of D&C relative to endometrial biopsy is the increased cost incurred in anesthesia and operating room fees.

HYSTEROSCOPY

Hysteroscopy is a procedure sometimes performed in conjunction with a D&C to determine the cause of abnormal bleeding (Figure 4.5). The hysteroscope is an endoscope that passes through the cervix and permits visualization of the endometrial cavity and tubal ostia. The presence of intrauterine polyps, myomas, adhesions, septae, or abnormal endometrial lesions can be determined in this manner. The small hysteroscopes (3 to 5 mm) are diagnostic, whereas the larger ones (8 to 10 mm) allow other instruments to be passed and operative procedures to be performed.

The cervical canal must be dilated to permit entry of the hysteroscope, and the uterine cavity must be distended with a medium such as carbon dioxide gas, dextran, or an electrolyte solution. Carbon dioxide gas is most frequently used for diagnostic hysteroscopy performed in the office setting. It is difficult to maintain a clear field with carbon dioxide if bleeding occurs, however; therefore, it is not useful for operative hysteroscopy. Similarly, electrolyte solutions are used only for diagnostic purposes, because they conduct electrical currents that may be used in operative procedure and are highly miscible with blood. Dextran is the ideal surgical medium because it does not conduct currents and is non-miscible with blood, allowing for a clear operative field.

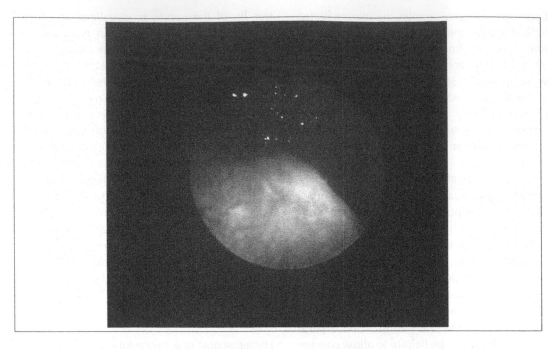

Figure 4.5   Hysteroscopic view of the endometrial cavity. The bubbles visualized are due to the distending media.

Indications for hysteroscopy include the following: (1) diagnosis of abnormal bleeding; (2) resection of polyps; (3) removal of small myomas, adhesions, or septae; (4) laser ablation of the endometrial lining; and (5) retrieval of lost intrauterine devices (IUDs). Contraindications include active infection, pregnancy, and heavy bleeding. Risks associated with hysteroscopy include infection, bleeding, uterine perforation, anesthetic risks, and risks from the distending media. Carbon dioxide, if infused rapidly or at high pressures, may result in gas embolism. Dextran has caused anaphylaxis in susceptible individuals and fluid and electrolyte imbalances.

HYSTEROSALPINGOGRAPHY

Like hysteroscopy, hysterosalpingography (HSG) can identify intrauterine lesions (Figure 4.6), but it also plays an important role in diagnosing tubal disease in the infertility patient. HSG is a radiographic study that images the endometrial cavity and fallopian tubes. Fluoroscopy permits visualization of the contrast material as it is injected through the cervix, distends the uterine cavity, and subsequently passes out through the fallopian tubes. HSG can identify intrauterine myomas, tubal occlusion, and congenital uterine anomalies such as septae or T-shaped uteri. This procedure can therefore be an important part of an infertility evaluation.

Contraindications for HSG include pregnancy, active infection, active bleeding, or allergy to the contrast media. Risks of the procedure include infection (a risk that can be reduced by administering prophylactic antibiotics), uterine perforation, and allergic reactions.

CLINICAL CORRELATION

E. F. underwent endometrial biopsy and was noted to have benign proliferative endometrium. Pelvic sonogram revealed that her uterine enlargement was due to uterine myomas. She was counseled on the therapeutic options available. Given her age, lack of desire for fertility maintenance, and the incapacitating nature of her bleeding, she elected to undergo a hysterectomy.

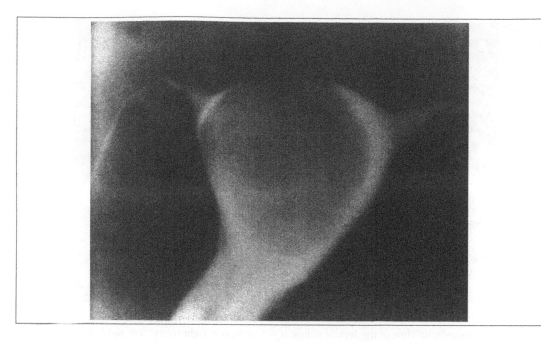

Figure 4.6 Hysterosalpingogram (HSG). There is a defect in the central portion of the uterus due to a large myoma (fibroid). Dye passes out the proximal end of both fallopian tubes.

HYSTERECTOMY

Hysterectomy is a surgical procedure that involves the removal of the uterus. It can be performed vaginally or abdominally. The vaginal approach permits quicker recovery than the abdominal approach. Conditions such as cancer, prior surgical difficulties, uterine size, and lack of descensus (relaxation of the uterus into the vagina) may dictate that an abdominal approach should be taken, however. The abdominal approach also permits exploration of the remaining organs in the abdomen. A hysterectomy can be total (removing the uterus and cervix) or subtotal (leaving the cervix in place).

Indications for hysterectomy include cancer of the uterus, uterine myoma that are symptomatic or greater than 12 weeks size, adenomyosis, or uterine prolapse. Contraindications include pregnancy (except in certain malignancies) and the desire to maintain fertility. The risks of hysterectomy are infection, bleeding, injury to adjacent organs such as the bowel and bladder, and anesthetic risks.

LAPAROSCOPY

Laparoscopy allows the clinician to both view and operate on the internal pelvic organs (Figure 4.7). While the patient is under general anesthesia, an infraumbilical puncture wound is made with a scalpel. Carbon dioxide gas is then used to distend the abdominal cavity, further elevating the abdominal wall away from the viscera. Next, a trochar and laparoscopy sleeve are inserted into the infraumbilical incision, through which the laparoscope is introduced for visualization of the abdomen. Multiple small trochars may be introduced if operative procedures are to be performed.

Laparoscopy is a valuable tool in the diagnosis of pelvic pain, treatment of endometriosis, removal of ovarian cysts or ectopic pregnancies, and sterilization procedures. The risks associated with it include bleeding, infection, and injury to other abdominal organs. Procedures done through the laparoscope often result in significant reduction in hospitalization and recovery time.

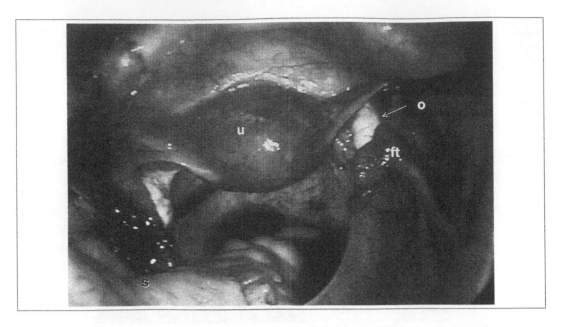

Figure 4.7   Laparoscopic view of the female pelvis. u = uterus; o = right ovary; ft = right fallopian tube.

SUMMARY

The evaluation of the gynecologic patient involves many diagnostic and therapeutic options. It is important that physicians be well versed in the indications, contraindications, risks, and alternatives to these procedures so that they can effectively counsel their patients on the available options.

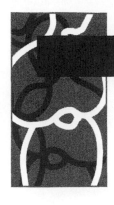

Anesthesia in Obstetrics and Gynecology

Young K. Shin

This chapter will discuss various anesthetics and analgesics for gynecologic procedures and obstetrical pain control. The choice of a particular anesthesia depends on the type of procedure planned, the risks to the patient, and the patient's desires.

CLINICAL CORRELATION

Mrs. AMO is a 49-year-old female with a diagnosis of cervical carcinoma. She is scheduled for a radical hysterectomy with lymphadenectomy. Significant medical history includes obesity, hypertension, and a history of heavy smoking. She takes dyazide and aldomet.

The main aims of preoperative evaluation and preparation is to maximize the patient's physical status for the surgical procedure and to reduce intraoperative complications (for example, hypoxia, hypotension, arrhythmias, and heart failure) and postoperative morbidity (for example, from infection, atelectasis, or pulmonary embolism). In addition, the preanesthetic goal is to acquaint the patient with anesthetic procedures and to dispel any misconceptions or fear about anesthesia.

The preanesthetic visit will focus on a review of concurrent systemic disease, medication, laboratory data, previous anesthetic experiences, adverse effects of anesthetics, and familial problems with anesthetics (Table 5.1). Physical examination will assess the upper air-

way to predict difficulties with endotracheal intubation. In particular, a short thyromental distance and poor visibility of the posterior pharyngeal wall may be predictors of such difficulties.

Cardiovascular and pulmonary disease have been the two major risk factors in the perioperative period. The patient with malignant hypertension, coronary artery disease, or chronic pulmonary disease may require preoperative medical consultation and appropriate treatments including cessation of smoking.

CHOICE OF ANESTHESIA

The decision about anesthetic techniques is based on the surgical requirement, the patient's physical status, her desires, and the anesthesiologist's skill. Although the majority of gynecologic surgery is performed under general anesthesia, avoidance of general anesthesia will reduce respiratory depression in patients with respiratory disease. In patients with ischemic or congestive heart disease, better hemodynamic stability may occur with regional anesthesia.

Regional anesthesia is contraindicated in patients with coagulopathy or who are taking anticoagulants because of a risk of hematoma formation in the epidural or subarachnoid space. It may also be avoided in patients with fixed cardiac output. Sympathetic blockade accompanying regional anesthesia can lead to hypotension and sudden cardiac decompensation in a patient with aortic stenosis.

Table 5.1   Preanesthetic Evaluation Checklist

_____   Preoperative diagnosis

_____   Proposed procedure

_____   Medical history: cardiac, pulmonary, renal, and so on

_____   Previous surgery/anesthetic experience/problems

_____   Family anesthetic problems

_____   Current medications

_____   Allergies

_____   Physical examination: vital signs, upper airway, heart, and so on

_____   Laboratory findings: Hct, platelets, chemistries, ECG, chest X ray

_____   Blood: type and screen, type and cross, autologous

_____   Consultation: cardiology, pulmonary medicine, and so on

PREMEDICATION

Almost all patients will have some preoperative anxiety or apprehension. Relief of anxiety can be achieved by an adequate preparation of the patient with reassurance and an informative discussion. Premedication with a variety of narcotics, sedatives, and tranquilizers may be given depending on the patient's emotional status and the magnitude of the surgical procedure. Midazolam hydrochloride (Versed), a benzodiazepine derivative, is used as a premedication drug and has an amnestic property.

INTRAOPERATIVE PATIENT MONITORING

Under all anesthetics, the patient's circulation, ventilation, oxygenation, and temperature should be monitored. ECG and automated blood pressure remain the standard monitors used intraoperatively to assess cardiac function. Pulse oxymetry can provide a means of noninvasive assessment of arterial blood oxygenation. Capnography confirms the correct placement of an endotracheal tube by identifying CO_2 in the expired gas and is used as a monitor to maintain normocarbia under general anesthesia.

ANESTHETICS

INTRAVENOUS ANESTHETICS

Intravenous agents such as thiopental, propofol, etomidate, midazolam, and ketamine are administered to induce and maintain unconsciousness in general anesthesia.

Thiopental (Pentothal) has potent respiratory and circulatory depressant effects. It reduces respiratory rate and tidal volume, and both blood pressure and heart rate decrease. Recovery is gradual, and will occur slowly if the patient is given repeated doses. Propofol (Diprivan) is a short-acting intravenous anesthetic agent for induction and maintenance of general anesthesia as well as sedation during local and regional anesthesia. Its cardiorespiratory depression is similar to that produced by thiopental. Its rapid distribution and elimination makes recovery significantly faster than with the use of thiopental.

SYNTHETIC OPIOIDS

A number of morphine-like agonists (Fentanyl, Sufentanil, Alfentanil), and agonist–antagonist opioids (Butorphanol, Nalbuphine) are currently used in anesthetic practice, where they are administered in the form of parenteral and intraspinal injection. All of these opioids produce a dose-dependent respiratory depression with relative stability of cardiovascular function. Naloxone (Narcan), an antagonist opioid, is used to reverse the respiratory depression associated with agonist opioids.

INHALATION ANESTHETIC GASES

The potency of inhalation anesthetic gases is expressed in terms of the minimum alveolar concentration (MAC) that is required to prevent movement in one-half of all patients exposed to a painful stimulus. Nitrous oxide (N_2O) is used as a supplement to other anesthetics because of its low potency (MAC is 101%). Halothane, enflurane, isoflurane, and sevoflurane are potent inhalational anesthetics. Hepatic dysfunction has been reported with halothane, however.

LOCAL ANESTHETICS

Local anesthetics are used for local infiltration, peripheral nerve blocks, and central neural blocks. These agents are classified based on their clinical properties (Table 5.2). Anesthesia for large nerve fibers, such as motor and proprioceptive fibers, requires a high concentration of local anesthetics like 2% lidocaine. A low concentration of 1% or 0.5% lidocaine is adequate for local infiltration. Epinephrine at a concentration of 1:200,000, when added to local anesthetics, prolongs the duration of anesthesia and reduces peak blood levels of local anesthetics.

Peripheral nerve blockades that are suitable for gynecologic procedures include paracervical block and pudendal nerve block, which provide anesthesia for the lower part of the vagina and perineum. Lidocaine 1% with epinephrine is adequate for these blocks with a maximum volume of 50 mL (500 mg).

POSTOPERATIVE PAIN MANAGEMENT

Adequate pain relief not only reduces the patient's suffering, but also improves her ability to ambulate, thereby reducing postoperative complications. Although a variety of treatment modalities are available, a more constant degree of analgesia can be achieved by the continuous infusion of narcotics.

PATIENT-CONTROLLED ANALGESIA

Patient-controlled analgesia (PCA) devices, which allow the patient to self-administer small bolus doses of drugs within lockout intervals, is routine management of postoperative pain after most surgical procedures.

EPIDURAL OPIOIDS

A variety of opioids have been administered intrathecally or epidurally by intermittent injection, continuous infusion, or patient-controlled techniques. Epidural Fentanyl produces a more rapid onset of action and less respiratory depression than does morphine. Continuous epidural infusion of Fentanyl provides good postoperative analgesia after hysterectomy.

Potential side effects of intraspinal opioids include nausea, vomiting, pruritus, and urinary retention. Diphenhydramine (Benadryl), given as 25 to 50 mg, may relieve pruritus. Frequent assessments of the patient's level of sedation and respiratory rate are necessary to minimize the serious respiratory depression.

KETOROLAC

Ketorolac tromethamine (Toradol) is a nonsteroidal analgesic with anti-inflammatory properties. Unlike opioids, it does not cause respiratory depression; therefore, it may be a useful alternative to opioids. A 30 mg intravenous or intramuscular dose is effective for moderate postoperative pain; the dose may be repeated every six hours.

CLINICAL CORRELATION

A preoperative pulmonary consultation was obtained for Mrs. AMO's expiratory wheezing, and pulmonary treatments including physical therapy and breathing ex-

---

Table 5.2 Local Anesthetics

Low potency with short duration of action (30–60 min)	Procaine (Novocain), 2-chloroprocaine (Nesacaine)
Moderate potency and duration of action (1–2 h)	Lidocaine (Xylocaine), mepivacaine (Carbocaine)
High potency, long duration of action (2–4 h)	Bupivacaine (Marcaine), ropivacaine (Naropin)

ercise began. Her blood pressure (140/80) was well controlled. ECG showed no myocardial ischemia. Potassium supplementation was given for her hypokalemia (serum potassium < 3.5 mEq/L). Difficulties with endotracheal intubation were anticipated because of poor visibility of the pharynx on examination. A continuous epidural technique in combination with propofol infusion was used for the radical hysterectomy, and epidural PCA with Fentanyl was initiated for postoperative pain control.

ANESTHESIA FOR SPECIFIC GYNECOLOGIC PROCEDURES

The following sections describe anesthetic issues related to specific gynecologic procedures.

Vaginal and Pelvic Floor Surgery

Vaginal and pelvic floor surgical procedures may require a steep Trendelenburg position in addition to lithotomy. The potential depressive effect of the steep Trendelenburg position on respiratory function is cause for concern among anesthesiologists, as the position decreases total lung volume and functional residual volume because of the pressure applied by the abdominal contents upon the diaphragm.

Laparoscopy

Laparoscopic examinations require pneumoperitoneum of carbon dioxide or nitrous oxide and the use of a steep Trendelenburg position. Excessive intra-abdominal pressure greater than 25 cm H_2O interferes with venous return to the heart.

Gynecologic Cancer Surgery

The anesthetic considerations in patients who have previously received chemotherapy involve effects of the chemotherapy on organ systems and its potential interaction with anesthetics. Adriamycin and cyclophosphamide may produce cardiomyopathy. Concomitant use of cyclophosphamide and a potent inhalation agent (halothane) can prove detrimental to myocardial function. Patients previously treated with bleomycin are at risk of developing postoperative respiratory failure secondary

to a pneumonitis associated with this chemotherapy.

Oncology procedures tend to be long in duration, and they are frequently associated with significant blood loss. Fluid and electrolyte balance, maintenance of hematocrit, correction of coagulopathy, and adequate tissue perfusion become critical in these patients.

ANESTHESIA FOR OBSTETRICS

The majority of nulliparous parturients (approximately 80%) receive regional analgesia for labor pain, and some 25% of infants are delivered by cesarean section. Thus anesthetic care should be readily available to parturients in labor and delivery suites.

Maternal Mortality Associated with Anesthesia

The incidence of maternal death is reported to be 9 in 100,000 live births in the United States. Approximately 5% to 10% of the deaths have been attributed to anesthetic mishap. Pulmonary aspiration of gastric contents and hypoxia resulting from failure to intubate during induction of general anesthesia are major causes of maternal death related to anesthesia. Consequently, careful airway assessment of the patient and appropriate measures for the prevention of aspiration (no food by mouth, antacids such as sodium citrate, or drugs to raise gastric pH such as ranitidine or metoclopramide) should be done on admission to labor and delivery.

Clinical Correlation

Mrs. BMO, a 29-year-old G1P0 at term gestation, was admitted to labor and delivery because of uterine contractions. Her medical history was insignificant, and this pregnancy was uncomplicated. She ate a sandwich two hours before her admission.

Analgesia for Labor Pain

Pain of labor results from the contraction of the uterine muscle and dilatation of the cervix during the first stage of labor. The pain travels along the nerves, enters the spinal cord at the level of the tenth, eleventh, and twelfth thoracic and first lumbar nerves (T10, T11, T12,

Table 5.3 Anesthetic Techniques for Labor and Vaginal Delivery

Systemic analgesia (IV or IM)	Narcotics (morphine, meperidine, Fentanyl)
	Sedative/hypnotics (benzodiazepines)
	Dissociative drugs (ketamine)
	Agonists/antagonists (nalbuphine)
Inhalation analgesia	Nitrous oxide
Regional anesthesia	Epidural block
	Spinal block
	Combined spinal-epidural block
Peripheral nerve block	Paracervical block
	Pudendal nerve block

L1), and projects to the cortex of the brain. During the second stage of labor, the pain also arises from the perineum, which travels along the pudendal nerve entering the sacral nerves of the spinal cord (S2, S3, S4). In addition to systemic administration of narcotics, several regional and peripheral nerve blocks are performed to block anatomical pathways to the pain (Table 5.3).

SYSTEMIC MEDICATIONS

The use of narcotics is often limited to the latent or early stages of labor, and adequate pain relief may be accompanied by some respiratory depression. Narcotics and general anesthesia are readily transferred to the fetus through the placenta, causing neonatal depression depending upon the amount of the drug and the timing of administration.

REGIONAL BLOCKS

Epidural block, subarachnoid block, and combined spinal-epidural block are performed using local anesthetics with or without a small dose of narcotics (Table 5.4). These techniques provide minimal sedation and avoid general

Table 5.4 Overview of Regional Techniques for Labor Analgesia

TYPE OF BLOCK	LOCATION	ANESTHETICS	AREA BLOCKED	COMPLICATIONS
Paracervical	Cervix Frankenhauser ganglion	Lidocaine	T10	Fetal bradycardia
Pudendal	Ischial spine Sacrospinous ligament	Lidocaine	S2–S4	Local anesthetic toxicity
Spinal	Subarachnoid L3–4	Bupivacaine Sufentanil Fentanyl	T10	Maternal hypotension Pruritus Fetal bradycardia Headache
Combined spinal epidural	Subarachnoid Epidural L3–4	Sufentanil Fentanyl Bupivacaine	T10	Maternal hypotension Fetal bradycardia Respiratory depression
Epidural	Epidural L3–4	Bupivacaine Ropivacaine Fentanyl	T10	Maternal hypotension

anesthesia in the case of cesarean delivery. Nevertheless, maternal hypotension resulting from vasodilation with sympathetic blockade can be a problem. It is essential to keep maternal blood pressure at normal level so as to ensure normal uterine blood flow and fetal oxygenation. Intravenous hydration with crystalloid solution, uterine tilt, frequent monitoring of blood pressure, and use of a vasopressor (ephedrine) are adopted. Epidural analgesia is associated with a prolongation of labor and an increase in instrument delivery and cesarean delivery. Pudendal block is done with local anesthetic and provides relief for operative vaginal deliveries (Figure 5.1).

A postspinal or epidural headache is a potential complication. Its incidence ranges from 2% to 7%, depending upon the size and shape of a needle. The incidence is lower with small pencil-point needles (25- and 27-gauge Sprotte or Whitacre). In most patients, autologous blood patch (20 mL of whole blood drawn from a vein in the arm) into the epidural space is effective in the alleviation of the headache.

Peripheral Nerve Blocks

Paracervical block is performed by an obstetrician and provides effective analgesia during the first stage of labor. It blocks sensory nerve fibers in the cervix. Unfortunately, its use has been complicated by frequent fetal bradycardia. Bilateral pudendal nerve blocks are useful for episiotomy in conjunction with local perineal infiltration.

Inhalation Anesthetics

Nitrous oxide 50% to 70% plus oxygen has analgesic effect for labor pain. Other volatile anesthetics may be administered for uterine relaxation.

Choice of Anesthetics for Obstetric Regional Blocks

Local anesthetics commonly used in obstetric anesthesia include 2-chloroprocaine (Nesacaine), lidocaine, bupivacaine (Marcaine), and ropivacaine (Naropin). It is worth noting that inadvertent intravenous injection of these local anesthetics may lead to maternal systemic toxicity and fetal or neonatal depression.

Narcotics frequently used for spinal or epidural blocks during the peripartum period include morphine, fentanyl, and sufentanil. Their potential side effects include pruritus, nausea and vomiting, urinary retention, and delayed respiratory depression with the use of morphine.

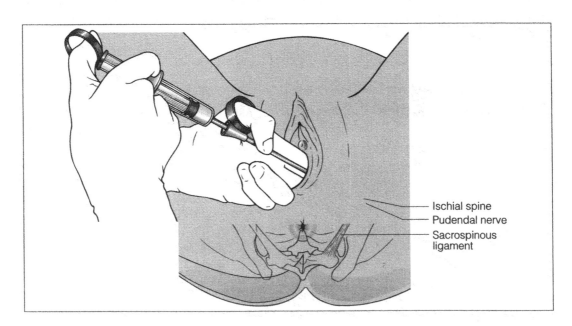

Ischial spine
Pudendal nerve
Sacrospinous ligament

Figure 5.1   Technique for transvaginal pudendal nerve block

Source: Callahan TL, Caughey AB, Heffner LJ. Blueprints in obstetrics and gynecology. Malden, MA: Blackwell Science, 1998:33.

CLINICAL CORRELATION

Vaginal examination of Mrs. BMO showed that the cervix was dilated to C/2. She was asking for pain medication for her contractions. Nubain 10 mg was administered intravenously with moderate relief of the pain for an hour. Next, an anesthesia consult was obtained for the use of epidural analgesia. Her platelet count was normal. Sodium citrate 30 mL, given orally, and metoclopramide 10 mg, given intravenously, were administered. To provide rapid hydration, 500 mL of dextrose-free lactated Ringer's solution was administered. A combined spinal-epidural anesthesia was performed with intrathecal 10 µg of Sufentanil and epidural infusion with bupivacaine 0.125% and Sufentanil 0.2 µg/mL at a rate of 10 mL/hour. Mrs. BMO was placed in the left lateral position to permit fetal heart rate and blood pressure monitoring, after which she reported complete relief of the pain. An infant was born by vacuum-assisted delivery, with Apgar scores 8 and 9 at 1 and 5 minutes, respectively. No headache was noted on a postdelivery visit.

ANESTHESIA FOR CESAREAN SECTION

Most elective cesarean deliveries are performed under regional blocks. A continuous epidural technique is less likely to produce maternal hypotension than is a spinal block to a T5 sensory level, and it provides effective analgesia for post-cesarean pain. In urgent situations, general anesthesia is the method of choice. Neonates born of mothers given general anesthesia have lower Apgar scores as compared with those infants delivered under regional anesthesia. Neurobehavioral scale of the neonate may also be depressed by general anesthesia for 24 hours postdelivery.

POST-CESAREAN PAIN MANAGEMENT

Poor management of the surgical pain puts mothers in distress, and it may deter early ambulation and infant nursing. Current techniques are either intravenous PCA or epidural PCA. Fentanyl is often chosen for epidural PCA.

SUMMARY

A thorough preoperative analysis of the patient's physical status can lead to a better outcome for surgery. Intraoperative monitoring of oxygenation and ventilation has been greatly improved by the use of pulse oximetry and end-tidal CO_2 monitoring. Regional anesthesia may be considered in high-risk gynecologic patients and is an excellent choice for alleviation of labor pain and cesarean anesthesia. PCA devices play a significant role in the management of postoperative pain.

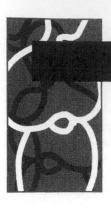

CHAPTER 6

Obstetric and Gynecologic Sonography

Cathy Spong and Thomas Pinkert

MECHANISM OF SONOGRAPHY

Ultrasonography is based on the system of submarine sonar in which pulses of energy are emitted into a body of water. When they meet a different density, they are reflected back to the transmitter, with the signal being proportional to the density of the object. Similarly, in obstetrics the sonogram emits sound waves either across the maternal abdomen or through the vagina; these sound waves travel across the filled bladder or amniotic fluid and reflect off of the pelvic structures and/or fetus. The transducer, which generates intermittent high-frequency sound waves, is connected to the maternal abdomen with a coupling agent (either gel or mineral oil). The coupling agent diminishes the loss of ultrasound waves at the interface between the transducer and the skin.

Real-time sonography requires the use of multiple-pulse-echo systems. When activated in sequence, these waves travel through the tissue and the energy is reflected (echoed) back to the transducer in proportion to the difference in tissue density. Using a multiple-pulse-echo system allows for detection of movement and other fetal activities, including breathing and vessel pulsations. Consequently, real-time sonography allows confirmation of fetal life through observation of cardiac activity, respiration, and active fetal movement.

The ultrasound probe's scanning frequency is measured in megahertz (MHz). Although a higher frequency gives better resolution, the trade-off is decreased penetration. A 3 to 5 MHz abdominal transducer allows sufficient penetration in most obstetric patients with adequate resolution.

Gynecologic and obstetric sonograms can be performed both abdominally and transvaginally. Transvaginal sonograms allow for better resolution of the uterus and adnexal structures as well as first-trimester gestations. Transabdominal ultrasound also gives excellent images of the pelvic organs and, as the pregnancy advances and moves out of the pelvis, is more useful for identification of fetal growth and anatomy. Throughout pregnancy, transvaginal sonography is useful for evaluation of cervical length and dilation.

INDICATIONS FOR OBSTETRIC SONOGRAM

Multiple indications exist for sonography during pregnancy (Table 6.1). In the first-trimester sonogram, identifying the viability and location of the gestation are critical elements. Evaluation of growth between sonograms is useful in fetuses with possible intrauterine growth restriction. The best sonographic estimate of gestational age is provided in the first trimester. In this trimester, sonogram estimates of age are accurate within 7 days; in the second trimester, they are accurate within 14 days; in the third trimester, they are accurate within 21 days. If multiple sonograms are performed

Table 6.1	Indications for Obstetric Sonogram

- Identification of pregnancy
- Evaluation of viability of pregnancy
- Location of pregnancy (intrauterine, ectopic, abdominal)
- Evaluation of size and interval growth of gestation
- Identification of multiple gestation
- Identification of placental location
- Evaluation of size and date discrepancies such as:
  - Size greater than dates
  - Size less than dates
  - Incorrect gestational age
  - Uterine myoma
  - Bicornuate uterus
  - Adnexal mass
  - Molar gestation
  - Hydramnios
  - Multiple gestation
  - Inaccurate dates
  - Blighted ovum
  - Oligohydramnios
  - Intrauterine growth restriction
- Calculation of estimated gestational age (uncertain last menstrual period)
- Detection of fetal anomalies
- Evaluation of amniotic fluid volume
- Evaluation of adnexae
- Evaluation of vaginal bleeding
  - Threatened abortion
  - Placenta previa
  - Placental abruption
  - Marginal sinus rupture
- Guidance for procedures
  - Amniocentesis
  - Percutaneous blood sampling/intrauterine transfusions
  - Placement of stents (i.e., posterior urethral valve syndrome)

throughout the pregnancy, the gestational age and due date should be estimated from the earliest sonogram.

INFORMATION OBTAINED FROM OBSTETRIC SONOGRAM

A wealth of information may be obtained from an obstetric sonogram (Table 6.2). The following measurements are commonly taken for assessment of gestational age:

- *Crown-rump length (CRL)* is used in the first trimester and measures from the top of the fetal head (crown) to the buttock of the baby (rump). Neither the limbs nor the yolk sac should be included in the CRL measurement. CRL is exclusively used as the predominant measurement until 12 weeks gestation (Figure 6.1).

- *Biparietal diameter (BPD)* measures across the head. To obtain this measurement, both the thalamus and the cavum septi pellucidum should be visualized. The measurement is taken from the outside of one of the sides of the cranium to the inside of the other and is perpendicular to the midline (Figure 6.2).

- *Head circumference (HC)* measures around the head in the same plane as the BPD, but the measurement goes only outside the fetal calvarium.

- *Cerebellum measurements* are taken as needed.

- *Abdominal circumference (AC)* is measured just below the fetal heart, with the stomach bubble and junction of the umbilical vein and portal sinus being visualized (Figure 6.3).

- *Humerus length (HUM)* and *femur length (FL)* are measurements of the long bones (Figure 6.4).

  Amniotic fluid volume is assessed by one of two measurements:

- *Amniotic fluid index (AFI)* is the measurement of the amount of amniotic fluid in the uterus. First, the maternal abdomen is divided into four quadrants (RUQ, RLQ, LLQ, and LUQ). Next, using the ultrasound transducer held perpendicular to the floor, the largest clear vertical pocket of amniotic fluid is calculated in centimeters. These pockets cannot contain extremities or loops

Table 6.2   Information Obtained From an
            Obstetric Sonogram

1. Number of fetuses
2. Fetal viability (heart tones, movement)
3. Fetal presentation: vertex, breech,
   transverse, compound
4. Gestational age and growth
5. Amniotic fluid volume
6. Placental location: fundal, anterior,
   posterior, lateral, low-lying, previa
7. Fetal anatomy
   a. Skull: shape and size
   b. Face
   c. Spine
   d. Four-chamber heart
   e. Bladder
   f. Stomach
   g. Kidneys
   h. Abdominal wall: size, defects
   i. Long bones
   j. Gender

the AFI. An AFI of less than 5 cm is defined as oligohydramnios (too little fluid); an AFI of more than 25 cm is polyhydramnios (too much fluid). A measurement of 8 to 25 cm is considered normal, whereas an AFI between 5 and 8 cm is borderline oligohydramnios.

- *Amniotic fluid volume (AFV)* is another method for calculating the amniotic fluid where the single deepest pocket of amniotic fluid is determined. If this pocket is greater than 2 cm, it is considered normal.

BASIC OBSTETRICAL SCAN

FIRST TRIMESTER ULTRASOUND

Scanning in the first trimester may be performed abdominally or vaginally. If abdominal scanning is performed and definitive information cannot be obtained, however, a vaginal scan should be performed. A pregnancy in the early first trimester is usually best documented with transvaginal sonogram, as less distance separates the transducer and the target. The location of the gestational sac should be documented and the number of gestational sacs (and embryos) identified. The uterus and adnexal structures should be evaluated to identify myomas and possible adnexal masses (Table 6.3).

of umbilical cord. In addition, the fetus cannot be pushed with the transducer to fill a counted pocket or open a new pocket. The sum of the four quadrants constitutes

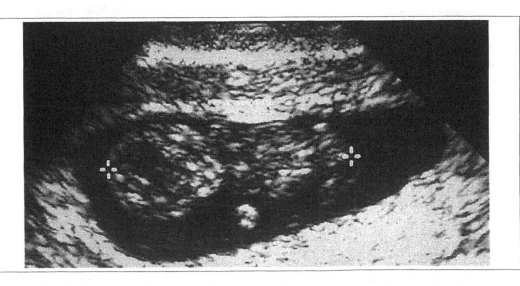

Figure 6.1   Sonogram demonstrating fetal crown-rump length. Gestational age is 10 weeks.

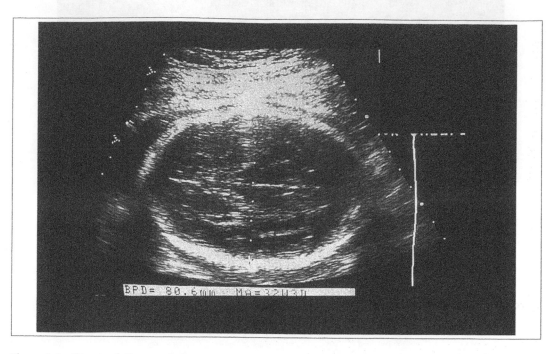

Figure 6.2   Biparietal diameter in later pregnancy

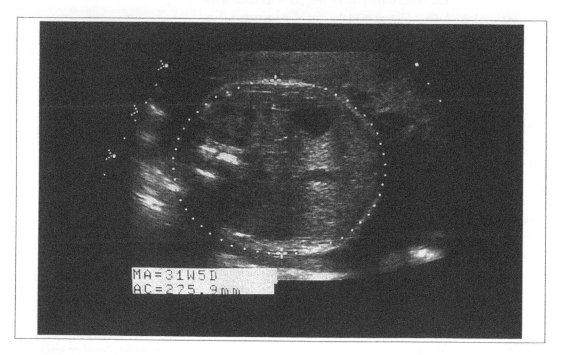

Figure 6.3   Measurement of fetal abdominal circumference

Figure 6.3   Measurement of fetal abdominal circumference

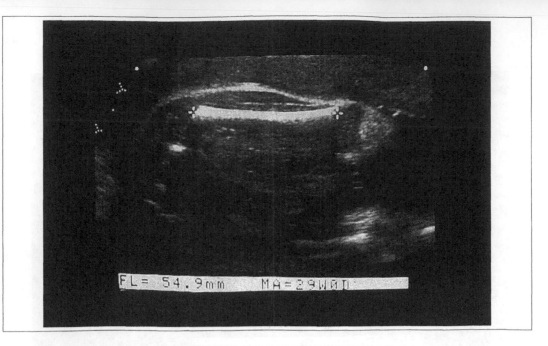

Figure 6.4 Measurement of fetal femur length

Table 6.3 Findings on First Trimester Obstetric Sonography

5 weeks	Gestational sac measures 4–5 mm
	Average beta-hCG is 400–800 mIU
	Early embryonic pole by fifth post-menstrual week
6 weeks	Yolk sac is one-third the size of the gestational sac
	Fetal heart rate visible by the end of the week
7 weeks	Fetal pole visible, measures 5–9 mm
	Amniotic membrane visible between yolk sac and fetal pole
	Gestational sac measures 15 mm
	Physiologic herniation of bowel at 7–12 weeks
8 weeks	Crown-rump length measurable
	Limb buds visible
9 weeks	Distinct body parts
	Brain structures
	Body movement visible
10 weeks	Measure biparietal diameter
	Visual abdominal organs, brain structures, and spine
11 weeks	Choroid plexus fills 75% of lateral ventricles
	Visualization of fetal heart, limbs, and facial structures
	Visualization of fetal hands and feet
12 and 13 weeks	Brain structures and facial contours well visualized
	Corpus callosum developed by the end of the thirteenth week

Note: For five to eight weeks, most observations are on transvaginal sonography only; after eight weeks, observations may be made by transabdominal sonography.

SECOND AND THIRD TRIMESTER ULTRASOUND

In the second and third trimesters, measurements of the fetus should be recorded to document fetal size (and evaluate growth if a prior scan was performed). In addition, the presenting part should be recorded as well as the location and grade of the placenta, amount of amniotic fluid volume, location of myomas, and documentation of fetal anomaly. Placental grading is a documentation of the extent of calcification within the placenta and reflects the age of the placenta. More extensive calcifications typically occur later in the pregnancy. Premature or excessive calcification of the placenta may be associated with maternal hypertension, diabetes, intrauterine growth restriction, or Rh isoimmunization (see Figure 19.2).

Anatomy that should be visualized includes the following structures:

- Head: choroid plexus (evaluate for position and cystic structures), size of lateral ventricles (normal is less than 10 mm), size of cisterna magna, measurement of nuchal skin fold
- Chest: cardiac axis, four-chamber view of fetal heart, right and left ventricular outflow tracts
- Abdomen/pelvis: stomach bubble, both kidneys, cord insertion site, fetal bladder
- Extremities: documentation of all four extremities
- Spine: evaluation in two planes, longitudinal and cross-section

INDICATIONS AND INFORMATION OBTAINED FROM A GYNECOLOGIC SONOGRAM

Gynecologic sonography focuses on the structures of the female pelvis so as to identify pelvic pathology. The uterus is scanned for size, the presence of masses, or a distortion of shape. The myometrium is examined to locate and characterize myomas or other masses. The endometrium is examined for thickness, echogenicity, and the presence of polyps. The adnexae are evaluated for tenderness, mobility, and the presence and characterization of any masses (Figure 6.5). In addition, the posterior cul-de-sac is evaluated for the presence of

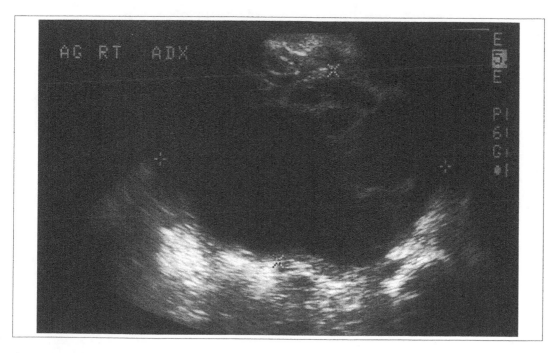

Figure 6.5   Ultrasound of a complex, multiseptated ovarian mass. Pathology was of a corpus luteum cyst and a mucinous cystadenoma.

fluid or masses in this region. The gynecologic sonogram may also review the kidneys and ureters to document lesions, hydronephrosis, or hydroureter.

SUMMARY

Ultrasound has probably had the greatest impact of any single advance in obstetrics. Prenatal diagnosis and therapy are greatly improved when this tool is used. Detection of ectopic versus intrauterine gestations is routine. Multiple gestations are no longer "discovered" in the delivery suite, but are detected from very early stages of gestation. The lack of radiation makes ultrasound an ideal method of performing serial radiologic studies throughout pregnancy. Also, this technique is a very efficient tool for detecting gynecologic pathology, and the unique proximity of the adnexae and the uterus to the vagina provides a portal through which transvaginal ultrasound can give very-high-resolution images of these organs. The obstetrician/gynecologist should be familiar with basic sonography. Indeed, most will choose to become adept at utilizing this technology to obtain more data on their patients.

PART II

Preventive
Health Care

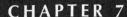
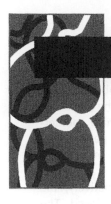

CHAPTER 7

Psychosocial Aspects of Women's Care

Alexander F. Burnett

This chapter deals with psychosocial aspects of women's care. Topics included in this chapter are substance abuse, stress management, and mood disorders as they relate to women. Unique to the field of obstetrics and gynecology are the issues of how substance abuse effects the unborn child and how pregnancy can influence or create mood disorders, such as post-partum depression.

SUBSTANCE ABUSE

Substance abuse in women has historically been ignored in comparison to the problems in men. The abuse by women of tobacco, alcohol, prescription drugs, and illicit drugs continues to rise, however, and physicians responsible for women's health must be prepared to identify patients at risk for substance abuse and provide meaningful treatment options for them. An attitude of openness and nonjudgment is critical in evaluating patients for these problems, as an extensive overlay of shame or fear may cause the patient to lie about the presence or extent of substance abuse.

CLINICAL CORRELATION

L. B. is a 35-year-old, gravida 3, para 1, abortus 2 female who comes to the office for yearly gynecologic examinations. Recently, she has been in to see her gynecologist approximately every three months with vague complaints of anxiety and restlessness. On several visits, she has indicated a desire to use tranquilizers to alleviate her anxiety. She reports a 20 pack-year history of smoking and states that she drinks socially but does not feel that it is a problem.

DETERMINATION OF SUBSTANCE ABUSE

Education of the patient is a critical step in treating substance abuse. The first part of education is identifying whether a problem exists. "Abuse" is broadly defined as the misuse or overuse of a particular substance. "Dependency" refers to a psychic craving for that substance which may or may not be accompanied by a physiologic dependence. "Tolerance" to a substance is a phenomenon of the body's reaction to continuous use of a substance such that there is a progressive decrease in that drug's effectiveness. Therefore, with tolerance, more of the substance is required over time to achieve the same effect.

When there is concern for maternal substance abuse and documentation is necessary (that is, to care for a newborn), blood or urine screening can be done. Commonly, these tests screen for barbiturates, cocaine, alcohol, nicotine, opiates, and any other drugs requested.

TOBACCO ABUSE

Tobacco is the number one abused drug in the United States. In 1989, total deaths in the

United States attributed directly to cocaine and heroin was estimated to be 6000; in contrast, in the same year deaths related to tobacco use numbered more than 60 times that figure. Young women continue to be the fastest-growing subset of new smokers in this country. Women's increased use of tobacco allowed lung cancer to surpass breast cancer as the leading cause of cancer death in women by 1986. Tobacco contributes significantly to the development of other cancers, including cancer of the uterine cervix, as well as to the development of heart disease, stroke, and chronic obstructive pulmonary disease.

The majority of cigarette abusers begin smoking in their mid- to late teens. For a number of years, advertising has aimed directly at the female market. Many of teenage and young adult women continue smoking in a belief that it will help to maintain their weight at a desirable level.

All patients should routinely be asked about tobacco use. The extent of smoking is usually quantified in terms of pack-years; for example, if a woman has smoked two packs per day for four years, she has a cumulative use of eight pack-years.

Alcohol Abuse

Alcohol abuse in women may be particularly difficult to diagnose because their patterns of drinking often differ from those observed with men. Female alcoholics tend to drink alone, and they will become alcoholics in a shorter time and with less volume of alcohol consumption than men. Historically, they have displayed less violent behavior, with less frequent encounters with the legal system than male counterparts. Women who come from families where alcohol was abused are at high risk for becoming alcoholics, as are survivors of sexual or physical abuse and women who are married to alcoholics.

All patients should be asked about alcohol consumption. Keep in mind that the female alcoholic is often older than her male counterpart; therefore, the elderly female patient must be questioned as well. One of the more useful and simple investigational tools is the TACE questionnaire (Table 7.1). Alternatively, the CAGE questionnaire may be employed. The CAGE includes four questions:

1. Have you ever cut down on your drinking?

2. Have people annoyed you by criticizing your drinking?

3. Have you ever felt bad or guilty about your drinking?

4. Have you ever had a drink first thing in the morning to steady your nerves or get rid of a hangover (eye-opener)?

A positive response on these questions suggests a problem with alcohol, with increased tolerance being the most sensitive indicator of abuse.

Prescription Drugs

Commonly prescribed drugs that can lead to abuse include the anxiolytics, such as benzodiazepines, narcotics, barbiturates, and amphetamines. The patient who repeatedly requests these medications over the phone, or the woman who is found to be receiving the same medications from several different sources, should give the gynecologist clues that substance abuse may be occurring. Narcotics should be prescribed in a diminishing fashion in the post-operative period. Patients with chronic pain should be evaluated by a pain service, which includes psychological evaluation if they continue to request narcotics.

The physician who prescribes these drugs

Table 7.1   TACE Questionnaire

T	Tolerance	How many drinks does it take to make you feel high?
A	Annoyed	Have people annoyed you by criticizing your drinking?
C	Cut down	Have you felt you ought to cut down on your drinking?
E	Eye-opener	Have you ever had to drink first thing in the morning to steady your nerves or to get rid of a hangover?

should keep accurate records of the amount given, the duration of use, and other sources that are supplying these agents.

ILLICIT DRUGS

The most commonly used illicit drugs in the United States include marijuana, cocaine, heroin, amphetamines, and hallucinogens. Difficulty exists in getting women to admit to illicit drug use for fear of prosecution, shame, and other factors. Questions about illegal drug use should be approached in a nonjudgmental manner. The first prenatal visit is often a unique opportunity to determine whether substance abuse is a problem because patients tend to be more honest about their behavior when it will also affect an unborn child.

CLINICAL CORRELATION

L. B. was asked about her alcohol consumption with the TACE questionnaire. She stated that often she felt sober even after several glasses of wine or cans of beer. Her husband had recently begun questioning her about the amount she drank. She stated, "He seems to bother me so much about it, I wish he would just mind his own business." In addition, she admitted to occasionally indulging in morning drinks. She denies any illicit drug use. She again reaffirmed her belief that if she could obtain a prescription for medication to relieve her anxiety, she wouldn't need to drink in the mornings. She mentioned several anxiolytics by name as a suggestion.

L. B.'s answers to the TACE questions suggest that she may have a problem with alcohol. It is difficult for the clinician to make the distinction between heavy alcohol abuse and alcoholism, so generally the physician's role is to educate the patient so that she may come to an understanding of her own alcohol consumption. The willingness of the patient to admit to a problem with alcohol will be directly related to how she perceives alcohol as interfering with other aspects of her life. Once the problem is identified, recommendations for intervention—such as therapy, referral to Alcoholics Anonymous, or referral to treatment centers—should be made.

In addition, the reproductive-age woman should be made aware of the possible consequences of alcohol consumption on pregnancy. Alcohol was first identified as a teratogen in 1968. Since then, much has been done to elucidate details about fetal alcohol syndrome (FAS). Diagnosis of FAS requires three criteria: (1) growth retardation, either prenatal or postnatal (failure to thrive); (2) central nervous system involvement; and (3) a characteristic facial dysmorphology. The degree to which these criteria are present is related to the amount of alcohol consumption, particularly in the period of organogenesis. In the United States, approximately 3 per 1000 live births display FAS. FAS is now believed to be the leading cause of mental retardation of a known etiology—more common than either Down syndrome or spina bifida.

STRESS MANAGEMENT

The American Academy of Family Physicians has estimated that two-thirds of office visits to family doctors are prompted by stress-related symptoms. "Stress" has been defined as a "relationship between the person and the environment that is appraised as taxing or exceeding his or her resources and endangering his or her well-being" (Lazarus, 1984). It may be differentiated from anxiety and burnout, even though the patient may frequently group these burdening sensations together. The woman who comes to the gynecologist with nonspecific complaints should be allowed to verbalize through open-ended questioning whether there are events or circumstances in her life that she feels are overwhelming. Questions about her work, relationships, family situations, and any other stressors should be posed in very general terms to allow her to express what she is feeling and to identify what she considers to be stressful. Patients who express a feeling of depression or who appear to be depressed should be asked directly about depression, and appropriate referrals should be made if indicated. In addition, women who show signs of more complicated neurotic or psychotic behavior should be referred to those well trained in the diagnosis and treatment of these disorders.

Management of stress in one's life may range from simple exercises intended to diminish the quality of stress to a complete reworking of one's life. For some patients, less radical interventions, such as meditation, exercise, and relaxation techniques, may be all that are required to make her life less stressful. Therapeutic intervention may include cognitive therapy with or without the addition of psychopharmacotherapeutics. These options should be presented to the patient in an open-ended manner, such as "Would you like to see a therapist to discuss some of the issues in your life?" Based on this questioning, the physician can then judge the amount of intervention desired by the patient.

The gynecologist is in a unique position to help in the recognition of emotional problems. Complaints regarding sexual difficulties, chronic pain, and generalized symptoms related to depression or anxiety all require a thorough physical work-up. Frequently, however, underlying stress may be contributing to the reported problem. An open-ended questioning about stressors in a patient's life may lead to alleviation of some of these complaints.

ANXIETY AND DEPRESSION

Anxiety and depression are common disorders among women, with as many as 2% experiencing anxiety and 25% experiencing clinical depression over their lifetimes. Issues related to pregnancy can be stressful, including infertility, pregnancy, and the post-partum period. Indeed, all of these issues may be stressors that accelerate anxiety or depression. Consequently, the obstetrician/gynecologist needs to be aware of symptoms of these disorders and be knowledgeable about those that require medical therapy and the common side effects of that therapy. In addition, any medication given to a reproductive-age woman requires knowledge of the potential effects on either the developing fetus or the newborn who is exposed to these drugs.

ANXIETY DISORDERS

Panic disorders are characterized by intense fear that is associated with at least four of the symptoms listed in Table 7.2. Typically, a panic disorder will be accompanied by agoraphobia or a fear of public places. Patients with this disorder may become increasingly unwilling to leave their homes. Other subsets of anxiety disorders include obsessive-compulsive disorders and post-traumatic stress disorder. It is unclear whether pregnancy exacerbates or improves symptoms of anxiety disorders, particularly if the patient has discontinued medi-

---

Table 7.2   Criteria for Generalized Anxiety Disorder

- For more than half the days in at least six months, the patient experiences excessive anxiety and worry about several events or activities.
- The patient has trouble controlling these feelings.
- Associated with this anxiety and worry, the patient has three or more of the following symptoms, some of which are present for more than half the days in the past six months:
  - Feelings of being restless, edgy, keyed up
  - Tiring easily
  - Trouble concentrating
  - Irritability
  - Increased muscle tension
  - Trouble sleeping (initial insomnia or restless, unrefreshing sleep)
- Aspects of another Axis I disorder do not provide the focus of the anxiety and worry.
- The symptoms cause clinically important distress or impair work, social, or personal functioning.
- The disorder is not directly caused by a general medical condition or by the use of substances, including medications.
- It does not occur only during a mood disorder, psychotic disorder, post-traumatic stress disorder, or a pervasive developmental disorder.

cation either prior to conception or early in pregnancy. Metabolites of progesterone may have a sedative effect and help reduce anxiety during pregnancy. It is clear that the post-partum period is a time when a high percentage of women with these problems will experience relapse or exacerbation of anxiety symptoms. High-risk patients may need to remain on medication throughout pregnancy and may require increased doses of medication in the post-partum period.

Commonly prescribed medications for anxiety disorders include tricyclic antidepressants (TCAs), monoamine oxidase inhibitors (MAOIs), selective serotonin reuptake inhibitors (SSRIs), and benzodiazepines. Patients with anxiety disorders without depression are at low risk for suicide; therefore, some clinicians advocate discontinuation of medication for anxiety disorders either prior to conception or upon diagnosis of pregnancy.

Unfortunately, only limited information is available regarding the effect of anxiolytic therapy on the developing fetus. The tricyclic antidepressants have not been documented to increase teratogenic risk. These drugs must be monitored in terms of their serum levels during pregnancy, as typically the volume of distribution is increased in the pregnant patient and dosages may need to be increased to maintain therapeutic levels. Pfizer operates a registry related to exposure to fluoxetine (Prozac) during conception; the data gathered to date have failed to show an increase in congenital defects with this drug. Some reports have indicated that increased perinatal complications may occur when fluoxetine is used in the third trimester, including increased premature birth, low birth weight, and poor neonatal adaptation. A long-term study of infants exposed to tricyclic antidepressants or fluoxetine during pregnancy failed to show any impact on global IQ, language development, or behavioral development up to seven years of age.

Although there is not sufficient information on MAOIs during pregnancy to correlate with specific complications, most physicians prefer to avoid use of these drugs due to their side-effect profile, which is less favorable than that of TCAs or SSRIs. Benzodiazepines have not been shown to increase the incidence of any congenital defects, but they are associated with withdrawal reactions in the neonate and "floppy infant syndrome" (characterized by hypotonia, sucking difficulties, hypothermia, lethargy, and cyanosis in the newborn). Some patients have been treated with antiepileptic drugs (carbamazepine, valproic acid) for anxiety; administration of these drugs is associated with increased risk of neural tube defects.

Depressive Disorders

One of the categories of depressive disorders listed in the DSM-IV is "major depressive episodes with post-partum onset." This condition is diagnosed when the episode occurs within four weeks after childbirth (Table 7.3). Three depressive diagnoses are associated with the post-partum period.

First, "maternity blues" is the most common psychiatric disorder associated with pregnancy, occurring in more than half of all new mothers. Typically, it begins about the third or fourth post-partum day and generally lasts less than one week. Symptoms include crying spells, insomnia, depressed mood, fatigue, anxiety, headache, and confusion. It is unclear what the etiology of maternal blues is, as studies have failed to document a specific hormonal change associated with this disorder.

Second, fatigue from a newborn and the overwhelming changes brought by the arrival of a new child is certainly a common complaint. This condition is generally self-limiting and does not require specific counseling or drug therapy.

Third, a less common but more severe diagnosis is post-partum depression. This condition is more frequently found if the patient has a prior history of post-partum depression or has suffered from depression or anxiety during the pregnancy. The criteria for this diagnosis match those for a major depressive episode. That is, in a two-week period, a patient must have five or more of the symptoms listed in Table 7.3, which represent a definite change from usual functioning. The criteria include either depressed mood or decreased interest/pleasure. If the patient is determined to be at risk for suicide, she should be immediately hospitalized in a psychiatric ward with 24-hour surveillance.

Commonly prescribed medications for depression include those discussed earlier, such as TCAs, SSRIs, and MAOIs. TCAs and SSRIs appear to be safe in pregnancy. If the patient is not at risk for suicide, it would be prudent to discontinue antidepressant medications prior to and during pregnancy as long as she can be closely monitored for signs of progressing depression. Lithium is commonly prescribed for patients with bipolar disorder (manic depression). This salt has been associated with significant cardiac anomalies in offspring of women taking it during pregnancy. In particular, Ebstein's anomaly has an increased prevalence associated with maternal ingestion. For those patients with severe depression unresponsive to medication, electroshock therapy has been performed during pregnancy.

The most severe form of postpartum depression is a major depressive episode with post-partum psychosis. This condition is very rare, being reported following only 0.1% to 0.2% of deliveries. It is characterized by rapid onset with delusional thinking. The woman may be either depressed or elated, have disorganized behavior, experience emotional ability, and develop hallucinations. Women with this degree of mental illness should be treated by specialists in psychiatry.

SUMMARY

The obstetrician/gynecologist may be the only health care provider a woman of reproductive age sees. The physician should be able to ask his or her patients about substance abuse and be able to refer them

---

Table 7.3 Criteria for Major Depressive Episode

- In the same two weeks, the patient has had five or more of the following symptoms, which are a definite change from usual functioning. Either depressed mood or decreased interest or pleasure must be one of the five.
  - Mood. For most of nearly every day, the patient reports depressed mood or appears depressed to others.
  - Interests. For most of nearly every day, interest or pleasure is markedly decreased in nearly all activities (as noted by the patient or by others).
  - Eating and weight. Although the patient is not dieting, there is a marked loss or gain of weight (such as 5% in one month) *or* appetite is markedly decreased or increased nearly every day.
  - Sleep. Nearly every day the patient sleeps excessively or not enough.
  - Observable psychomotor activity. Nearly every day *others* can see that the patient's activity is speeded up or slowed down.
  - Fatigue. Nearly every day there is tiredness or loss of energy.
  - Self-worth. Nearly every day the patient feels worthless or inappropriately guilty. These feelings are not just about being sick; they may be delusional.
  - Concentration. As noted by the patient or by others, nearly every day the patient is indecisive or has trouble thinking or concentrating.
  - Death. The patient has had repeated thoughts about death (other than the fear of dying), or about suicide (with or without a plan), or has made a suicide attempt.
- These symptoms cause clinically important distress or impair work, social, or personal functioning.
- They don't fulfill the criteria for a mixed episode.
- This disorder is not directly caused by a general medical condition or the use of substances, including prescription medications.
- Unless the symptoms are severe (defined as severely impaired functioning, severe preoccupation with worthlessness, ideas of suicide, delusions or hallucinations, or slowed psychomotor activity), the episode has not begun within two months of the loss of a loved one (bereavement).

Criterion for Post-partum Onset

- An episode of the disorder begins within four weeks after childbirth.

to the appropriate places for help. Many health complaints are stress related, and the physician should be able to help patients identify stressors in their lives and provide suggestions or referrals to try to cope with these stresses. As a primary care provider, the ob/gyn needs to be able to identify mental illness such as anxiety or depression and can prescribe a variety of pharmacologic and non-pharmacologic therapies for these conditions. The obstetrician needs to realize that the immediate post-partum period can be particularly stressful and can exacerbate previously existing mental illness or uncover previously undiagnosed mental illness. Judicious referral to the appropriate psychiatrist or psychologists will also benefit our patients.

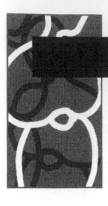

CHAPTER 8

Preventive Screening Guidelines

D. A. Dessouky

Obstetricians and gynecologists have long assumed the responsibility for the primary health care of their patients in addition to taking on a role as specialists in obstetrics and gynecology. Frequently, women have a better rapport with their obstetricians/gynecologists than with their other primary care physicians because of their long relationship with their doctors.

HEALTH CARE FOR WOMEN

Most women are conscientious about their yearly visits to their obstetricians/gynecologists, and many visit these care givers even more frequently. In general, women tend to seek treatment from their physicians more often than men do. It is therefore prudent for obstetricians and gynecologists to address these needs properly and to use the annual visit as a time to promote primary-preventive health care for women in addition to gynecologic care. To this end, obstetricians and gynecologists should be able to perform excellent health screening through taking of a history, physical examination, and appropriate tests. Counseling and intervention, consulting, and recommendations for immunization should complete the task.

OBJECTIVES

Promoting primary health care, rather than treating advanced or neglected diseases, should be a major objective of health care. By identifying risk factors in each age group, disease screening and discovery become more efficient. Preventive services should prove both beneficial and cost-effective. The World Health Organization has identified guidelines for good screening tests; these guidelines are listed in Table 8.1.

PREVENTIVE SERVICES

Preventive health care services include the following:

- *Screening.* Through history taking, physical examination, and proper laboratory testing, disease could be detected before it becomes symptomatic.

- *Counseling.* Counseling and behavioral intervention attempt to provide advice to change certain high-risk behaviors. Reducing risk activity may, in turn, reduce exposure to injury and disease. Examples of these services include counseling about tobacco, alcohol, and drug abuse; discussion of risky sexual behavior and contraception to reduce unwanted pregnancy and sexually transmitted diseases; and referrals to social and psychological help for women who are victims of domestic violence.

Each age group will have specific needs that should be addressed. The following sections describe these age-related considerations.

Table 8.1   Guidelines for a Good Screening Test (WHO)

- The condition to be screened is an important cause of morbidity, disability, or mortality.
- The natural history of the disease being screened should be well known, with effective treatments available for early disease.
- Screening tests should have a high sensitivity and specificity for detecting the screened disease.
- The screening tests must be acceptable to the target population and their health care providers, and appropriate follow-up of positive findings must be ensured.

ADOLESCENT POPULATION (AGES 13–18)

Screening

In this age group, history taking should inquire about causes of morbidity and mortality such as violent behavior (car accidents, suicide, homicide), sexual behavior (sexually transmitted diseases, partners, adolescent pregnancy), alcohol and drug use/abuse, and family relationships (child abuse, depression). Physical examination should include a secondary sexual characteristic evaluation. Laboratory evaluations may include cholesterol, tuberculosis, gonorrhea, Chlamydia, human papillomavirus, human immunodeficiency virus (HIV), and/or syphilis testing. Pap smears and pelvic examinations are required at age 18 or when the patient becomes sexually active.

Counseling

Counseling should address prevention of unwanted pregnancy (contraceptive options), prevention of sexually transmitted diseases (barrier protection and partner selection), dietary behavior, exercise programs, injury prevention (helmets and safety belts), family relationships (depression, abuse, suicide), and tobacco, alcohol, and other drug use.

Immunization

Immunization in this age group includes vaccination against tetanus-diphtheria (booster between years 14 to 16), measles, mumps, rubella, and hepatitis B.

ADULT POPULATION (AGES 19–39)

Screening

Many of these women share the same health problems associated with the adolescent age group—that is, tobacco, alcohol, and drug abuse; sexually transmitted diseases; unwanted pregnancy; and problematic interfamily relationships. In addition, members of this age group have other special heath needs. History taking should include inquiry into cardiovascular-vascular disease; high-risk sexual behavior (HIV); cerebral vascular accidents; family history of breast, ovarian, and uterine cancer; domestic violence; and sexual dysfunction. (The American Cancer Society guidelines for cancer screening are provided in Table 8.2.) Physical examination should include breast, abdomen, and pelvic examination. Laboratory tests include a Pap smear every year and a lipid profile every five years, or sooner depending on family history of cardiovascular disease. Mammography, HIV testing, rubella titer, sexually transmitted disease testing, and fasting blood sugar should be done on high-risk patients.

Counseling

Counseling should include high-risk sexual and other behaviors, contraceptive options, fitness, domestic violence, job satisfaction, and stress.

Immunization

Immunization in this age group includes a tetanus-diphtheria booster every 10 years, MMR, hepatitis B, influenza, and pneumococcal vaccines.

MIDDLE-AGE POPULATION (AGES 40–64)

Screening

Health care in this age group should address the physiologic changes that accompany aging. The leading causes of death in women are vascular disease, cancer, and pulmonary disease. Other chronic illnesses, such as osteoporosis and hypertension, cause prolonged morbidity, lead to poor quality of life, and contribute to the rapid increase in health care costs. History tak-

Table 8.2   American Cancer Society Screening Guidelines

TEST OR PROCEDURE	BEGIN AT AGE	FREQUENCY
Digital rectal exam	40	Yearly
Fecal occult blood testing	50	Yearly
Flexible sigmoidoscopy	50	Every 5 years
Pap smear	18*	Yearly†
Pelvic examination	18–40	Every 1–3 years†
	Over 40	Yearly
Self breast examination	20	Monthly
Breast examination	20–40	Every 1–3 years
	Over 40	Yearly
Mammography	40 and over	Yearly

*Or at time of initiation of sexual activity, whichever comes first.
†Frequency depends on risk factors such as degree of sexual activity and number of partners.

ing should make note of any injury from physical activity, medications, hormone replacement therapy, and injury prevention measures. Physical examination should include neck adenopathy, breast, abdomen pelvic and rectal examination in addition to the general examination. Laboratory tests should include fecal occult blood test and sigmoidoscopy in addition to a Pap smear, mammography, and lipid profile (Figure 8.1).

COUNSELING

Counseling and behavioral intervention should be directed at sexual function and infection, contraception, exercise, diet, retirement planning, injury prevention, hormone replacement therapy, lifestyle and stress, and tobacco, alcohol, and drug abuse.

IMMUNIZATION

Immunization in this age group includes a tetanus-diphtheria booster every 10 years, annual influenza and pneumonia vaccines, and hepatitis B vaccines.

ELDERLY POPULATION (AGES 65 AND OLDER)

Screening

This segment of the population is growing steadily. By 2040, the population is predicted to include 50 million elderly women who need a special kind of health care that is designed to promote health and prevention—rather than

treatment—of disease. The needs of this age group are not only physical, but also psychological and economic. History taking should be directed to consumption of medications, lifestyle, causes of depression (neglect and abuse), hygiene, diet, and exercise. Physical examination should include visual acuity, hearing, and signs of neglect and abuse. Laboratory tests are similar to those performed for patients aged 40 to 64.

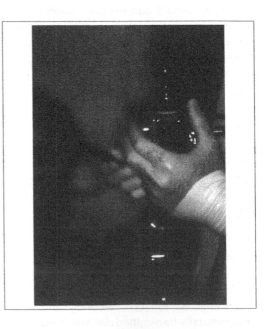

Figure 8.1   Flexible sigmoidoscope

COUNSELING

Counseling and intervention should include education in fitness, diet, hygiene, sexual function, injury prevention (accidents are the sixth leading cause of death in the elderly, and half of these accidents involve falls), lifestyle, and interfamily relationships. Causes of death in this age group are cardiovascular, coronary, cerebral-vascular, pulmonary, cancers, and accidents.

IMMUNIZATION

Immunization in this age group includes influenza, pneumonia, and hepatitis B, in addition to other periodic vaccines.

SUMMARY

Emphasis on primary-preventive health care for women should be a goal for obstetricians and gynecologists. Diet and exercise have known benefits against cardiovascular disease, which is the leading cause of death in women in the United States. Cessation of smoking has proven benefits against stroke and vascular disease as well as lung and other cancers. Modification of high-risk behaviors, such as alcohol and drug abuse, reduces violent behavior (car accidents, other accidents, firearm use), which accounts for three-fourths of all adolescent deaths. Chemoprophylaxis may promote health in the elderly. Proper hygiene and safe sexual behaviors may reduce the patient's risk of sexually transmitted diseases, infertility, chronic pelvic pain, and unwanted pregnancy. Cancer screening (breast, cervical, colorectal) and promotion of a healthy lifestyle may reduce the woman's risk of prolonged morbidity and mortality from cancers.

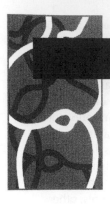

CHAPTER 9

Human Sexuality

Alexander F. Burnett

Knowledge of human sexuality is critical to many different types of physicians. The ability to detect abuse of a child, knowledge of the changing sexual physiology of the adolescent, understanding of the reproductive physiology during the reproductive years, and appreciation of the sexuality in the elderly are some examples of how sexuality can be manifested in any clinical practice. Because the field of obstetrics and gynecology deals with the female genital organs, issues of sexuality are commonplace. The gynecologist is expected to be knowledgeable in the physiology of sexual response and be able to identify sexual problems and provide solutions. An open and accepting attitude in discussion of sexual matters is critical for patient care, regardless of the physician's personal views on certain sexual issues. The gynecologist should be familiar with the various modes of sexual expression (such as heterosexuality, homosexuality, and bisexuality) and should be competent to address concerns occurring with each of these modes of expression. Signs of sexual abuse should be identified in the physical examination if they are present. Finally, the physician is responsible for initiating the dialog with the patient to allow her to express her sexual concerns or questions.

CLINICAL CORRELATION

T. F. is a 26-year-old, gravida 0, white female who is seen in your office for her annual examination and refill of oral contraceptive pills. She has been married for three years. Her menstrual history is normal on the oral contraceptives. During questioning, she admits that intercourse with her husband has become less pleasurable over the past one and a half years, concomitant with increasing pain at the time of intercourse. When further questioned about her sexual health, she states that she has never had an orgasm with her husband and feels sex is a duty for her. She reports coitarche at age 18 when she was under the influence of alcohol. She states that she has had four other sexual partners and that all of her sexual experiences prior to marriage occurred under the influence of alcohol. She denies experiencing orgasm with any of her previous partners. She does state, however, that she loves her husband very much and wishes things were better sexually.

The approach to dealing with a sexual problem begins with its identification. Again, sensitivity and acceptance are critical characteristics to display when discussing the often sensitive issues of sexuality. An understanding of the normal phases of sexual response is important in counseling patients. Masters and Johnson performed the key investigation into this field by observing hundreds of women and couples during sexual encounters and determining the normal physiology of sexual response. They determined that the female response cycle has four phases (Table 9.1):

1. *Excitement Phase.* The initial phase of sexual response may last a few minutes to several hours. During this period, vasocongestion and myotonia occur. Vasocongestion results in increased size of the breasts, clitoral engorgement, and enlargement of the labia. Myotonia results in nipple erection. Vaginal secretions occur during this phase as a transudate is released from the vaginal walls that provides lubrication for intercourse and helps to buffer the acidity of the vagina to a more neutral pH, which is more favorable to sperm survival. The upper two-thirds of the vagina lengthens and distends.

2. *Plateau Phase.* Sexual tension increases during the plateau phase, which generally lasts only 30 seconds to 3 minutes. Skin flushing occurs in the majority of women, generally beginning at the epigastrium and expanding to the breasts. The breasts continue to enlarge. The clitoris elevates and retracts behind the clitoral hood. The outer one-third of the vagina continues to become engorged and diminishes in diameter, creating the orgasmic platform. The uterus and cervix are displaced upward into the pelvis, and the cervix begins to swell.

3. *Orgasmic Phase.* In this shortest phase, there is a release of the vasocongestion and myotonia developed in prior phases. This release is focused strictly in the pelvis. No changes occur in the skin, breasts, clitoris, labia majora, and upper two-thirds of the vagina during this phase. The labia minora contract, with contractions affecting the lower third of the vagina. These muscle contractions occur in 0.8-second intervals and may occur 3 to 15 times. Uterine contractions also occur, with the strongest contractions occurring during pregnancy and masturbation.

4. *Resolution Phase.* During this phase, the body returns to the unstimulated state. This phase has the widest variation in time, occurring as quickly as 15 minutes after orgasm or, if orgasm is not achieved, as long as one day. The vaginal secretions and

semen may pool in the posterior vagina in the supine state, and the cervix rapidly descends to this region and remains patulous for approximately 10 minutes.

Sexual dysfunction in women is due to either of two causes: (1) an inability to have intercourse secondary to vaginismus (a rare condition where the pubococcygeus muscle contracts and restricts admission of the penis) or (2) an inability to achieve orgasm (the more common of the two causes). The easiest way for a woman to achieve orgasm is through masturbation; some women, however, may have religious or personal interdictions to this behavior. The anorgasmic patient should be queried if she ever has or has had orgasms and what type of stimulation brought them about. If she previously was orgasmic and more recently became unable to achieve orgasm, she should be asked about what situations in her life have changed and perhaps brought about this difference. In most circumstances, orgasm requires clitoral stimulation, which can occur during intercourse through penile thrusting that causes movement of the clitoral hood or through direct stimulation with the hand or symphysis pubis. Contrary to Freudian thought, there is no physiologic distinction between a "vaginal orgasm" and a "clitoral orgasm."

Poor communication and lack of knowledge may be the most common elements responsible for sexual dysfunction. Indeed, few physiologic conditions directly relate to female sexual dysfunction. Many women may have fears about expressing their desires to their partners or be ignorant of those processes that will adequately fulfill them sexually. Studies have shown that relationships where the couple is cohabiting (whether married or not) have a higher degree of sexual satisfaction, probably relating to more extensive communication between the partners. In addition, a feeling of security in a sexual relationship has a positive effect on female sexual response. Women who are anorgasmic have greater difficulty in discussing sexuality with their partners and have more negative attitudes toward masturbation and increased guilt feelings associated with sex. Differentiation between primary orgasmic dysfunction (those who have never experienced orgasm) and secondary orgasmic

Table 9.1 Phases of Female Sexual Response

	VAGINA	LABIA	CLITORIS	UTERUS	BREASTS	OTHER
Excitement	Lubrication, elongation, and distention	Thinning and flattening in the nulliparous; venous distention in the multiparous	Increase in size of the glans	Elevation away from bladder and vagina	Nipple erection; venous engorgement; increase in size	
Plateau	Vasocongestion of anterior third of vagina (orgasmic platform); increase in width and depth	Increased labial diameter; color changes: pink to red in nulliparous bright red to dark red in the multiparous	Elevation and retraction of the clitoral body	Elevation of the cervix	Aerolar engorgement; engorgement of tissues around the nipple	Sex flush of the skin of chest; perspiration; myotonia; tachycardia; hyperventilation; increased blood pressure
Orgasm	Lengthening of the vaginal cul-de-sac; vaginal contractions			Contractions		Hyperventilation; rhythmic muscular contractions; tachycardia; increased blood pressure; distention of the external urethral meatus; contraction of the external rectal sphincter and pelvic floor muscles
Resolution	Return to unstimulated size	Return to usual color and thickness	Descent to unstimulated position	Return to usual position		Disappearance of sex flush; return of normal muscle tone, normal heart rate, and blood pressure

Source: Adapted from Masters WH, Johnson VE. Human sexual response. Boston: Little, Brown, 1966.

dysfunction (those who situationally no longer have orgasms) is important in determining the patient's level of awareness of her sexual response and in deciding possible interventions.

Ideally, sexual therapy should involve both partners. The American College of Obstetricians and Gynecologists (ACOG) technical bulletin on sexual dysfunction specifies a nine-step technique for partners to perform to overcome primary orgasmic dysfunction:

1. Increase self-awareness by examining the body and genitals.

2. Explore the genitals with her fingertips.

3. Identify sensitive areas of the genitals that produce pleasurable feelings.

4. Manually stimulate the pleasure-producing areas.

5. Increase the intensity and duration of stimulation and increase psychologic stimulation by means of sexual fantasy.

6. If after completing step 5 an orgasm has not been reached, use a vibrator on or around the clitoris to increase stimulation.

7. Once masturbation has resulted in orgasm, masturbate with the partner present to demonstrate effective and pleasurable techniques of stimulation.

8. Guide the partner in manual stimulation through nonverbal communication (for example, place a hand on top of the partner's hand).

9. Once high levels of arousal and, possibly, orgasms have occurred in step 8, engage in intercourse. The so-called bridge technique, in which the clitoris or clitoral area is manually stimulated during intercourse, can be helpful.

Physicians should be aware that while heterosexual relationships are the predominant sexual union, women who are homosexuals may also experience sexual dysfunction. Alternative sexual lifestyles such as bisexuality, transsexuality, and transvestism may also present difficulties in sexual function. Again, it is critical that the physician be nonjudgmental of habits different from his or her own so as to be of maximum benefit for the patient.

Other critical points in assisting patients with their sexuality come at times of physiologic changes in life. The onset of menarche as a signal of the transformation of a girl into a reproductively functioning woman can be a frightening experience during which basic education in the physiology of these changes may help make the transition smoother. It may also be an ideal opportunity to begin a discussion of the topics of sexual activity and contraception. Again, it is not the physician's role to place moral values on sexual behaviors or abstinence; rather, it is his or her responsibility to provide education about sexuality and some of the potential consequences of sexual activity. Sexually transmitted diseases and safe sexual practices should be mentioned so that if the patient does decide to become sexually active, she can provide herself with the best defense against contracting these illnesses.

Pregnancy generally results in decreased frequency in sexual relations, particularly during the first trimester, when couples fear it will be dangerous for the pregnancy, and during the third trimester, when discomfort may play a role. Nevertheless, some couples report normal or even increased sexual relations during pregnancy, with no ill effects on the developing fetus. Certain situations will prohibit sexual relations, such as premature labor or premature rupture of membranes. Many women find pregnancy a time when they have increased desire for nurturing physical contact, such as holding, rather than sexual relations that are orgasmically focused.

Finally, menopause is also a time of great physiologic change that can affect a woman's sexuality.

CLINICAL CORRELATION

B. C. is a 56-year-old white female who had her last menstrual period at age 52. Since the time of menopause, she has noted decreased sexual relations with her husband of 32 years. She specifically complains of a lack of desire for sex and indicates that when she does have intercourse, she is unable to achieve adequate vaginal lubrication for comfortable relations. She no longer experiences hot flushes.

The loss of estrogen production by the ovaries at menopause has multiple physiologic effects on the woman. Estrogen, by definition, is responsible for cornification of the vaginal epithelium, and lack of estrogen eventually results in vaginal atrophy in many women. This termination can contribute to difficulty in producing adequate lubrication of the vagina for intercourse. Some couples benefit greatly by using commercially available lubricants. Unless contraindicated for some other reason, post-menopausal replacement with estrogen is generally recommended to alleviate these symptoms. As the post-menopausal woman often has an increased production of androgens relative to estrogens, her libido may increase at this time. Occasionally, women with decreased sexual desire in the post-menopausal years respond very well to testosterone as a stimulant for the libido. A decrease in sexual function in the post-menopausal woman may also occur secondary to her partner's inability to have intercourse or lack of desire for sexual relations.

CLINICAL CORRELATION

B. C., who previously underwent a hysterectomy, is prescribed both estrogen and testosterone. After approximately four weeks, she notices a significant increase in her desire for sexual relations. In addition, she finds intercourse much more pleasurable with the thickening of her vaginal mucosa and increased ability at lubrication that has occurred since she began taking the medication.

Other conditions that can severely alter a woman's sexuality include the development of systemic illnesses and cancer. Cancer of the sexual organs, including breast cancer or pelvic cancer, can cause significant changes in body image and result in a woman feeling as though she has lost her sexuality. Breast cancer patients frequently report alterations in their sexuality after diagnosis and treatment of their disease. Patients with pelvic cancers who are treated with surgery or radiation may find intercourse painful or experience vaginal agglutination. Although most women want their physicians to discuss the effect on sexuality that their treatment will have, very few physicians readily discuss these topics. Counseling the patient and her partner prior to therapy about the sexual implications of such therapy may help to prevent the onset of significant sexual dysfunction.

SUMMARY

The obstetrician/gynecologist is in a unique position of directly caring for women's genital organs and therefore has the responsibility to investigate her sexual function or sexual problems. Open, frank communication about sexuality without value judgements by the gynecologist will enable patients to express their concerns about these very personal issues. The gynecologist should be prepared to educate the patient on alterations of sexuality, which can be anticipated with pregnancy, surgery, menopause, and gynecologic cancer therapy. The gynecologist should also be able to educate the woman on identifying sexual dysfunction, its causes, and strategies to alleviate the dysfunction.

CHAPTER 10

HIV in Obstetrics and Gynecology

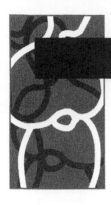

Eva A. Olah

In recent years, there has been a rapid increase in the number of women infected with the human immunodeficiency virus (HIV) in the United States. Since the acquired immunodeficiency syndrome (AIDS) was first described in 1981, this disease has spread in epidemic proportions throughout the world. By 1995, 18% of adult cases of AIDS reported to the Centers for Disease Control and Prevention (CDC) involved women. In 1993, the definition of AIDS in women was expanded to include HIV-infected persons with pulmonary tuberculosis, recurrent bacterial pneumonia, invasive cervical cancer, or CD4+ lymphocyte counts lower than 200 per milliliter (Table 10.1). In many metropolitan areas of the United States, HIV disease is the leading cause of death of reproductive-age women. This infection has struck minority women particularly hard—in fact, the leading cause of death among African American women ages 25–44 in 1993 was HIV disease. Currently, the most common mode of transmission of HIV to women is through heterosexual contact with a partner who most likely contracted the virus from intravenous drug use.

Approximately 85% of all HIV-infected women are members of the reproductive-age group. According to the CDC, in 1994 the median age of women with AIDS was 35. The prevalence of HIV infection in women giving birth in the United States in 1993 was about 1.6 per 1000. As a consequence, it behooves the obstetrician/gynecologist to take an active role in identifying these women and in providing counseling and treatment in an effort to prevent transmission of the disease to their partners and children.

VIROLOGY

HIV is a retrovirus that codes for a reverse transcriptase enzyme that allows the viral RNA to be transcribed to DNA. After transcription, the DNA is integrated into the genetic material of the host cell. HIV preferentially infects cells with the CD4+ antigen, as this antigen serves as a receptor for the virus. Targeted cells include T cells, macrophages, and some neural cells.

The following body fluids have been documented to carry free virus: plasma, cerebrospinal fluid, tears, urine, sweat, saliva, vaginal and cervical secretions, and breast milk. The virus may be found intracellularly in saliva, peripheral mononuclear cells in blood, semen, vaginal and cervical secretions, and bronchial fluid.

After the initial infection, a person may remain asymptomatic or perhaps develop a mononucleosis-like illness. Antibodies can be found as soon as 6 to 12 weeks after the infection or may take up to six months to develop following exposure. Progression from HIV-positive status to AIDS varies from person to person.

CLINICAL CORRELATION

A. W. is a 22-year-old, gravida 0, female who presents with a history of eight weeks'

Table 10.1   CDC 1993 Classification System for HIV Infection for Adolescents and Adults

CD4+ T-LYMPHOCYTE CATEGORY	CLINICAL CATEGORY		
	A	B	C
> 500 cells, > 29% CD4+	A1	B1	C1
200–499 cells, 14%–28% CD4+	A2	B2	C2
< 200 cells, < 14% CD4+	A3	B3	C3

Clinical Category A

Acute (primary) HIV infection, persistent generalized lymphadenopathy (PGL), and asymptomatic HIV-infected patients

Clinical Category B

Symptomatic conditions occurring in an HIV-infected adolescent or adult, but not A or C conditions. Examples include:

Candidiasis, vulvovaginal: persistent, frequent, or poorly responsive to therapy
Candidiasis, oropharyngeal: thrush
Cervical dysplasia, moderate or severe, carcinoma in situ
Constitutional symptoms, such as fever or diarrhea lasting longer than one month
Hairy leukoplakia, oral
Herpes zoster (shingles) involving at least two distinct episodes or more than one dermatome
Idiopathic thrombocytopenic purpura
Listeriosis
Pelvic inflammatory disease, particularly if complicated by turboovarian abscesses
Peripheral neuropathy

Clinical Category C

AIDS indicator conditions:

Candidiasis of bronchi, trachea, or lungs
Candidiasis, esophageal
Cervical cancer, invasive
Coccidioidomycosis, disseminated or extrapulmonary
Cryptosporidiosis, chronic intestinal (> 1 month duration)
Cytomegalovirus disease (other than liver, spleen, or nodes)
Cytomegalovirus retinitis (with loss of vision)
Encephalopathy, HIV-related
Herpes simplex: chronic ulcers (> 1 month duration) or bronchitis, pneumonitis, or esophagitis
Histoplasmosis, disseminated or extrapulmonary
Isosporiasis, chronic intestinal (> 1 month duration)
Karposi's sarcoma
Lymphoma, Burkitt's (or equivalent)
Lymphoma, immunoblastic (or equivalent term)
Lymphoma, primary of brain
Mycobacterium avium complex or *M. kansaii,* extrapulmonary
M. tuberculosis, any site, pulmonary or extrapulmonary
Mycobacterium, other or unrelated species, extrapulmonary
Pneumocystis carinii pneumonia
Pneumonia, recurrent
Progressive multifocal leukoencephalopathy
Salmonella septicemia, recurrent
Toxoplasmosis of brain
Wasting syndrome caused by HIV

amenorrhea. She has recently become sexually active with a new partner and wishes to be tested for pregnancy and sexually transmitted diseases, as she has used condoms only sporadically. Her past medical, surgical, and family histories are unremarkable. Although her review of systems was remarkable for mild nausea without vomiting and mild lethargy, the patient has not experienced any change in weight, fevers, chills, or other complaints. Her social history is remarkable for occasional tobacco use, but she denies any drug or alcohol use. On physical examination, she is noted to have a grayish-white vaginal discharge with an inflamed nulliparous cervix. There is no cervical motion tenderness and the remainder of the examination is normal.

Cultures are performed for gonorrhea, Chlamydia, and bacteria. Serum is drawn for a pregnancy test. When a sample of the vaginal discharge is placed on a microscope slide with potassium hydroxide, the analysis reveals copious vaginal candida. After the examination she was counseled on testing for HIV, hepatitis, and syphilis. Her written consent was obtained prior to testing for the presence of HIV antibodies. She was asked to return in one week for results of her tests and was told to begin with over-the-counter vaginal antifungal therapy.

COUNSELING THE PATIENT

It is important to appropriately counsel the patient before testing for HIV. She should be aware of the types of activities that will place her at risk for infection with HIV. This knowledge will enable an HIV-positive woman to be tested and begin therapy for the disease. For an HIV-negative woman, this information may encourage her to alter her lifestyle and adopt safe-sex practices, including limiting the number of sexual partners and utilizing condoms with penetrative sex.

A female patient also needs to be made aware that the test may occasionally give false-negative results, especially if exposure to the virus occurred too recently for her to develop antibodies. If she has engaged in high-risk behavior during the past six months and the test is negative, she should be counseled to stop the high-risk behavior and get retested in six months.

If the HIV test returns a positive result, the patient needs to be informed of the clinical ramifications and prognosis of HIV infection and educated on methods to prevent viral transmission to others. The patient should notify those persons at risk of exposure to the virus, including health care workers and sexual partners.

CLINICAL CORRELATION

A. W. returned to the office for her test results and was surprised to find out that she was pregnant. She was also informed that her HIV test was confirmed to be positive. After a long counseling session, she and her obstetrician outlined a comprehensive plan for her prenatal care, involving frequent evaluation of her CD4 counts, observation for opportunistic infections, and zidovudine therapy beginning at 15 weeks gestation.

HIV IN PREGNANCY

In 1993, 1.6 of every 1000 women who gave birth were infected with HIV. In addition, approximately 85% of all pediatric AIDS cases are known to result from perinatal transmission of the virus. These statistics have caused clinicians to examine the effects of HIV infection on pregnant women, the effects of pregnancy on HIV progression, and the risk and prevention of transmission of HIV disease to the fetus.

Because pregnancy is a relatively immunocompromised state in itself, concerns were initially raised that pregnancy would accelerate the progression of HIV infection. Research has since shown that this does not appear to be the case. Nevertheless, it remains important to observe these women closely for signs of opportunistic infections throughout pregnancy.

PERINATAL TRANSMISSION

Perinatal transmission of the HIV virus has been documented to occur at rates ranging from 13% to 40%. Infection can take place as early as the eighth week of gestation, although it is estimated that 50% of transmission occurs during labor and delivery. Infants with cord-blood samples that test negative for virus have been known to seroconvert shortly after birth, suggesting post-partum transmission. Intrapartum infection has been further documented by studies that showed a higher incidence of infection in first-born twins when delivered vaginally, presumably due to a greater exposure to vaginal secretions. Cesarean delivery has now been shown to be protective against HIV transmission and should be scheduled prior to the onset of labor. Data also reveal that the likelihood of prenatal transmission of HIV is influenced by maternal viral load, which suggests that perhaps this level should be monitored and dictate changes in the medical management during pregnancy in the future.

As noted earlier, the presence of the virus has been confirmed in breast milk, and vertical transmission by breast-feeding has occurred. Therefore, current recommendations are to restrict breast-feeding if the mother is HIV-positive.

During pregnancy, treatment with zidovudine (ZDV) should be started as soon after the fourteenth week of gestation as possible. Zidovudine (formerly known as AZT) inhibits the reverse transcriptase enzyme of the HIV virus, thereby blocking its replication. The treatment of HIV during pregnancy with ZDV was established by the AIDS Clinical Trials Group (ACTG) protocol 076. The patients participating in this protocol were pregnant women with CD4 counts greater than 200/mL who had not previously received the drug. The ZDV-treated mothers had an 8.3% transmission of virus to their infants versus 25.5% for a matched, placebo-treated group. The CDC recommends therapy for all HIV-positive women during pregnancy (Table 10.2).

HIV-infected women are also at risk for contracting opportunistic infections. The pregnant HIV-positive woman should be screened for toxoplasmosis and should have monthly complete blood counts, liver enzyme studies, and CD4 counts. In patients with CD4 counts of less than 200/mL, prophylaxis for *Pneumocystis carinii* with trimethoprim-sulfamethoxazole should be initiated. Aerosol pentamidine may be substituted in patients who are allergic to sulfonamides.

During delivery, universal precautions should be utilized with all patients. After delivery, the woman should receive follow-up care from an infectious diseases specialist. The infant should have repeated HIV antibody testing. The presence of HIV antibodies for longer than 15 months after delivery signifies infection in the infant.

Guidelines for treatment during pregnancy will continue to change, as therapeutic guidelines for nonpregnant women are rapidly evolving. Highly active antiretroviral therapy (HAART) is very active in diminishing viral load, which is a critical factor in mother-to-child transmission of the virus. Animal studies with protease inhibitors have failed to show that this class of drugs is teratogenic; however, no human data are available on this issue. Some studies have suggested that maternal ingestion of vitamin A can reduce the mother-to-child transmission. It is not year clear what role vitamin A will play in pregnancy, but caution is advised as vitamin A does have

Table 10.2   CDC Recommendations for HIV-Positive Pregnant Women

• Anterpartum:	100 mg ZDV orally 5 times per day beginning at 15 weeks gestation continued throughout pregnancy
• Labor and delivery	Intravenous loading of 2 mg/kg ZDV over 1 hour followed by continuous infusion of 1 mg/kg/h until delivery
• Post-partum	Newborn given ZDV syrup orally at 2 mg/kg every 6 hours for the first 6 weeks of life, beginning 8–12 hours after birth

teratogenic potential when consumed in high doses.

HIV IN THE GYNECOLOGICAL PATIENT

Although the prevention of pregnancy and the transmission of HIV to the fetus are important issues, the gynecologic care of the HIV patient requires attention as well. The courses of several diseases can be altered by HIV infection, including pelvic inflammatory disease (PID), vulvovaginal candidiasis, and cervical intra-epithelial neoplasia (CIN). According to recommendations issued by the CDC, women with PID who are HIV-positive should be hospitalized for administration of intravenous antibiotics. Although such women appear to be infected with the same organisms as HIV-negative women, immunocompromised patients cannot be treated adequately on an outpatient basis. Recurrent vulvovaginal candidiasis can pose a significant problem for the HIV-infected woman, occasionally requiring oral treatment with fluconozole to adequately treat or prevent outbreaks.

The immunocompromised patient is at risk for viral infections, including infection with the human papillomavirus, which is associated with the development of condyloma, cervical dysplasia, and carcinoma (Figure 10.1). HIV-infected women have a higher incidence of cervical dysplasia than their HIV-negative counterparts, when other risk factors for cervical disease are taken into account. It is recommended that these women undergo Pap smears of their cervix every 6 months. Several studies have questioned the sensitivity of Pap smears in detected dysplasia in HIV-positive women, which suggests that either more frequent cytology or routine use of colposcopy may be warranted.

SUMMARY

As the rate of HIV infection among women continues to climb, obstetricians and gynecologists are becoming more involved in this epidemic. Physicians must take an active role in educating patients about high-risk behaviors that place them or their offspring in danger of infection with this virus.

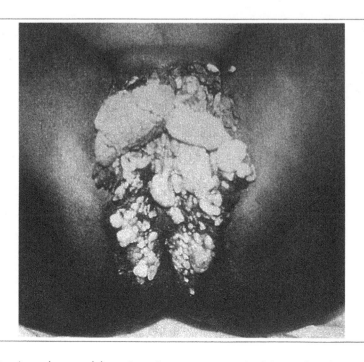

Figure 10.1   Extensive vulvar condyloma in an immunocompromised (HIV-infected) woman

In addition, obstetricians should have a basic understanding of managing an HIV-infected mother through pregnancy and should know which drug therapy will reduce the risk of transmission of the virus to her infant. The gynecologist should know which gynecologic symptoms may relate to a diminished immune system, how to counsel their patients on HIV testing, and what to do if the test results are positive.

PART III

Obstetrics

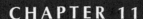

CHAPTER 11

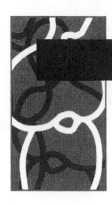

Maternal/Fetal Physiology

Alexander F. Burnett

Significant changes occur to a woman as she progresses through pregnancy. The fetus and placenta develop so as to extract the necessary nutrients to allow the gestation to grow. Knowledge of the normal changes that occur in pregnancy is important, especially when these changes affect pre-existing illnesses (Table 11.1).

CLINICAL CORRELATION

P. T. is a 22-year-old female who had her last menstrual period six weeks ago. She has been married for two years and recently discontinued taking oral contraceptive pills in an effort to conceive. She is very regular, with her menses occurring every 28 days. In the past two weeks, she has experienced breast tenderness and occasional morning nausea. She recently took a home pregnancy test, which gave a positive result.

MATERNAL CHANGES IN PREGNANCY

Morning sickness is quite common, occurring in as many as 70% of all pregnancies. Most women experience this condition initially between 4 and 8 weeks gestation, and generally the symptoms abate by 14 weeks gestation. In most cases, morning sickness is a self-limiting entity that rarely causes significant electrolyte or fluid imbalances. Its exact etiology is unknown, although human chorionic gonadotropin (hCG) levels are believed to play a role. Although an exact correlation does not exist between the hCG level and the degree of nausea or vomiting, morning sickness does chronologically parallel the rise, peak, and fall of hCG during pregnancy. Early in pregnancy, hCG levels double approximately every 48 hours. Urine pregnancy tests will often be positive by the time of the missed menstrual period.

In severe forms of nausea and vomiting, morning sickness may persist well beyond the first trimester as hyperemesis gravidarum, which can have significant effect on the gestation in terms of nutrition to the mother and fetus, dehydration, and ketosis. Parenteral replacement of fluids and calories may be required as well as hospitalization. Hyperemesis may persist for the entire pregnancy. Hyperemesis may also be a sign of a molar gestation, a condition in which there may be abnormally high hCG levels associated with abnormal placental tissue (see Chapter 55 for more detail).

Breast tenderness and/or heaviness is often evident by 4 weeks gestation. The breasts will enlarge over the entire course of pregnancy due to ductal growth, stimulated by estrogen, and alveolar hypertrophy, stimulated by progesterone. The cervix will take on a bluish discoloration due to increased blood flow to this region—a condition known as Chadwick's sign. Skin changes due to increased levels of alpha-

Table 11.1 Maternal Physiologic Changes in Pregnancy

ORGAN/SYSTEM	CHANGES	CONSEQUENCES
Gastrointestinal tract		
Stomach	Decreased tone and motility	
Small intestine	Decreased motility	Longer transit time
Colon	Increased water absorption	Constipation
	Decreased motility	
Integument		
Skin	Spider angiomata, palmar erythema	
	Striae, hyperpigmentation of nipples, areolae, axillae, face (chloasma), and midline of lower abdomen (linea nigra)	
Hair	Increased loss first 2–4 months post-partum	
	Returns to normal in 6–12 months	
Renal		
Kidneys	Ureterocalyceal dilatation	Increased incidence of pyelonephritis
	Increased renal plasma flow, GFR	Decreased BUN/creatinine
	Increased renin and angiotensinogen	
	Increased glucose excretion	
	Increased amino acid excretion	Increased UTIs
Cardiovascular		
Heart	Increased heart rate and stroke volume	Increased cardiac output
	Decreased systemic vascular resistance	
	Decreased mean arterial pressure	
	Output to uterus increases from 1%–2% to 17% of C.O.	
	No change in flow to brain, kidneys, skin, or coronary arteries	
	S3 and systolic ejection murmur common by midpregnancy	
Peripheral	Increased ankle edema	
Hematologic	Increased plasma volume; increase in RBC volume but not as great	Decreased hematocrit
	Increased WBCs	
	Increased coagulation factors (I-fibrinogen, VII-X)	Increased thromboembolic risk, particularly in post-partum
	Increased iron requirements with some increase in iron absorption	
Glucose metabolism	Decreased tissue sensitivity to insulin (due to hPL)	
Ocular	Increased corneal thickness, decreased intraocular pressure	
Skeletal	Relaxation of ligaments of symphysis pubis and sacroiliac joints	
Breasts	See Chapter 30	

melanocyte–stimulating hormone include hyperpigmentation of the nipples and areolae, umbilicus, perineum, and midline of the lower abdomen (linea nigra). Some women also develop a rash on the face, known as chloasma of pregnancy.

Cardiovascular changes over the course of pregnancy include a 33% (on average) increase in cardiac output due to increases in both stroke volume and heart rate. Plasma volume increases by 50% over the pregnancy, and red cell volume increases by 20% to 30%, leading to a relative decrease in hematocrit. Blood flow to the uterus increases from 1% to 2% of cardiac output in the nonpregnant and first-trimester woman to 17% by term. Late in pregnancy, the gravid uterus can completely occlude the inferior vena cave when the mother is in a supine position. The increase in overall cardiac output allows blood flow to the kidneys, brain, and coronary arteries to remain unchanged over pregnancy. Systemic vascular resistance falls over pregnancy, and arterial blood pressure will fall by approximately 10 mm Hg for systolic and diastolic pressure over the first 24 weeks. Thereafter, the blood pressure gradually rises, returning to pre-pregnancy levels by term. If the blood pressure rises significantly above pre-pregnancy levels, it may indicate that the mother is developing pre-eclampsia.

Pulmonary changes during pregnancy include an increase in tidal volume (the amount of breath inspired and expired with a normal breath) with a decrease in expiratory reserve (Figure 11.1). The chest volume increases, as does diaphragmatic excursion, despite the increased mass of the uterus in the abdomen. Progesterone appears to be responsible for the increased tidal volume, as it increases the sensitivity of the respiratory center to CO_2 and perhaps stimulates the respiratory center directly.

Nutritional requirements increase over the gestation as well. The average woman requires approximately 300 kcal/day increase in calories during pregnancy (Table 11.2). Weight gain should be in the range of 20 to 30 pounds. Protein, folate, iron, and vitamin requirements also increase, and most women are advised to take prenatal vitamins and iron supplements.

CLINICAL CORRELATION

P. T. is instructed to begin taking prenatal vitamins and iron. She returns in 6 weeks, stating that she still has nausea in the mornings and occasionally vomits; overall, however, this symptom is lessening. Her weight has increased by 3 pounds. Examination now reveals the uterus to be consistent with a 12-week gestational size and fetal heart

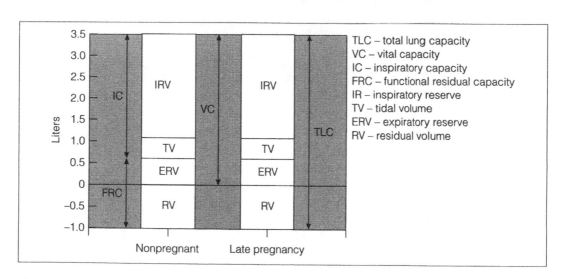

Figure 11.1 Respiratory changes with pregnancy

Source: Callahan TL, Caughey AB, Heffner LJ. Blueprints in obstetrics and gynecology. Malden, MA: Blackwell Science, 1998:2.

Table 11.2 Recommended Daily Dietary Allowances for Nonpregnant, Pregnant, and Lactating Women

	NONPREGNANT WOMEN (YR)					PREGNANT WOMEN	LACTATING WOMEN
	11–14	15–18	19–22	23–50	51+		
Energy (kcal)	2400	2100	2100	2000	1800	+300	+500
Protein (g)	44	48	46	46	46	+30	+20
Fat-soluble vitamins							
Vitamin A activity (RE)	800	800	800	800	800	1000	1200
(IU)	4000	4000	4000	4000	4000	5000	6000
Vitamin D (IU)	400	400	400	—	—	400	400
Vitamin E activity (IU)	12	12	12	12	12	15	15
Water-soluble vitamins							
Ascorbic acid (mg)	45	45	45	45	45	60	80
Folacin (µg)	400	400	400	400	400	800	600
Niacin (mg)	16	14	14	13	12	+2	+4
Riboflavin (mg)	1.3	1.4	1.4	1.2	1.1	+0.3	+0.5
Thiamin (mg)	1.2	1.1	1.1	1	1	+0.3	+0.3
Vitamin B_{12} (mg)	1.6	2	2	2	2	2.5	2.5
Vitamin B_6 (µg)	3	3	3	3	3	4	4
Minerals							
Calcium (mg)	1200	1200	800	800	800	1200	1200
Iodine (µg)	115	115	100	100	80	125	150
Iron (mg)	18	18	18	18	10	+18	18
Magnesium (mg)	300	300	300	300	300	450	450
Phosphorus (mg)	1200	1200	800	800	800	1200	1200
Zinc (mg)	15	15	15	15	15	20	25

Source: Gabbe SG, Niebyl JR, Simpsen JL. Obstetrics: normal and problem pregnancies, 2nd ed. New York: Churchill Livingstone, 1991:196.

tones are detected by Doppler. An ultrasound in the office reveals a singleton intrauterine pregnancy with crown-rump length consistent with 12 0/7 weeks. All measurements are consistent with the dates of her last menstrual period, and her estimated date of confinement is calculated.

Detection of fetal heart tones by Doppler should occur by 11 to 12 weeks gestation. Failure to detect the heart tones at that time may indicate either a problem with the pregnancy (for example, ectopic pregnancy, fetal demise, or molar gestation) or a problem with dates. The latter issue can quickly be resolved by using ultrasound, which is accurate in dating to plus or minus one week in the first trimester. Early establishment of dates is critical for determining adequate growth throughout gestation and timing of delivery. Quickening, or the maternal feeling of fetal movement, normally occurs around 19 to 20 weeks during the first gestation, and about two weeks earlier in subsequent gestations. Later in pregnancy, maternal detection of frequency of fetal movement can be an important indicator of fetal well-being.

Eventually, the size of the gestation will cause postural changes that almost universally lead to low back pain. These postural changes are necessary to maintain the center of gravity over the legs while the uterus grows. The ligaments of the symphysis pubis become more lax over pregnancy due to the hormone relaxin, and often the woman's gait may become more unsteady. Striae occur in the skin of approximately 50% of pregnant women, reflecting the stretching of the skin during gestation rather than excessive weight gain. There is no treatment to prevent these marks from developing.

FETAL AND PLACENTAL PHYSIOLOGY

The placenta forms from tissue present within the blastocyst stage. The trophoblastic (placental) tissue is composed of two types of cells: (1) the cytotrophoblast, which consists of cuboidal cells, and (2) the syncytiotrophoblast, which consists of multinucleated cells that form the leading edge of invasion into maternal vessels. As the placenta matures, villi develop that form the exchange unit with the maternal surface. The trophoblast serves to transport substances from the maternal circulation to the fetal circulation. The terminal villi are bathed in maternal blood and eventually coalesce on the fetal side of the placenta to form the fetal vessels (usually one umbilical vein and two umbilical arteries) (Figure 11.2).

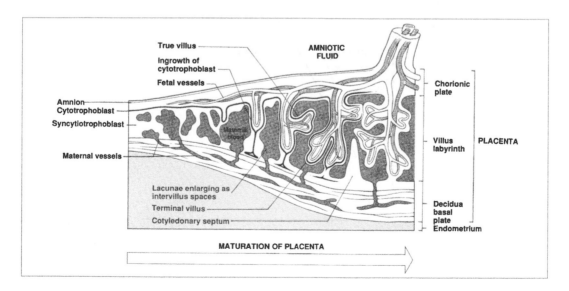

Figure 11.2   Morphology of the placenta

Source: Gabbe SG, ed. Obstetrics: normal and problem pregnancies, 2nd ed. New York: Churchill Livingstone, 1991:63.

Transfer of materials across the placenta can occur by many mechanisms. For example, respiratory gases pass between the two circulations by simple diffusion. Fetal hemoglobin has an oxygen dissociation curve to the left of maternal hemoglobin; therefore, for any given oxygen tension, the fetal blood will have higher oxygen saturation. This concentration largely reflects the ability of fetal hemoglobin to bind 2,3-diphosphoglycerate (2,3 DPG), which increases the oxygen affinity of fetal hemoglobin (Figure 11.3). Glucose is transferred to the fetus via a facilitated transport involving a specific plasma membrane protein. Amino acids are transferred by transport-specific membrane proteins as well; unlike with glucose, however, movement of these acids is largely sodium-dependent. Water transfer is determined by the filtration coefficient for water and the colloid osmotic pressure gradients. The syncytiotrophoblast contains receptors for insulin, immunoglobulin, transferrin, and low-density lipoprotein; these receptors promote endocytosis of these molecules for transfer.

In addition to specialized hemoglobin, the fetal circulation utilizes several mechanisms that are essential for development of the fetus. The circulatory system of the fetus is discussed in detail in Chapter 28. For now, it is suffices to say that the formation of urine by the fetus is important in maintaining amniotic fluid balance. The fetus's gastrointestinal tract absorbs very small amounts of glucose, lactate, and amino acids. Bilirubin elimination is maintained by the placenta well into the third trimester, and often the immaturity of the newborn liver results in neonatal jaundice. The fetal adrenal gland is proportionally larger than its counterpart in the adult. Dehydroepiandrosterone sulfate (DHEAS)—the major output of the fetal zone of the adrenal gland—is converted in the placenta to estriol and then secreted into the maternal circulation. Consequently, maternal levels of estriol during pregnancy have been used as an indicator of fetal well-being. More recently, estriol levels have been added to the "triple screen" for the presence of trisomy 21 in early pregnancy.

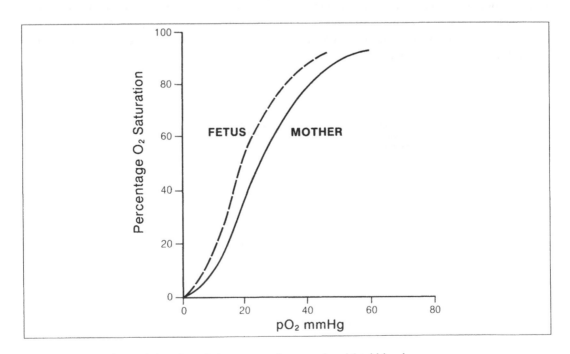

Figure 11.3   Oxyhemoglobin dissociation curves of maternal and fetal blood

Source: Gabbe SG, ed. Obstetrics: normal and problem pregnancies, 2nd ed. New York: Churchill Livingstone, 1991:109.

EFFECTS OF PHYSIOLOGIC CHANGES OF PREGNANCY

As discussed in Chapter 23, physiologic adaptations to pregnancy can significantly affect preexisting maternal disease. For example, the changes in plasma blood flow and cardiac output can unduly stress a sick heart. The pulmonary changes will have profound effects on women with primary pulmonary hypertension or women with significant intrinsic pulmonary disease such as asthma, bronchitis, or emphysema. Diabetics will tend to have worse control of their blood sugar during gestation due to the development of a relative insulin resistance during pregnancy. In certain circumstances, some diseases improve during pregnancy, only to be followed by an exacerbation in the post-partum period. This observation is true for many autoimmune diseases, for example.

SUMMARY

Recognizing the outstanding changes in maternal physiology during pregnancy are important for understanding the normal signs and symptoms of pregnancy and thereby detecting problems. The feto-placental unit must establish itself early in gestation to provide the nutrients for the growing gestation. This system is designed to provide for all of the fetus's needs without completely stripping the mother of her ability to function and survive.

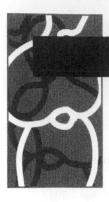

CHAPTER 12

Preconception and Antepartum Care

Alexander F. Burnett

PRECONCEPTION CARE

Good health prior to conception can diminish maternal and fetal morbidity and mortality. It is important to know how certain medical conditions can affect pregnancy as well as how pregnancy can affect the mother's preexisting medical conditions. The time prior to conception is a period when education of the couple may have significant ramifications for pregnancy outcome.

CLINICAL CORRELATION

A. B. is a 22-year-old female, gravida 0, who has recently married and is interested in beginning a family. She is a healthy woman with the exception of insulin-dependent diabetes mellitus diagnosed four years ago. Her blood sugars are maintained in a healthy range, and she has no complications of diabetes at this time. Her husband has no medical problems. Their families do not have any dominant diseases. Her husband has a cousin with cystic fibrosis. The couple visit her obstetrician to understand what potential risks A. B. may have in becoming pregnant.

The maternal history prior to conception should include a thorough medical, surgical, obstetrical, social, and family history. Medical conditions that are affected by pregnancy include diabetes, heart disease, hypertension, asthma, renal disease, and autoimmune diseases (see Chapter 23). The preconceptual visit offers an opportunity to discuss how the physiologic changes of pregnancy will play out in terms of these illnesses. Certain diseases, such as primary pulmonary hypertension or diabetes with extensive end-organ damage, may be contraindications to pregnancy in that a high mortality may be associated with carrying a pregnancy. Other illnesses, such as autoimmune diseases and renal failure, may make conception difficult. Treatment of still other conditions may involve drug therapy that is potentially teratogenic to the developing fetus.

Genetic anomalies should be discussed in relation to particular characteristics of the couple. For instance, heritable genetic illnesses present in the family may require extensive genetic counseling prior to conception to determine the risks for the couple. As women get older at the time of conception, their risk of genetic abnormalities increases, particularly for Down syndrome. In addition, certain individuals may be at risk for specific illnesses such as sickle cell disease, Tay-Sachs, and thallassemias.

Prior reproductive history should be discussed with patients. In particular, prior ectopic gestation increases the risk of ectopic gestation in the future. Information on previous miscarriages, including the gestational age of miscarriage, should be noted. Repetitive first-trimester abortions may indicate genetic, anatomic, or endometrial anomalies that warrant further investigation. Later-gestation losses may also be due to uterine anomalies.

Immunity to rubella and hepatitis should be discussed, and any appropriate immunizations performed. The woman should be assessed for risk of infection with human immunodeficiency virus and, if she is positive for this infection, educated on its potential effects on offspring. Social habits should be discussed and education provided on the need to reduce or eliminate smoking, alcohol, and drug use prior to conception.

CLINICAL CORRELATION

A. B. is briefed on the potential impact of diabetes on pregnancy. Tight control during the preconceptual period and early in conception is important to reduce the incidence of diabetes-related birth defects. Good control over pregnancy will reduce macrosomia. A. B. is told that pregnancy reduces glucose tolerance and her insulin requirements will likely increase over the course of the gestation. A plan to coordinate care with her endocrinologist is suggested if she desires to conceive.

PRENATAL CARE

Thoughtful care of the woman during her pregnancy will improve her likelihood of delivering a healthy child. Good prenatal care decreases the risk of premature delivery as well as serious maternal complications of pregnancy. Education during this time can help prepare a woman for childbirth and for the changes that her body is expected to experience through pregnancy and post-partum period. Generally, health screening—including Pap smear, cervical cultures, blood testing, physical examination, and monitoring of vital signs—can uncover preexisting health problems and lead to a diagnosis earlier in the pregnancy, when new problems can develop.

CLINICAL CORRELATION

A. B. returns to her physician's office in six months, reporting that seven weeks have passed since her last menstrual period. She took a home pregnancy test two weeks ago that gave a positive result. She has noted some breast tenderness but only minimal nausea. She denies any abdominal pain or cramping.

Examination of the cervix reveals a bluish discoloration. The uterus is minimally enlarged and the right ovary is approximately 6 cm. When a transvaginal ultrasound is performed, it reveals a singleton intrauterine gestation with heart motion noted. A right ovarian simple cyst is present, consistent with a corpus luteum cyst of pregnancy. Crown-rump length measurement is 11 mm, consistent with 7½ weeks gestational age.

A full panel of prenatal labs is performed, including a hepatitis B antibody titer and a hemaglobin A1c. A. B. is given a container and instructions for collecting a 24-hour urine sample for creatinine clearance determination. She is instructed to return in one week to review the early laboratory test results and to make an appointment with her endocrinologist in one week as well.

Diagnosis of pregnancy is assumed when a woman with regular menses having unprotected intercourse misses a menstrual period. Over-the-counter urine-based pregnancy tests can detect less than 50 mIU/mL serum hCG levels, which is consistent with a four- to five-week gestation, or about the time of the first missed menses (Table 12.1). In contrast, serum pregnancy tests can detect hCG levels of 5 mIU/mL or less, which are found prior to the first missed menses. Subjective symptoms of pregnancy include breast tenderness and nausea, although many women remain asymptomatic.

The initial prenatal visit calls for a complete history and physical examination, including genetic history, psychosocial history, and medical history. The physical examination should note the patient's initial weight, blood pressure, any physical abnormalities, and size of the uterus. Cultures of the cervix for gonorrhea, Chlamydia, and group B streptococcus, as well as a Pap smear, are routinely performed. Routine prenatal lab work includes a

Table 12.1 HCG Values and Sonography in Early Pregnancy

GESTATIONAL AGE	MEAN HCG VALUE (IU/L)	SONOGRAPHIC FINDINGS
4 weeks	1885	TVS: gestational sac
6 weeks	12,870	TVS: yolk sac
7 weeks		TVS: cardiac motion
8 weeks	56,010	
10 weeks	108,800	

Source: Adapted from Hay DL. Placental histology and the production of human choriogonadotropin and its subunits in pregnancy. Br Ob Gyn 1988;95:1268, and Common Problems.

type and screen to detect blood type and the presence of antibodies, hemoglobin, plus blood tests for rubella, syphilis, and hepatitis. HIV testing should be offered with appropriate counseling. A urine dipstick and culture should be taken as well.

Early visits should screen for factors that may identify a pregnancy at high risk for complications. This effort includes identifying women at the extremes of the reproductive ages—that is, teen pregnancy and pregnancy in women older than age 35. Teen pregnancy is associated with less frequent prenatal visits and higher risk of pre-eclampsia and preterm labor. Pregnancy is women older than age 35 is associated with increased risk of genetic defects and requires the patient to be asked about genetic screening. The older gravida is also at increased risk for pre-eclampsia and for thrombotic phenomena associated with gestation.

With particular medical conditions, additional tests may be performed, such as tests for glucose, hemoglobin A1c, and renal function monitoring with diabetic patients, drug levels in patients who require continuous medication such as for seizure prevention, or thyroid function monitoring in patients with a history of thyroid disease.

Repeat prenatal visits in uncomplicated pregnancies should take place every 4 weeks up to 28 weeks gestational age, every two weeks from 29 to 36 weeks, and then weekly thereafter, as indicated in Table 12.2. With complications or significant medical conditions, more frequent visits will be required. At each visit, at a minimum weight, blood pressure, and fetal growth should be measured.

Fetal heart tones should be detectable by Doppler prior to week 12. Measurement of maternal serum alpha-fetoprotein levels is offered at 15 to 16 weeks gestation to detect neural tube defects and may be included as part of triple screening (along with hCG and estradiol) for Down syndrome. In nondiabetic patients, glucose screening by one-hour glucola testing is done at 28 weeks (discussed in Chapter 28). For the Rh-negative mother without prior sensitization, RhoGAM is given prophylactically at 28 weeks.

Total weight gain over pregnancy is generally about 20 to 30 pounds. Underweight women may gain as much as 40 pounds; overweight women should limit weight gain to a maximum of 25 pounds. Generally, women gain 3 to 6 pounds in the first trimester and then between 0.5 and 1 pound per week until term. Inadequate weight gain may indicate a risk for a low-birth-weight infant or signal inadequate nutritional intake by the mother. Excess weight gain may be an indication of edema, which can occur as part of pre-eclampsia (discussed in Chapter 23).

Pregnant women generally require about 300 additional kcals of nutrition per day. Substantial increases in a woman's need for calcium, phosphorus, iron, folic acid, and vitamin D occur during pregnancy. Most prenatal formula vitamins with iron will cover these requirements, as well as the requirements for the lesser increases in trace elements. Taking mega-doses of vitamins and minerals is discouraged, as some—particularly vitamin A— have been associated with an increase in birth defects.

Table 12.2 Recommendations for All Women for Prenatal Care

	PRECONCEPTION OR FIRST VISIT	WEEKS								
		6–8	14–16	24–28	32	36	38	39	40	41
History										
Medical, including genetic	X									
Psychosocial	X									
Update medical and psychosocial		X	X	X	X	X	X	X	X	X
Physical examination										
General	X									
Blood pressure	X	X	X	X	X	X	X	X	X	X
Height	X									
Weight	X	X	X	X	X	X	X	X	X	X
Height and weight profile	X									
Pelvic examination and pelvimetry	X	X								
Breast examination	X	X								
Fundal height			X	X	X	X	X	X	X	X
Fetal position and heart rate			X	X	X	X	X	X	X	X
Cervical examination	X									

Table 12.2 *(Continued)*

	PRECONCEPTION OR FIRST VISIT	WEEKS								
		6–8	14–16	24–28	32	36	38	39	40	41
Laboratory tests										
Hemoglobin or hematocrit	X	X		X		X				
Rh factor	X									
Pap smear	X									
Diabetic screen				X						
MSAFP			X							
Urine										
Dipstick	X									
Protein	X									
Sugar	X									
Culture		X								
Infections										
Rubella titer	X									
Syphilis test	X									
Gonococcal culture	X	X				X				
Hepatitis B	X									
HIV (offered)	X	X								
Illicit drug screen (offered)	X									
Genetic screen	X									

Activity levels can remain where the mother is comfortable, although most women experience a need for increased rest. Long-term strenuous exercise should be lessened during pregnancy. Although sexual activity need not be reduced during pregnancy, changes in comfort and sexual desire often occur. Women at risk for preterm labor may need to restrict intercourse if it has been associated with increased uterine contractions.

Live attenuated-virus vaccines are not given during pregnancy; in contrast, inactivated-virus vaccines, toxoids, or tetanus immunoglobulin appear safe in these patients. Although there is no evidence of congenital rubella syndrome in offspring of women inadvertently given rubella vaccine during pregnancy, this vaccine is generally given after gestation if the woman is not already immune. Yellow fever and oral polio vaccines are safe to give during gestation.

Other frequent symptoms that may occur with pregnancy include heartburn, constipation, hemorrhoids, urinary frequency, round ligament pain from uterine stretching, backache, and occasionally syncopal sensations due to poor venous return secondary to compression of the vena cava from the enlarging uterus.

CLINICAL CORRELATION

A. B. returns in one week to review her lab tests performed to date. She has seen her endocrinologist, who has altered her insulin regimen to maintain tighter control of her blood sugar over the course of the day. Her hemoglobin A1c is 6.0, indicating good glucose control during early pregnancy when organogenesis is occurring. The remainder of her test results are normal. She is instructed to return in four weeks and will see her endocrinologist every two weeks during gestation.

As the pregnancy progresses, patients should be educated on the signs of labor. They should be instructed to call for vaginal bleeding, regular uterine contractions, rupture of membranes, or lack of fetal movement. Encour-

agement of breast-feeding should occur over the pregnancy. Preparation for childbirth often incorporates classes where a woman and her partner learn about the process of labor and delivery, the various alternatives for the birthing environment, options regarding pain control, and other obstetric procedures such as episiotomy, cesarean delivery, and assisted vaginal delivery. The patient should be allowed to discuss her desires for the birthing process during her prenatal care, and these preferences should be noted in the prenatal record.

Each visit will assess growth of the fetus in terms of fundal height of the uterus. Significant alterations from normal growth may signal intrauterine growth restriction, macrosomia, or abnormalities of amniotic fluid (oligohydramnios or polyhydramnios). Abnormalities of growth require further attention. Ultrasound should be used liberally whenever any concern arises.

As the pregnancy reaches the third trimester, the fetal position is noted on each visit. The patient should be informed about this position in case spontaneous labor occurs at a time when the clinic record is unavailable. For example, if the woman calls to complain of rupture of membranes in the middle of the night and was noted on office examination the day before to have her fetus in a nonvertex position, this fact may increase the urgency with which she should come to the hospital, as she has a higher risk of cord accidents or labor difficulties.

SUMMARY

Preconceptual care is important for identifying risks for ensuing pregnancies and offering an opportunity to reduce these risks prior to conception. Prenatal care is important for improving birth outcome. Careful monitoring of basic maternal and fetal changes over the gestation may detect abnormalities early, when intervention to improve outcome is still possible. Throughout the course of the gestation, education is critical to reduce maternal anxiety and improve compliance with prenatal care.

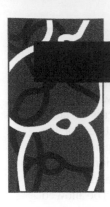

CHAPTER 13

Genetic Counseling

Michele B. Prince, Michele E. Martin,
and Alexander F. Burnett

Genetic counseling is an allied health profession that combines the science of medical genetics with the art of counseling. As defined by the American Society of Human Genetics in 1975,

"Genetic counseling is a communication process which deals with the human problems associated with the occurrence, or the risk of occurrence, of a genetic disorder in a family. This process involves the attempt by one or more appropriately trained persons to help the individual or family to (1) comprehend the medical facts, including the diagnosis, probable course of the disorder, and the available management; (2) appreciate the way heredity contributes to the disorder, and the risk of recurrence in specified relatives; (3) understand the alternatives for dealing with the risk of recurrence; (4) choose the course of action which seems to them appropriate in view of their risk, their family goals, and their ethical and religious standards, and to act in accordance with that decision; and (5) to make the best possible adjustment to the disorder in an affected family member and/or to the risk of recurrence of that disorder."

Today, issues of genetic risks for development of adult illnesses, such as certain cancers, also has come under the purview of genetic counselors.

PRENATAL AND PRECONCEPTUAL GENETICS COUNSELING

In obstetrics and gynecology, patients can be referred for genetic counseling prior to conception, at any point during the ongoing pregnancy, or following a pregnancy loss. Genetic counselors prefer to see patients prior to conception, when a discussion of potential risk factors and options for prenatal testing can occur without the additional stress of decision making during pregnancy.

Patients are referred to a genetic counselor for many reasons (Table 13.1), although the majority of prenatal patients are seen for advanced maternal age (35 years and older) due to an increased risk for chromosome abnormalities such as Down syndrome in their offspring, as shown in Table 13.2. An increasingly more common reason for referral in the population of patients younger than 35 years of age is the maternal serum multiple marker screen (or triple screen of maternal levels of hCG, estriol, and alpha-fetoprotein), which provides a risk refinement for Down syndrome and open neural tube defects (Table 13.3). Maternal estriol levels are an indirect indicator of fetal well-being. Almost all of the maternal estriol originates from placental conversion of fetal 16 alpha-OH DHEAS to estriol; therefore, depressed maternal estriol levels may indicate poor adrenal cortex function in the fetus. Maternal serum alpha-fetoprotein (MSAFP) is measured at 16 to

Table 13.1   Reasons for Referrel to a Prenatal Genetic Counselor

- Maternal age 35 years or greater
- Positive maternal serum multiple marker screen
- Abnormal ultrasound findings in current pregnancy
- Exposure to potential teratogens
- Medical condition that poses increased risk for birth defects (diabetes, epilepsy)
- Multiple miscarriages
- Previous pregnancy loss with birth defect or genetic abnormality
- Family history of genetic disease, birth defect, or mental retardation
- History of chromosome abnormality
- One parent who carries a chromosome rearrangement
- Increased risk for genetic disease based on ethnicity
- Parent(s) known carrier(s) of a single-gene disorder

Table 13.2   Incidence of Down Syndrome Relative to Maternal Age

MATERNAL AGE	RISK FOR DOWN SYNDROME
20	1/1667
21	1/1667
22	1/1429
23	1/1429
24	1/1250
25	1/1250
26	1/1176
27	1/1111
28	1/1053
29	1/1000
30	1/952
31	1/909
32	1/769
33	1/625
34	1/500
35	1/385
36	1/294
37	1/227
38	1/175
39	1/137
40	1/106
41	1/82
42	1/64
43	1/50
44	1/38
45	1/30
46	1/23
47	1/18
48	1/14
49	1/11

Source: Adapted from Hook EB. Rates of chromosomal abnormalities of different maternal ages. Ob Gyn 1981;58:282; Hook EB, Cross PK, Schreinemachers DM, et al. Chromosomal abnormality rates at amniocentesis and live-born infants. JAMA 1983; 249:2043.

18 weeks gestation and reported as a multiple of the median value for normal pregnancies at that time of gestation. Elevated levels of MSAFP are associated with open neural tube defects (Table 13.4), whereas diminished levels are associated with Down syndrome.

CLINICAL CORRELATION

A. G. is a 31-year-old, gravida 1, female in good general health who has experienced an uncomplicated pregnancy to date and who had a reliable last menstrual period date. She has undergone a maternal serum "triple" screen performed at 16 weeks gestation in her obstetrician's office, where she also received a pamphlet about the screen. A week later, the obstetrician receives a report from the laboratory indicating that the risk for Down syndrome in her fetus is greater than A. G.'s age-related risk of 1/796 at term. The risk of Down syndrome is reported as 1/59 based on the assessment of the multiple of the median for

---

Table 13.3   Maternal Serum Triple Screen for Genetic Anomalies

Down syndrome associated with:

1. Decreased maternal serum alpha-fetoprotein: median 0.8 MoM* (about 20% lower than median of normal pregnancy)

2. Increased hCG: median > 2.5 MoM

3. Decreased maternal estriol: median 75% of normal

Down syndrome detection rates are 55%–60% with triple screen

*MoM = multiples of the median.
Source: Adapted from Ross HL, Elis S. Maternal serum screening for fetal genetic disorders obstetrician. Obstet Gynecol Clin N Am 1997;24:33.

---

alpha-fetoprotein (AFP), beta-hCG, and unconjugated estriol. The other component of the screen—risk assessment for open neural tube defects—is negative, indicating a substantially reduced risk for this birth defect. The obstetrician telephones the patient with the results, recommending that she schedule an appointment for genetic counseling and an amniocentesis at the medical center affiliated with her practice. The patient is informed that amniocentesis is available because of the increased risk of Down syndrome, but is not mandatory.

PRINCIPLES AND PRACTICE OF GENETIC COUNSELING

Genetic counselors strive to present information in a nondirective, value-neutral manner that takes into account the patient's or couple's psychosocial, religious, and ethnocultural context. This attitude fosters an environment of patient autonomy in decision making, especially in the areas of prenatal diagnosis and pregnancy termination for abnormal results. At times, genetic counselors serve as interpreters of often complex technical information and concepts, explaining the accuracy, risks, benefits, and limitations of the available medical procedures and genetic tests.

Table 13.4   Causes for Elevated MSAFP

- Underestimation of gestational age
- Multiple gestation
- Fetal demise
- Fetal anomalies
  - Neural tube defects
  - Ventral abdominal wall defect (gastroschisis, omphalocele)
  - Rh immunization, cystic hygroma, fetal edema
  - Urinary tract abnormalities
  - Dermatologic disorders (epidermolysis bullosa)
  - Atresia of the gastrointestinal tract
- Maternal disorders
  - Tumor of liver, yolk sac
  - Acute viral hepatitis
  - Blood group sensitization (Rh, KELL)
  - Lupus autoantibody
- Placental
  - Hemangiomas of placenta, umbilical cord
  - Placental lakes
  - Retroplacental bleed

CLINICAL CORRELATION

A. G. arrives for genetic counseling with her husband several days after receiving the triple screen results from her doctor. The couple expresses their concerns about the results and their need for more information regarding the implications and options for further testing.

The primary information-gathering tool is the genetic pedigree. A detailed family and medical history is obtained, resulting in a multigeneration pedigree with symbols representing each individual and any significant health conditions (Figure 13.1). Specific questions about each family member include age, general health, presence of chronic illness, genetic disease, birth defects, mental retardation or learning problems, mental health history, and reproductive history. In addition, the patient and her partner are asked about their ethnic backgrounds and whether their relationship is consanguineous (Figure 13.2). A pregnancy history is also obtained, including information on exposures to alcohol, tobacco, illicit drugs, prescription medications, over-the-counter medications, and environmental or occupational hazards. The resulting pedigree allows for easy documentation and assessment of the patterns of transmission of any problems in the family and serves as an oral and visual communication tool throughout the session.

As noted previously, the pedigree and

evaluation should take into account the ethnic background of the couple. Certain ethnic groups are more susceptible to particular heritable conditions. For example, Ashkenazi Jews have an increased incidence of Tay-Sachs disease (decreased serum hexosamidase-A). African Americans are susceptible to sickle cell anemia; Mediterraneans have an increased incidence of beta-thalassemia, and Southeast Asians have an increased incidence of alpha-thalassemia. Northern European Caucasians are at increased risk for cystic fibrosis.

CLINICAL CORRELATION

A. G. and her husband are both 31 years old and in good general health. This pregnancy is the first for both of them. Their family history is negative for birth defects, mental retardation, or genetic disease. Both are of Northern European Caucasian ancestry and deny consanguinity. The genetic counselor explains that the background risk for birth defects in the general population is 3% to 4%. Based on the family and medical

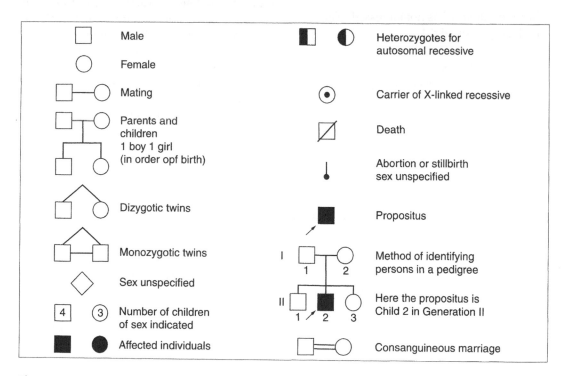

Figure 13.1 Symbols used in pedigree charts

Source: Creasy RK, Resnik R, eds. Maternal-fetal medicine, 4th ed. Philadelphia: W. B. Saunders, 1999.

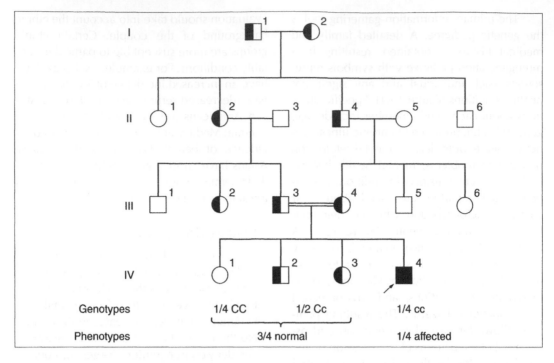

Figure 13.2 Pedigree of autosomal recessive trait (cystic fibrosis)

Source: Creasy RK, Resnik R, eds. Maternal-fetal medicine, 4th ed. Philadelphia: W. B. Saunders, 1999.

histories, their risk is not increased relative to the background risk.

Options for prenatal diagnosis are described, with information being provided regarding risks, benefits, and limitations. The ensuing genetic testing—whether chromosomal or DNA based—is also discussed and its accu-racy and limitations described. Most prenatal genetic diagnoses are confirmed by examining the fetal DNA from cells obtained by amniocentesis (Table 13.5). Many diagnoses require culturing the amniocytes, which extends the time to receive the diagnosis. Early in gestation, fetal cells may be obtained by chorionic villus sampling, which aspirates fetal villi. This testing can be done as early as nine weeks gestational

Table 13.5 Abnormalities Detected by Amniocentesis

DISORDER	MOLECULAR DEFECT	METHOD OF STUDY
Cystic fibrosis	CFTR	PCR for 32 mutations
	Gene mutation	RFLP
Fragile X	Triplet base-pair expansion of FMR-1 gene	PCR, Southern blot
Sickle cell anemia	Beta-globin gene mutation	PCR
Hemophilia A	Factor VIII gene mutation	Southern blot, linkage analysis
Rhesus D incompatibility	RhD gene deletion	Multiplex PCR

Source: Adapted from Gupta GK, Bianchi DW. DNA diagnosis for the practicing obstetrician. Obstet Gynecol Clin N Am 1997;24:123.

age, when termination for genetic abnormalities is more acceptable to some women. All of the tests that can be performed on amniocytes can be done with fetal villi as well. In contrast, tests that require amniotic fluid, such as measurement of alpha-fetoprotein, require amniocentesis.

CLINICAL CORRELATION

Maternal serum triple screen is explained in detail to A. G. and her husband. Based on the 1/59 risk for Down syndrome identified by the screening, a level II sonogram and amniocentesis are considered medically indicated. These procedures are described in detail. The risks (< 1/200 for procedure-related miscarriage), benefits, and limitations of amniocentesis for prenatal diagnosis are reviewed. General concepts about chromosomes and nondisjunction as the mechanism for trisomy 21 (Down syndrome) are explained.

The prenatal genetic counseling session often immediately precedes an appointment for sonogram and/or amniocentesis. Genetic counselors may be present for these procedures to provide continuity and ongoing support.

CLINICAL CORRELATION

A. G. and her husband have a level II sonogram performed. The fetus is confirmed to be 17 weeks gestational age by measurements, which corresponds with the last menstrual period. The sonogram reveals an "echogenic bowel" where the fetal bowel has greater echogenicity than the surrounding bone. The obstetrician explains that this finding has been associated with digestive system pathology, chromosome abnormalities, cystic fibrosis (CF), and congenital infection (see Table 13.5). Amniocentesis is performed, with the removal of 20 cc of clear amniotic fluid for chromosome and AFP analysis. Fluid is also sent for virology for cytomegalovirus (CMV) cultures. A. G. and her husband are provided with more information about echogenic bowel and cystic fibrosis.

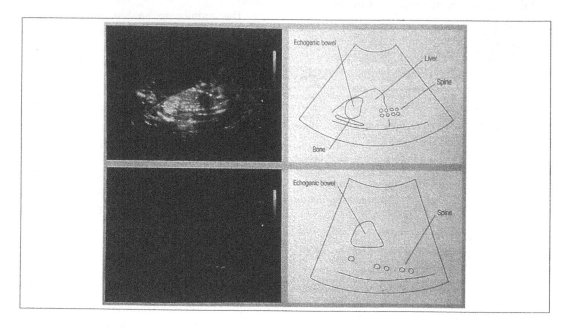

Figure 13.3   Fetal echogenic bowel demonstrated on ultrasound

Source: Eddleman KA, Stone JL, Berkowitz RL. Fetal echogenic bowel: the bottom line. Contemp Ob Gyn 1998;43:53–69.

Echogeneic bowel can be a normal transient physiologic variation, or it may be indicative of underlying pathology (Figure 13.3). The risk of CF is 3% to 13% and the risk of chromosome abnormalities is 25% to 30% when sonogram identifies echogenic bowel in the second trimester (Table 13.6). Cystic fibrosis is a genetic disease that is inherited in an autosomal recessive manner. (Recessive inheritance and the 25% risk of an affected offspring when both parents are carriers should be explained in detail to the patient.)

Caucasians of Northern European ancestry with no family history of CF have about a 1 in 25 risk of being a CF carrier. Gene testing for CF by DNA mutation analysis is available, with approximately 90% of CF-causing mutations being identifiable. The absence of one of these mutations does not completely eliminate the risk of being a CF carrier, however, although it reduces this risk by 90%. Blood or buccal cell samples from the parents can be analyzed to ascertain their carrier status. Three possible scenarios result from this information:

1. Both parents are negative for mutations by DNA analysis, which greatly reduces the risk of having an affected offspring. Prenatal diagnosis is not indicated in this scenario.

2. Both parents are identified as CF carriers, meaning that there is a 25% risk of the offspring having the disease. Prenatal testing on amniocytes can then be done.

3. One parent is a carrier and the other is negative for known DNA mutations. This scenario is the most complicated because of the risk—albeit small—that the negative parent may have an unidentified mutation that could result in having a child with the disease.

CLINICAL CORRELATION

The chromosome analysis reveals a normal 46, XX karyotype and normal amniotic fluid AFP. The CMV cultures are negative. The CF carrier testing of the parents reveals that A. G. carries the most common CF mutation, DF508. Her husband is negative for the 32 CF mutations analyzed. The couple is relieved about the results of the chromosome test, but confused about the results of CF analysis. Because a small risk exists that the husband carries an unidentified mutation, it is estimated that the risk of the child having CF is about 1/250. Although DNA mutation analysis of fetal chromosomes can document whether DF508 mutation is present, confirming that the fetus is at least a carrier, it is impossible to tell whether the child will have the disease. The fetus will be affected with CF only if the DF508 mutation is inherited from A. G. and an unknown mutation is inherited from the father.

The amniocyte analysis reveals that the fetus has the DF508 mutation. The parents are informed that their chance of having a child with CF is between 13% and 43%. The couple decide to continue the pregnancy. They inform their pediatrician of the possibility that their baby may have CF and arrange to have sweat testing performed after birth. Follow-up sonograms are recommended during this pregnancy to monitor the echogenic bowel. If this finding resolves by term, it is less likely that the child is affected with CF.

Table 13.6   Differential Diagnosis of Echogenic Bowel on Second Trimester Sonogram

- Normal transient physiologic variant of fetal development
- Primary gastrointestinal pathology
- Chromosome abnormalities
- Cystic fibrosis
- Congenital infection

CANCER GENETICS

The role played by the genetic counselor has recently expanded as additional genetic markers for familial cancers have been identified. Many common cancers are associated with putative genetic mutations (Table 13.7). Patients who are referred for genetic counseling are those with a family history of cancer or

Table 13.7 Genes Implicated in Cancer Susceptibility

CANCER OR CONDITION	GENE	LOCATION
Breast, ovary	BRCA1	17q21
Breast	BRCA2	13q12–13
Li-Fraumeni	p53	17p13
Breast	AT	11q22–23
Retinoblastoma	Rb	13q14
Lynch/HNPCC	MLH1	3p21.3–23
	PMS1	2q31–33
	PMS2	7p22
Melanoma	MLM	9p21
Neurofibromatosis	NF1	17q11.2
von Hippel-Landau	VHLS	3p25

those who may themselves have cancer and wish to know whether they have genetic defects. The majority (more than 90%) of cancers are sporadic and not familial; hence, the likelihood of having a genetic alteration is low. Genetic counselors will take an extended pedigree for family cancer history to determine the risk to the individual and the likelihood that a mutation is present (Table 13.8).

CLINICAL CORRELATION

P. F. is a 37-year-old, gravida 4, para 4, white female who seeks genetic testing for the ovarian cancer gene. Her pedigree is significant for multiple cancers, including a maternal grandmother who died from

Table 13.8 Principles of Familial (Genetic) Cancers

- Early age of onset
- Increased bilateral involvement, where applicable
- Patterns of multiple primary cancers
- Premonitory physical signs or biomarkers
- Mendelian inheritance (autosomal dominant)

ovarian cancer at age 65, two paternal aunts with breast cancer diagnosed in their seventies, a father with colon cancer diagnosed at age 47 and surgically cured, and, most recently, a mother who has undergone surgery and chemotherapy for advanced ovarian cancer diagnosed at age 54. P. F. is in good health, has no medical problems, is currently taking no medications with the exception of oral contraceptives, and has regular gynecologic examinations with normal Pap smears. She has had four normal, spontaneous, vaginal deliveries without complications. She does not use tobacco or illicit drugs, and uses alcohol rarely. She has no physical complaints.

As with prenatal counseling, cancer genetics counseling begins with a pedigree. Cancers that are known to follow a familial pattern include colorectal cancer, breast cancer, ovarian cancer, endometrial cancer, and some less common cancers, including retinoblastoma and melanoma. As the number of affected individuals (particularly first-degree relatives) increases, so does the likelihood that a genetic alteration is present in the family. Familial cancers tend to occur at earlier ages; therefore, there is increased risk for a genetic alteration when breast cancer is occurring premenopausally as opposed to post-menopausally. Note that cancers on both the maternal and paternal sides of the family are important for genetic considerations. Most familial cancers are associated with autosomal dominant transmission with variable degrees of penetration.

For ovarian cancer, three syndromes have been identified to date that display a familial inheritance. First, the Lynch II syndrome is characterized by increased incidence of colorectal, ovarian, endometrial, and less common gastrointestinal cancers. Second, the most common familial, ovarian cancer syndrome is the breast-ovary cancer syndrome, in which both of these tumors have a high incidence, particularly in premenopausal women. Lastly, the least common familial ovarian syndrome is site-specific ovarian cancer syndrome.

Genetic counseling begins with risk assessment of cancer genes on the basis of the pedigree. Options for early detection and screening, if available, should be discussed with the patient. The patient should be counseled regarding the availability of genetic testing, the costs of such testing, and the ramifications of a positive result. Prophylactic measures, such as bilateral oophorectomy or bilateral mastectomy, can be discussed, although no data definitively prove that such measures eliminate the possibility of developing these cancers. For instance, women with a strong family history of ovarian cancer who undergo prophylactic oophorectomy may still be at risk for the development of a primary peritoneal carcinoma that behaves identically to primary ovarian cancer. The patient at risk for ovarian cancer should be informed of possible measures to decrease that risk, including prolonged oral contraceptive use and multiple pregnancies, both of which have resulted in decreased incidence of this cancer.

CLINICAL CORRELATION

P. F. is told that the presence of ovarian cancer in her grandmother and mother is suggestive of a genetic alteration. Typically, each subsequent generation develops the cancer at a younger age when the mutation is present. Based on the pedigree, the estimated risk of a genetic alteration may be as high as 50%. Potential screening measures, including regular pelvic examinations, CA-125 serum testing, and transvaginal sonography of the ovaries, have been advocated by some, but as yet have not proven to decrease the mortality from this disease. The facts that P. F. has had four full-term pregnancies and has used oral contraceptives for more than five years confer a decreased risk for ovarian cancer, compared to women with no pregnancies or oral contraceptive use. Prophylactic oophorectomy is discussed with P. F. as an option to decrease ovarian cancer; this procedure is occasionally performed in women at risk who have completed childbearing and are particularly anxious to have their ovaries removed. Finally, the testing for gene alterations associated with ovarian cancer is discussed.

The two genes that are currently identified as being associated with breast and ovarian cancer are BRCA1 and BRCA2. These genes likely code for tumor suppressor proteins in their wild or nonmutated state. BRCA1 and BRCA2 are located on chromosomes 17 and 13, respectively. Because each has had multiple mutations within the DNA identified, in most circumstances the patient's DNA for the respective genes must be entirely sequenced to identify a mutation. This sequencing is a time-consuming and expensive task. The most efficient method of detecting these gene mutations is to sequence a known affected family member, such as P. F.'s mother, for a mutation. If one is found, then subsequent patients are tested only for that specific mutation, which decreases the time and expense of further testing. If the patient is found to be negative for the cancer mutation, continued screening may still be advocated because unidentified genes may be involved. If the patient undergoes genetic testing and is found to possess a cancer mutation, she must be counseled on options of screening, prophylactic surgery, or observation.

CLINICAL CORRELATION

P. F.'s mother undergoes testing for mutations of BRCA1 and BRCA2. After several weeks, the results are returned and indicate a single defect of BRCA1 (185delAG). In the meantime, P. F. has undergone a pelvic examination, CA-125 testing, and transvaginal ultrasound, all of which were normal. She elects to have specific testing done on her DNA for the 185delAG mutation. When the results are returned two weeks later, they are negative for this mutation. P. F. elects to have semiannual examinations with transvaginal sonography to allay her anxiety.

SUMMARY

Cancer genetics is a rapidly evolving area of medicine, with new markers being found frequently. Currently, it is unclear how one should proceed after positive results are found or whether the testing should even be done. Positive results have implications for the patient's social and economic future; therefore, confidentiality is critical. At present, genetic testing for cancer susceptibility should be performed only under a research setting, where the information can be collected to help determine future directions of such testing.

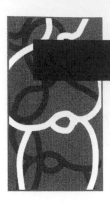

CHAPTER 14

First Trimester Bleeding

Brian D. Acacio

First trimester bleeding is an anxiety-provoking event. Women fear the uncertainty of what their bodies are experiencing and are concerned about the future of their pregnancy. Following a logical approach in evaluating a pregnant woman with bleeding may not only affect the outcome of the pregnancy, but will also help reassure the patient (Table 14.1). Bleeding in the first trimester can vary dramatically in presentation. It can be mild, as in the case of the "placental sign"—that is, bleeding at the site of implantation of the fertilized ovum. Alternatively, it can present as profuse hemorrhage, either internally from a ruptured ectopic gestation or externally from an incomplete abortion that continues to bleed. In these situations, immediate attention is required and surgery is warranted for hemodynamic instability. The vast majority of bleeding in the first trimester is *not* an obstetric emergency and, in fact, is quite common. Approximately 30% to 40% of all pregnant women will spot or bleed in the first trimester. Half of these pregnancies will end in spontaneous abortion (miscarriage).

ABORTION

The term "abortion" is commonly misconstrued as an elective termination of pregnancy. The need for proper terminology and understanding of their definitions is important (Figure 14.1).

CLINICAL CORRELATION

L. F. is a 21-year-old, gravida 1, para 0, female whose last menstrual period was six weeks ago. She purchased a home pregnancy test from her local pharmacy two weeks prior to seeing the physician, which gave a positive result. She has notified her obstetrician/gynecologist's office and has been counseled to begin taking prenatal vitamins and iron supplementation if she is not already doing so. An appointment was scheduled in four weeks for a confirmation visit and comprehensive history and physical examination. Furthermore, L. F. was instructed to call sooner if she had any vaginal bleeding or lower abdominal pain.

At her current office visit, she presents with a complaint of "crampy" lower abdominal pain and vaginal spotting (lighter than her menses) for the past eight days. A repeat urine qualitative hCG test confirms a positive result. Vital signs are stable. On physical examination, L. F. is noted to be mildly anxious with no evidence of rebound or guarding abdominal tenderness. A bimanual pelvic exam reveals a slightly enlarged, nontender uterus approximately six to eight weeks in gestational size. A speculum examination reveals a scant amount of bloody cervical discharge from the os, yet no gross cervical lesions. The cervical os is closed. A transvaginal ultrasound is performed and reveals an intra-

Table 14.1   Differential Diagnosis of First
Trimester Bleeding

- Threatened abortion
- Inevitable abortion
- Incomplete abortion
- Complete abortion
- Missed abortion
- Ectopic gestation
- Molar gestation (GTD)
- Cervicitis
- Cervical neoplasia

uterine sac and pole as well as a 1.6 cm. A
corpus luteum cyst is found on the right
ovary.

The diagnosis of threatened abortion is
made when vaginal bleeding occurs before the
twentieth week of gestation, no evidence of an
extrauterine pregnancy exists, and the cervical
os is closed. Unless evidence of hemodynamic
instability is found, the woman should be reassured and no additional therapy initiated. Rh
status should be determined and Rh immunoglobulin (RhoGAM) administered if an Rh-negative result is obtained, as is the case of any
vaginal bleeding in pregnancy. A threatened
abortion becomes inevitable when the cervical os is dilated. When only a portion of the
products of conception have been expelled
and the cervical os is dilated, this condition is
called an incomplete abortion. In these circumstances, the woman should be offered an
evacuation of the remaining products of conception. A complete abortion is defined as the
case in which all of the fetal and placental tissue having been expelled and the cervical os is
closed, with little or no bleeding.

Rarely, the diagnosis of missed abortion
can be made when a dead fetus is retained in
utero for several weeks. Such a patient may or
may not have previously presented with a
threatened abortion. The reason why some
abortions end spontaneously while others do
not remains unclear. In some cases, missed
abortions have been linked to the use of

progestational agents in the treatment of
threatened abortions. In the case of a missed
abortion, the woman should be counseled of
her risk of serious coagulation defects, such as
severe hypofibrinogemia, and should undergo
a dilation and curettage for definitive treatment.

In the past, septic abortion was the most
common cause of death in young reproductive-age women. Its higher incidence preceded
the *Roe vs. Wade* decision, which legalized
elective terminations. Currently, septic abortion complicates spontaneous abortions in approximately 0.5 per 100,000 cases (Table
14.2). Broad-spectrum antibiotics, including
anaerobic coverage, should be administered to
the patient with this condition. When adequate
levels of antibiotics in the serum have been
reached (after approximately two hours), the
uterus should be evacuated.

Historically, recurrent abortion has been
defined as three successive losses. Current
practices calls for an etiology to be sought after
two successive first-trimester losses or one sec-
ond-trimester loss. After karyotyping has ruled
out a parental chromosomal abnormality, the
only other cost-effective treatments are as follows: (1) testing for antiphospholipid antibodies; (2) empirical treatment with exogenous
progesterone for a presumptive luteal-phase
defect; and (3) prophylactic cervical cerclage,
if a history of cervical incompetence is suspected (Table 14.3).

Antiphospholipid antibody syndrome is
most commonly associated with systemic lupus
erythematosis. These patients have increased
levels of abnormal antibodies, such as lupus
anticoagulant or cardiolipin antibody (IgG and
IgM antibodies), which are associated clinically with thromboses in the utero-placental
vasculature. When suspected, treatment consists of aspirin and heparin during pregnancy.
Luteal-phase defects occur when there is insufficient progesterone production by the ovary,
which causes the endometrium to be out of the
optimum phase for implantation when fertilization occurs. As a result, the endometrium does
not support the early pregnancy.

ECTOPIC GESTATION

An ectopic pregnancy is any gestation located
outside of the uterine cavity. It is sometimes re-

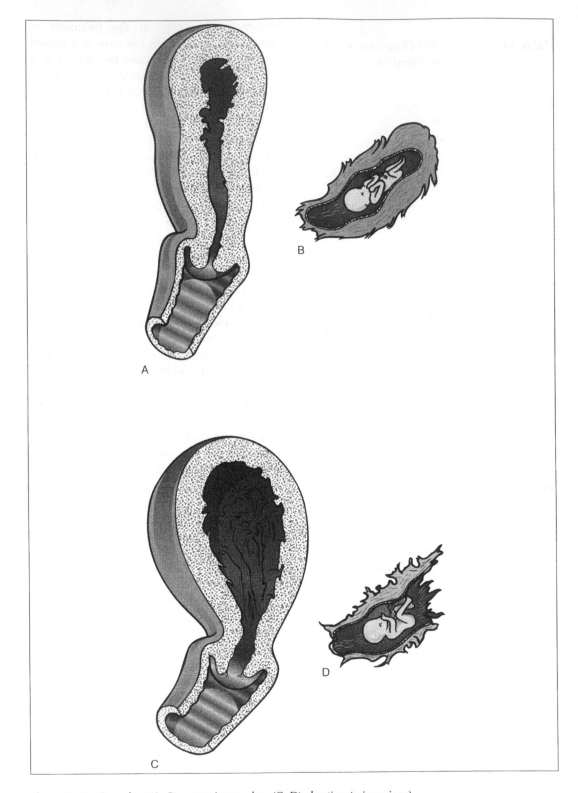

Figure 14.1 Complete (A, B) versus incomplete (C, D) abortion (miscarriage)

Source: Callahan TL, Caughey AB, Heffner LJ. Blueprints in obstetrics and gynecology. Malden, MA: Blackwell Science, 1998:12.

Table 14.2 Recurrence Risks for Counseling Women with Repeated Spontaneous Abortions

	PRIOR ABORTIONS	RISK (PERCENTAGE)*
Women with liveborn infants	0	12
	1	24
	2	26
	3	32
	4	26
Women without liveborn infants	2 or more	40–45

*Recurrence risks are slightly higher in older women and those who smoke or drink alcohol.

ferred to as a "tubal" pregnancy, because the fallopian tubes are the site of more than 95% of such gestations. Ectopic gestations complicate 1% to 3% of all pregnancies in the United States. Ectopic pregnancy is covered in detail in Chapter 47.

MOLAR GESTATION

A molar gestation or gestational trophoblastic disease (GTD) refers to the spectrum of proliferative abnormalities of the trophoblast associated with pregnancy. The first sign of this disorder is often abnormal bleeding in early pregnancy. Molar gestation is discussed in further detail in Chapter 55.

CERVICITIS

Acute cervicitis in pregnancy can occasionally be the etiology of vaginal bleeding and is one reason for a speculum examination with direct visualization of the cervix. Women will commonly report post-coital bleeding as the presenting symptom. A wet-mount evaluation will often reveal the source as trichomoniasis, bacterial vaginosis, or candidiasis. Pregnancy-induced physiologic eversion of the cervical transformation zone can occasionally become irritated during coitus and lead to a scant amount of vaginal bleeding in pregnancy (Figure 14.2).

CERVICAL NEOPLASIA

All pregnant women should have a first trimester Pap smear to screen for cervical dysplasia and cancer. The incidence of abnormal cytology in pregnancy is equal to the incidence in nonpregnant women (approximately 3%). Carcinoma in situ occurs in approximately 1.3 per 1000 pregnancies and invasive carcinoma in roughly 1 per 2200 gestations. In the case of intraepithelial neoplasia or carcinoma in situ,

Table 14.3 Causes of Recurrent Abortion

Chromosomal	Translocations, inversions, aneuploidy
Uterine	Luteal-phase defects
	Uterine cavity synechiae
	Cervical incompetence
	Acquired uterine defects (leiomyomas, septae, DES changes)
Lupus anticoagulant activity and antiphospholipid antibodies	Increased thrombosis at implantation site

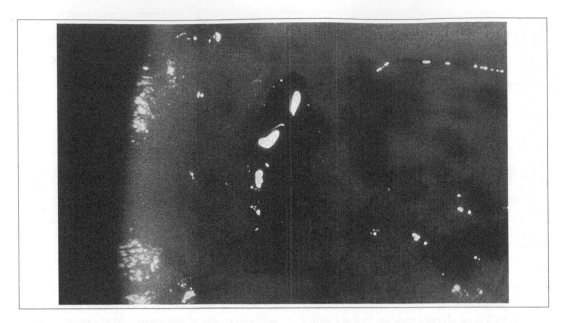

Figure 14.2 Cervicitis secondary to *Trichomonas* vaginal infection, described as a "strawberry cervix"

the patient is observed and delivered, with a final evaluation being made and any necessary therapy beginning approximately six weeks after delivery. Cervical cancer in the first trimester is problematic. The woman needs to decide whether to continue the pregnancy and delay definitive surgical/radiation therapy or undergo an elective termination and immediate treatment. Further information on cervical dysplasia and carcinoma can be found in Chapter 49.

SUMMARY

First trimester bleeding is the most common complication of consequence in pregnancy. With a few simple tests, its etiology and diagnosis become clear. In many cases, reassurance is all that is necessary to allay a woman's fears, not only for herself, but for her pregnancy as well.

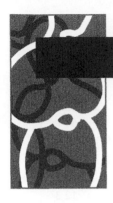

CHAPTER 15

Multiple Gestations

Alexander F. Burnett

Multifetal gestations account for fewer than 1% of all births; their contribution to perinatal morbidity, however, is substantially higher. Unique maternal and fetal difficulties are associated with twins and other multiple gestations.

The spontaneous rate of twin gestations varies among different populations and with advancing maternal age. More recently, the advent of superovulation has significantly increased the incidence of multifetal gestations, including those involving more than two fetuses.

TWINS

Twins may be monozygotic (identical) or dizygotic (fraternal), depending on whether the offspring are the result of a single fertilized ovum that splits very early or the result of two separate ova being fertilized, respectively. Dizygotic twins account for approximately 70% of all twins. Although the incidence of dizygotic twinning varies with different populations, monozygotic twins have a fairly constant prevalence—approximately 4 per 1000 worldwide. In some populations, dizygotic twins are associated with an incidence of 45 per 1000 births. In the United States, the rate is about 8 per 1000 births (Table 15.1).

As women age, they have a greater chance of bearing twins. The incidence of twinning is 3 per 1000 births for women younger than 20

years old, climbing to 14 per 1000 births for women 35 to 40 years old.

Spontaneous triplets are born much less frequently, occurring in about 1 in 8000 births. Multizygotic gestations are usually the result of ovarian stimulation.

CLINICAL CORRELATION

P. L. is a 31-year-old G3P2002 white female who comes to the office for her first prenatal visit eight weeks after her last menstrual period. She has noted much more nausea with this pregnancy than with her previous two and occasionally experiences morning vomiting. She denies any other problems to date. Examination reveals normal blood pressure. Her obstetrical examination reveals a uterus that is approximately 12 weeks size and soft. An office ultrasound confirms two separate gestational sacs holding separate fetuses with documented heartbeats. Sonographic measurement of the fetuses reveals both to be consistent with eight weeks gestation.

Sonography, particularly early in pregnancy, is extremely accurate in diagnosing twin gestations. Prior to the era of sonography, twins were diagnosed presumptively on the basis of uterine enlargement greater than that normally associated with the pregnancy dates (generally observed in the second trimester) and the presence of two separate fetal heart

Table 15.1   Twin Rates per 1000 Births by Zygosity

COUNTRY	MONOZYGOTIC	DIZYGOTIC	TOTAL
Nigeria	5.0	49	54
United States			
African American	4.7	11.1	15.8
White	4.2	7.1	11.3
England and Wales	3.5	8.8	12.3
India (Calcutta)	3.3	8.1	11.4
Japan	3.0	1.3	4.3

Source: Adapted from MacGillivray I. Epidemiology of twin pregnancy. Semin Perinatol 1986;10:4.

tones on auscultation or Doppler of the uterus. As the gestation advances, Leopold maneuvers should accurately diagnose the presence of twins. With maternal triple screening for Down syndrome or neural tube defects, normal twin gestations will have hCG levels and alpha-fetoprotein levels higher than singleton counterparts at that particular gestational age.

The fetal sacs in twin gestations are determined by the type of twinning and the age of gestation when twinning occurs, as shown in Figure 15.1. With dizygotic twins, because each develops from a separate fertilized ovum, each fetus has its own placenta, amnion, and chorion. If the blastocysts are implanted very close to one another, however, the placentas may appear to fuse together, although vascular anastamoses between the gestations does not occur. In monozygotic twins, three separate placental arrangements may occur. If the cleavage of the fertilized ovum occurs within 2 to 3 days of fertilization, each twin will develop its own amnion and chorion (diamniotic, dichorionic). Cleavage that occurs after three days cannot split the chorionic cavity, so the twins will be diamniotic, monochorionic—that is, they will share the same placenta. Cleavage between 8 and 13 days gestation does not allow splitting of the amnion or the chorion; as a result, the twins will be monoamniotic, monochorionic. Such twins will float within the same amniotic sac and are at high risk for cord entanglement with in utero death. If cleavage occurs between 13 and 15 days after fertilization, the resulting conjoined twins will be monoamniotic, monochorionic. Twinning

cannot occur after 15 days gestation. Ultrasound diagnosis of whether twins are dizygotic or monozygotic can be made with certainty only if the twins are monochorionic, monoamniotic or conjoined (monozygotic twins).

Maternal changes secondary to twin gestation are due to increased uterine size and fetal requirements. Caloric intake should be increased by at least 500 to 600 kcal/day to compensate for the increased nutritional requirements. Genetic screening should be performed as for any singleton gestations, with the previously mentioned caveat that triple screening values will normally differ from those for single gestations.

Multiple sonograms are undertaken throughout the pregnancy to document interval growth of the fetuses. Intrauterine growth retardation is more common in twins. If one twin is more than 20% larger in estimated fetal weight than the other, this difference may be indicative of twin-twin transfusion syndrome, where vascular anastamoses preferentially supply blood and nutrients to one fetus.

If genetic amniocentesis is indicated, commonly one sac is entered and amniotic fluid is removed. A small amount of indigo carmine is then injected. Next, the other sac is entered and documented to be separate by lack of dye in the fluid, and a separate amniotic fluid sample is taken.

The most frequent perinatal complication of twins is preterm labor, which as many as 70% of women experience. It is not clear whether bedrest reduces the incidence of preterm labor in twins; nevertheless, it is a fre-

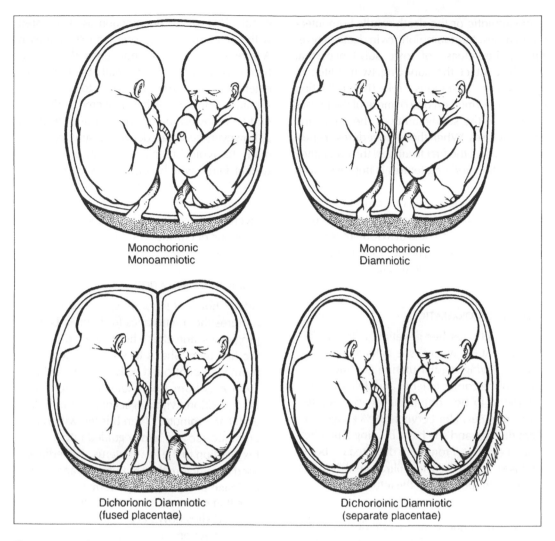

Monochorionic
Monoamniotic

Monochorionic
Diamniotic

Dichorionic Diamniotic
(fused placentae)

Dichorioinic Diamniotic
(separate placentae)

Figure 15.1 Placentation in twin pregnancies

Source: Gabbe SG, ed. Obstetrics: normal and problem pregnancies, 2nd ed. New York: Churchill Livingstone, 1991.

quent recommendation. Tocolytics may be used if preterm labor develops. In such a case, one must determine that the etiology of the premature labor is not infectious, which would be a contraindication to tocolysis.

CLINICAL CORRELATION

P. L. returns in 4 weeks and shows good interval growth of fundal height since her 8-week visit. Her blood pressure remains normal. Repeat sonography is performed, measuring both twins at 12 weeks. Adequate amniotic fluid is observed around the fetuses, and two amniotic sacs are clearly evident. The triple screen evaluation do not place either of her fetuses at excess risk of having a neural tube defect or chromosomal anomaly. The plan with P. L. will be routine visits every 3 to 4 weeks with sonography up to 28 weeks, when she will begin visits every 2 weeks, and then every week starting at 34 weeks.

Approximately 4% of twin gestations are complicated by the death of one or both fetuses. If the death of one fetus occurs prior to 20 weeks gestation, there is generally not a hazard to the other twin's survival, unless the twins are monoamniotic or the death results from infectious causes. Monoamniotic twin death may result in the release of toxic substances that directly contact the surviving twin. Often in multizygotic gestations, selective reduction will be performed on one or more of the fetuses to increase the survivability of the remaining fetus or fetuses. When these procedures are performed during the first trimester, the pregnancy outcome for surviving fetuses is improved with minimal toxicity to the survivors. With four or more fetuses, pregnancy outcome in terms of delivery of viable babies is improved by reducing the uterine load to less than four fetuses. Debate continues over whether triplet gestations benefit from reduction to twins.

CLINICAL CORRELATION

P. L. continues her gestation without difficulty. At 36 weeks, she calls to say that she is having regular uterine contractions. When she comes to labor and delivery, she is found to be contracting every three to four minutes. Her cervix is 80% effaced, 3 cm dilated, and she has a bulging amniotic sac. Fetal heart tones are detected on both fetuses and a bedside ultrasound is performed for position of the fetuses.

By convention, twins are designated as twin A and twin B, with twin A being that fetus with the presenting part lowest in the uterus. Three combinations in position may be noted:

- Twin A and twin B may both be vertex (head first).

- Twin A may be vertex and twin B non-vertex.

- Twin A nonvertex and twin B either vertex or nonvertex (Figure 15.2).

Approximately 45% of twins at term are vertex/vertex, of whom 80% can be anticipated to be born vaginally. There may be a long delay of even several hours between delivery of the two fetuses; this delay is not cause for concern unless twin B shows signs of distress. When twin A is nonvertex, a cesarean delivery should be performed. If twin A is breech and twin B is vertex, then there is a risk of the twins locking heads as they come down the birth canal. This rare phenomenon is associated with a fetal mortality greater than 30%. If twin A is vertex and twin B is nonvertex, the second twin may be delivered vaginally by internal or external version from nonvertex to vertex presentation after twin A has delivered. If the second twin has estimated weight less than 2000 g, however, cesarean delivery is advocated by many to avoid breech extraction of a lower-weight fetus, which is associated with an increase in morbidity and mortality. Gestations involved more than two fetuses are uniformly delivered via cesarean delivery, with very rare exceptions occurring in some triplet births.

CLINICAL CORRELATION

After 3 hours of labor, P. L. spontaneously ruptures the membranes for twin A. Labor progresses, and after 6 hours she is pushing the first twin. She is taken to the delivery room for a controlled delivery of the twins. Twin A is born 20 minutes later from an LOA position, with Apgars of 6 at 1 minute and 9 at 5 minutes. Twin B is felt within its amniotic sac and gently guided into a vertex position to the lower uterus. A needle is used to puncture the amniotic sac and slow drainage of the fluid is performed, making sure that neither a fetal part nor the umbilical cord slips down before the head. Uterine contractions become strong again once the head is firmly applied to the cervix, and 7 minutes later twin B is delivered from an LOP position with Apgars of 7 at minute and 9 at 5 minutes. The placenta delivers 12 minutes later and reveals separate, but fused placentas. The vessels from both placentas appear normal. Oxytocin and manual stimulation are provided to help the uterus contract and stop bleeding.

Due to uterine distention with multiple gestations, uterine atony post-delivery and subsequent hemorrhage is increased. One should be prepared with oxytocin, prostaglandins, and massage as needed to help the uterus contract. In some cases of multizygosity, the uterine muscle is stretched beyond the ability to contract down again, and a hysterectomy must be performed to control bleeding.

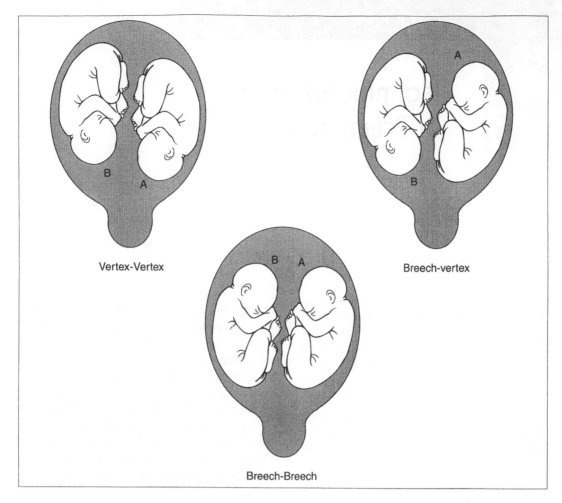

Vertex-Vertex

Breech-vertex

Breech-Breech

Figure 15.2   Positions of twins in utero at term

SUMMARY

Multiple gestations represent a small portion of pregnancies, but are responsible for a high percentage of perinatal complications. Maternal changes from pregnancy are increased with multiple gestations. Premature labor and delivery are the major causes of fetal morbidity and mortality. Post-partum hemorrhage is the major cause of maternal morbidity. In some cases of multizygosity, selective termination may be performed to improve pregnancy outcome. Twin delivery may be either vaginal or cesarean, depending on the presentation of the twins, the size of the twins, and the experience of the obstetrician.

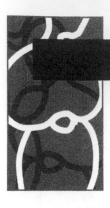

CHAPTER 16

Isoimmunization in Pregnancy

Alexander F. Burnett

Isoimmunization occurs when there is an incompatibility between the maternal and fetal blood antigens that results in maternal antibodies being produced against the fetal red blood cells. The incidence of this condition has fallen dramatically in the past 40 years as knowledge, prevention, and treatment options for this disease have increased. In the past, fetal and neonatal mortality in an affected pregnancy were greater than 50%. Today, the mortality rate is approximately 10% for affected pregnancies.

The sensitization of the mother can occur after any type of gestation that produces fetal red cells that are antigenic to the mother. Consequently, prophylaxis is required in affected women following ectopic gestations, abortions, or term pregnancies.

CLINICAL CORRELATION

T. B. is a 28-year-old female, gravida 3, para 1101. It is 12 weeks since her last menstrual period, and she comes into the office for her first prenatal visit. T. B.'s prior pregnancies have included an ectopic diagnosed at 10 weeks that was removed via the laparoscope two years ago and a term normal spontaneous vaginal delivery of a living, female infant four years ago. The father of her first pregnancy was different than the father of the ectopic or this pregnancy. The initial evaluation reveals normal blood pressure and vital signs, her weight is increased 2 lb relative to her pre-pregnancy weight, and she has no complaints. Her uterus is 10 to 12 weeks size, and fetal heart tones are heard by Doppler. Two days later, her blood test results indicate that T. B. is Rh-negative. She recalls not receiving Rh-immune globulin (RhoGAM) with the first pregnancy because the father was Rh-negative as well. She is not sure whether she received RhoGAM with the ectopic, but does not believe she did. Her prior records are requested.

RED CELL ANTIGENS

When fetal blood group antigens are inherited from the father but not possessed by the mother, a maternal immune response may occur that creates antibodies against the fetal red blood cells. The fetal cells gain access to the maternal circulation via transplacental passage. Their presence may be particularly increased with events such as abruption, placental removal, D&C for miscarriage or abortion, or iatrogenic procedures such as amniocentesis or chorionic villus sampling. The maternal antibodies (mostly IgG) readily cross into the fetal circulation and cause destruction of the fetal red blood cells (erythroblastosis), leading to anemia and hydropic changes, such as pericardial effusion or edema of the skin or scalp.

The Rhesus antigen (Rh) is a surface antigen on the red blood cells that can elicit an immune response. The antigen may be one of several produced by three genetic loci on chromosome 1. Each locus (designated C, D, and E) has two major alleles, designated C, c, D, and E, and e. The most significant of these antigens is the D antigen. By convention, Rh-positive indicates the presence of D antigen and Rh-negative indicates the absence of D antigen on red cells. For Rh incompatibility to occur, the following conditions must be met:

1. The fetus must be Rh-positive and the mother must be Rh-negative.

2. Enough fetal blood must be transferred into the maternal system to generate an immune response.

3. The mother must generate the immune response.

For this reason, only Rh-negative women are at risk for isoimmunization of their fetus.

Incompatibility of ABO blood groups may cause problems for the newborn but does not cause erythroblastosis. Thus this discrepancy does not require detection during pregnancy. In fact, ABO incompatibility reduces the likelihood of Rh incompatibility, probably by leading to more rapid clearance of the fetal blood cells from the maternal circulation.

The incidence of Rh-negative varies with different populations (Table 16.1). In the Caucasian population of North America, approximately 15% of all people are Rh-negative. In Asian populations, the percentage of Rh-negative persons is much lower. Among the Basques, between 25% and 40% are Rh-negative. Among Rh-positive men, 60% are heterozygous and 40% are homozygous for the

D antigen. Statistically, without even knowing the paternal blood type, an Rh-negative woman has a 60% chance of bearing an Rh-positive fetus.

Not all pregnancies with an incompatibility in Rh antigen will result in maternal immune response because of the variable degrees of fetal bleeding into the maternal circulation. An estimated 20% of incompatible pregnancies lead to maternal sensitization. Once the mother is sensitized, the immune response will become more pronounced with each subsequent exposure. Therefore, a woman with a previously affected pregnancy has an increased risk of severity of isoimmunization with each successive Rh-positive fetus.

Rh-IMMUNE GLOBULIN

RhoGAM is an anti-Rh antibody preparation formulated in the 1960s that effectively prevents Rh sensitization. The passive administration of this antibody prevents active immunization by the respective antigen. On an early prenatal visit, all women should undergo ABO blood group testing, Rh typing, and an antibody screen (indirect Coombs test). If anti-D antibodies are detected, the woman should be considered sensitized and is not a candidate for RhoGAM prophylaxis. If she is Rh-negative and anti-D-antibody-negative, then she is a candidate for prophylaxis.

The standard dose of RhoGAM is 300 µg, although lower doses may be adequate. It is recommended that the woman receive RhoGAM within 72 hours of delivery or termination of gestation if the fetal blood type is Rh-positive or unknown. With this dosing, however, 1% to 2% of women may nevertheless develop sensitization despite post-partum administration of RhoGAM. Therefore, it is also recommended that Rh-negative women without anti-D antibodies receive RhoGAM at 28 weeks gestation to decrease the likelihood of sensitization occurring prior to delivery.

The standard dose of RhoGAM is designed to neutralize as much as 30 cm^3 of fetal blood in the maternal circulation. If an event occurs that raises concerns about bleeding of more than 30 cm^3, more RhoGAM may be needed. Testing of the maternal blood for fetal

Table 16.1	Prevalence of Rh Negativity by Race	
RACE	**PERCENT Rh NEGATIVE**
Caucasian	15
African American	8
African	4
Native American	1
Asian	<<1

blood cells can allow quantifying of the fetal bleeding. When the quantity exceeds 30 cm^3, RhoGAM should be given at 10 µg/mL blood. The quantity of fetal red blood cells in the maternal circulation may be determined by an acid elution (Kleihauer-Betke stain), which rids the blood of maternal hemoglobin but not fetal hemoglobin (Figure 16.1).

CLINICAL CORRELATION

T. B. has a positive antibody to D antigen found in her blood. The titer of the antibody is 1:8 by indirect Coombs test. Typing of her husband reveals him to be homozygous D; therefore, the fetus must be Rh-positive. Because antibodies have already formed (likely from sensitization occurring with the prior ectopic gestation), T. B. is not a candidate for RhoGAM prophylaxis. It is explained to her that her antibodies could potentially destroy her fetus's erythrocytes with a subsequent manifestation of anemia or hydrops. If these conditions are severe, intrauterine transfusion may be necessary to save the fetus's life. Review of T. B.'s past records confirms that she did not receive RhoGAM with her ectopic pregnancy.

MANAGEMENT OF ISOIMMUNIZATION OF PREGNANCY

Once a woman has been determined to be sensitized, she is managed differently during her pregnancy. Titers of maternal antibodies are determined on the first prenatal visit and then again at 20 weeks and every 4 weeks thereafter. When the titer is greater than or equal to 1:32 by indirect Coombs test, amniocentesis or percutaneous umbilical cord blood sampling should be considered. If the mother has had a prior pregnancy affected by isoimmunization, such as prior neonatal exchange transfusion, early delivery, or intrauterine transfusion, antibody titers do not need to be obtained, as the physician will plan to intervene with amniocentesis or umbilical cord sampling regardless of the maternal titers. In subsequent pregnancies, this testing should begin four to eight weeks prior to the advent of difficulties with the last pregnancy.

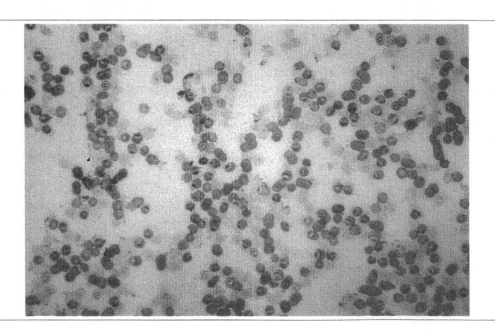

Figure 16.1 Kleihauer-Betke stain of maternal peripheral blood smear. The smear is eluted with an acidic buffer that results in fading of maternal hemoglobin (Hb A) and maintenance of fetal hemoglobin (Hb F). The cells that stain for hemoglobin are the fetal red blood cells; the "ghost" red blood cells are maternal. The amount of fetal hemorrhage is calculated by the percentage of fetal red blood cells seen.

With a rise in maternal titers, amniocentesis may be performed to assess the degree of fetal hemolysis. The amniotic fluid is passed through a spectrophotometer, with the technician looking for a change in optical density of the fluid at 450 nm wavelength, called the OD 450. This change will correlate with the amount of bilirubin in the amniotic fluid and indirectly correlate with the degree of fetal hemolysis. Liley detailed normal values over the course of pregnancy for OD 450. Deviations may fall into zone I, zone II, or zone III, depending on the degree of change from normal (Figure 16.2). The higher the change in OD 450, the higher the zone, and consequently the higher the risk to the fetus. Readings in zone III suggest very severe hemolysis and high likelihood of fetal death within 7 to 10 days. Readings in zone I are reassuring. Zone II readings suggest a risk between those associated with zone I and zone III readings

and require amniocentesis to determine the hemolysis trend. If it is progressively worsening, intervention is indicated.

Umbilical cord blood sampling is a direct way to measure fetal hematocrit and degree of anemia (Figure 16.3). This blood sample can also be analyzed to determine the fetal blood type and thereby confirm that the fetus is at risk. The disadvantages of umbilical cord sampling are its potential for boosting the amount of fetal blood in the maternal circulation and an increased (although small) risk for pregnancy loss as compared with amniocentesis. The therapeutic advantage of umbilical cord sampling derives from the technique of transfusion of the fetus in utero. Recommendations for transfusion occur when the fetal hematocrit is less than 25%; transfusions seek to raise the hematocrit to approximately 45%. Repeat transfusions may be necessary, with a loss of approximately 1% of fetal erythrocytes occurring each day.

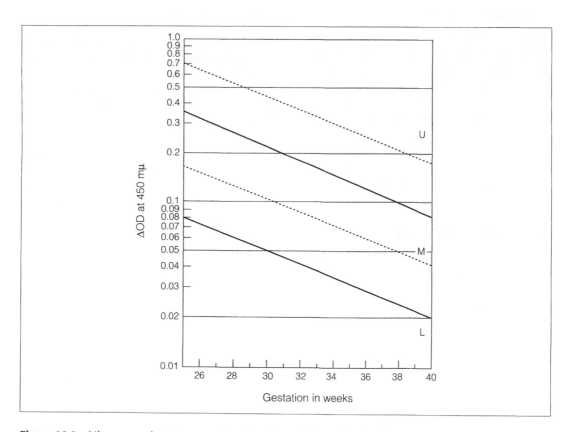

Figure 16.2   Liley zones depicting severity of fetal hemolysis with red cell isoimmunization

Source: Callahan TL, Caughey AB, Heffner LJ. Blueprints in obstetrics and gynecology. Malden, MA: Blackwell Science, 1998:55.

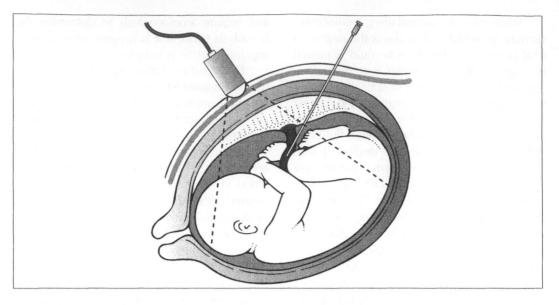

Figure 16.3   Drawing of percutaneous umbilical blood sampling (PUBS)

Source: Queenan JT, ed. Management of high risk pregnancy, 3rd ed. Boston: Blackwell Science, 1994:65.

> **CLINICAL CORRELATION**
>
> At 20 weeks gestation, a repeat of maternal antibody titers returns positive at 1:32 by indirect Coombs test. T. B. undergoes ultrasound, which reveals a normal-appearing female fetus with no evidence of hydrops. Amniocentesis is performed. The fluid is sent to the lab in a dark bag to prevent photo-oxidation of the bilirubin. The OD 450 gives readings in zone I. Repeat ultrasound is scheduled in four weeks.

ULTRASOUND FINDINGS

Findings on ultrasound that are suggestive of severe anemia include an increased size of the fetal liver, increased placental thickness, pericardial effusion, polyhydramnios, and visualization of both sides of the fetal bowel (bowel edema). Some researchers suggest that fetal echocardiography is sensitive enough to detect significant anemia by noting the presence of small pericardial effusions. They use this sign as an indication for amniocentesis and/or umbilical cord blood sampling, rather than initiating amniocentesis prior to the emergence of physical sequelae in the fetus.

For the pregnancy that continues with iso-immunization, ongoing care includes fetal heart rate monitoring. A sinusoidal heart rate pattern is indicative of severe anemia and possibly significant cardiac failure. Nonreassuring signs on monitoring indicate the need for delivery or transfusion.

The choice of delivery is influenced by the degree of hydrops (Figure 16.4). Severely hydropic fetuses are most often delivered by cesarean delivery, not only to prevent potential birth trauma, but also to manage the delivery in a controlled manner with the necessary neonatal personnel alerted and available. The newborn may require exchange transfusions to improve anemia. Newborn survival is determined by the degree of prematurity and the significance of the hydrops. The process will begin to abate at birth, as maternal antibodies are no longer present. Exchange transfusions may be required to diminish the risk of heart failure in the newborn.

> **CLINICAL CORRELATION**
>
> At 24 weeks, the fetus begins to show signs of anemia, with a small pericardial effusion being noted. Repeat amniocentesis reveals a D OD 450 reading in the middle of zone II. One week later, an umbilical cord blood sampling is performed that shows a fetal

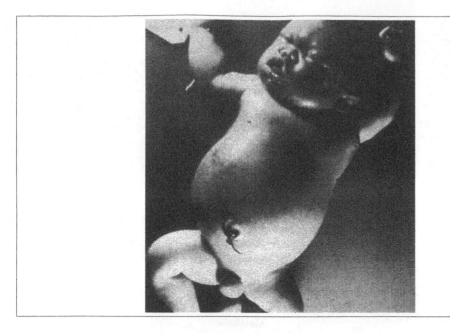

Figure 16.4   Infant with severe hydrops fetalis. Note the extensive edema.

Source: Gabbe SG, Niebyl JR, Simpson JL, eds. Obstetrics: normal and problem pregnancies, 2nd ed. Philadelphia: Churchill Livingstone, 1991:981.

hematocrit of 24%. A transfusion is performed to raise the hematocrit to 45%. The fetus requires two subsequent transfusions over the pregnancy to maintain the hematocrit at more than 25%. With the transfusion, the pericardial effusion resolves, and the fetus displays no other signs of hydrops on ultrasound. At 35 weeks, a cesarean delivery is performed after the amniocentesis reveals a mature lecithin–sphingomyelin ratio signifying pulmonary maturity. T. B. delivers a female infant with Apgars of 5 at one minute and 7 at five minutes. The baby is monitored closely in the neonatal intensive care unit and recovers uneventfully. T. B. has expressed a desire for permanent sterilization during this pregnancy, and this procedure is performed at the time of cesarean delivery.

Other blood antigens that can cause isoimmunization and erythroblastosis include Kell and Duffy. Lewis antigens on the red cells most commonly lead to antibody formation after D antigen presence. Fortunately, Lewis antigens are predominantly of the IgM type and are poorly expressed by fetal red blood cells. As a result, they do not lead to erythroblastosis.

Although ABO blood group incompatibilities do not cause fetal erythroblastosis, they may cause increased fetal bilirubin that the immature liver of the newborn handles only poorly. The most severe consequence of elevated bilirubin in the newborn is deposition of bilirubin in the brain, where it may be neurotoxic. Aggressive therapy with phototherapy—and, in some cases, exchange transfusions—is warranted to prevent this complication.

Nonimmune hydrops fetalis is a condition of fetal edema not due to isoimmunization. Its most common causes include cardiac failure, chronic anemia, hypoproteinemia, decreased venous return, infections, and malformations. Ascites, pleural effusions, pericardial effusions, or skin edema may be diagnosed on ultrasound (Table 16.2). The majority of fetuses affected by nonimmune hydrops have polyhydramnios (excess amniotic fluid). In many cases, no therapy is effective. Those fetuses who die usually succumb to cardiac failure.

Table 16.2 Causes of Nonimmune Hydrops

Cardiovascular
Left heart hypoplasia
Right heart hypoplasia
Transposition of the great vessels
VSD
ASD
Tetralogy of Fallot
Tachyarrhythmias
Bradyarrhythmia
High-output failure
Cardiomyopathy

Chromosomal
45,X
Trisomy 21
Trisomy 18
Trisomy 13

Chondrodysplasias
Thanatophoric dwarfism
Osteogenesis imperfecta
Achondrogenesis

Twin Pregnancy
Twin–twin transfusion syndrome
Acardiac twin

Hematologic
Alpha-thalassemia
Parvovirus B19 infection
Fetomaternal transfusion
G6PD deficiency
In utero hemorrhage

Thoraces
Diaphragmatic hernia
Intrathoracic mass
Chylothorax
Pulmonary neoplasia
Bronchogenic cyst

Infections
CMV
Toxoplasmosis
Parvovirus B19 (fifth disease)
Syphilis
Herpes
Rubella

Metabolic
Gaucher disease
GM1 gangliosidosis

Urinary
Urethral stenosis or atresia
Posterior urethral valves
Congenital nephrosis
Prune belly syndrome

Gastrointestinal
Malrotation of the intestines
Midgut volvulus
Meconium peritonitis
Hepatic fibrosis
Cholestasis
Biliary atresia

Source: Adapted from Creasy RK, Resnick R, eds. Maternal–fetal medicine, 4th ed. Philadelphia: W. B. Saunders, 1999:773.

SUMMARY

Isoimmunization during pregnancy is becoming less common as prophylaxis of appropriate mothers with RhoGAM continues to be effective in preventing sensitization. Those women who do become sensitized fare better today due to the technology of intrauterine transfusions via the umbilical cord. It is critical to ascertain a woman's Rh status and antibody status so that effective prophylaxis, monitoring, or treatment may be performed.

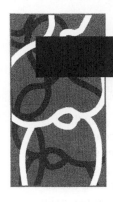

CHAPTER 17

Fetal Growth Abnormalities

Alexander F. Burnett

Fetal growth abnormalities are significant contributors to morbidity and mortality. Consequently, routine monitoring of fetal growth is an integral part of prenatal care. The detection of abnormalities in growth will have implications for diagnosis, intervention, and prevention of various pathologic situations that may affect both mother and fetus. Alterations in growth are often the first sign that prompts investigation of these pathologic conditions. Thus measurement of fetal growth throughout the prenatal period is critical for detecting fetal well-being.

CLINICAL CORRELATION

L. C. is a 37-year-old female, gravida 4 para 3, whose fetus is currently 32 weeks gestational age by dates and a 10-week sonogram. L. C. was last seen at 24 weeks gestation. At that time, the examination revealed a singleton fetus in breech presentation with heart tones in the 150s and palpable fetal movement. The fundal height was 22 cm, which was 2 cm higher than the height found at L. C.'s examination at 20 weeks. She was referred for an ultrasound, but did not keep the appointment and has missed two subsequent prenatal visits. L. C. has a history of substance abuse but has been through a rehabilitation program and had a negative toxicology screen at 14 weeks. Today the fetus is in vertex presentation with heart tones in the 150s and palpable fetal movement. The uterine fundal height is 28 cm. The remainder of the examination is negative, with a maternal blood pressure of 130/70 and maternal weight gain of 5 lb since L. C.'s last visit. A toxicology screen is performed, and an ultrasound is scheduled that afternoon at the perinatal center in the hospital.

GROWTH RESTRICTION AND SMALL FOR GESTATIONAL AGE

Growth abnormalities are defined as excessive growth (macrosomia) or diminished growth, called either small for gestational age (SGA) or intrauterine growth restriction (IUGR). The newborn who is below the tenth percentile in birthweight is defined as growth-restricted. Nevertheless, it is important to differentiate those infants who are merely constitutionally small (SGA) from those who fail to develop to their growth potential (IUGR). The difference between SGA and IUGR may be subtle but significant in that constitutionally small newborns are not at increased risk for poor outcome, whereas those showing growth restriction are at increased risk. Growth restriction is not common, accompanying some 3% to 7% of all gestations. This problem is, however, significantly related to poor perinatal outcomes, with approximately 20% of stillborn infants being growth-restricted.

The difficulty of distinguishing SGA versus

IUGR is further complicated in that fetal weight cannot be accurately determined via sonography, which makes prenatal diagnosis problematic. Nomograms have been developed for sonographically measurable parameters that define the distribution of percentiles over normal pregnancies (Figure 17.1). In situations where fetuses are expected to be smaller, such as with multiple gestations, the nomograms may not apply. In addition, the only way to define growth is to take measurements during at least two separate instances during gestation and determine the interval change over time. When a fetus is below the tenth percentile for a particular parameter consistently over time but manages to maintain appropriate interval growth between the time periods, one may consider SGA more strongly.

Conversely, when a fetus early in gestation is within the normal parameters for growth but falls below the tenth percentile later in gestation, the suspicion for IUGR will increase.

When comparing dates and growth, it is important to establish dates as accurately and as early as possible. First trimester sonograms are superior in reliably establishing gestational age when compared to second or third trimester studies. This further supports the necessity of early prenatal care.

IUGR has many etiologies, as indicated in Table 17.1. These causes can be related to fetal, placental, or maternal contributions. Fetal factors associated with IUGR include genetic abnormalities such as trisomy 21 or 18, dwarfism, congenital anomalies such as Potter's syndrome or cardiac problems, and multiple ges-

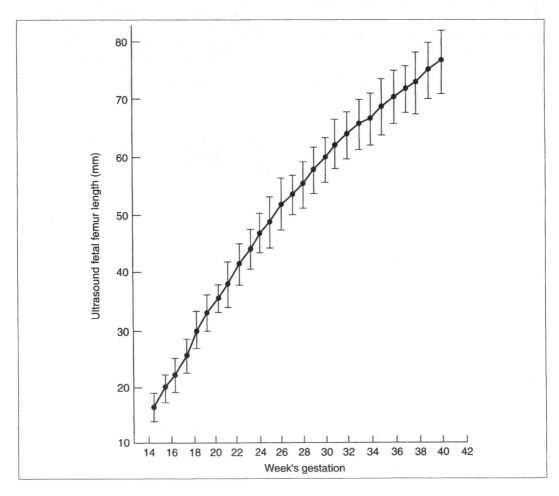

Figure 17.1 Nomogram for femur length versus weeks gestation

Source: Queenan JT. Management of high-risk pregnancy. Boston: Blackwell Scientific Publications, 1994:77.

Table 17.1 Etiologies of Intrauterine Growth Restriction

Fetal

Genetic abnormalities

    Trisomy 21 or 18

    Dwarfism

Congenital abnormalities

    Potter's syndrome

    Cardiac malformation

Multiple gestation

Placental

Decreased placental mass

    Abruption

    Infarction

    Multiple gestation

Intrinsic placental disease

    Poor implantation site

    Malformations (single umbilical artery, velamentous cord insertion)

    Vascular disease

Decreased placental flow

    Maternal vascular disease

    Postural hypotension

    Hyperviscosity

Maternal

Decreased nutrition

    Starvation

Decreased oxygen availability

    Hemoglobinopathy

    Cyanotic heart disease

    Smoking

Drug ingestion

    Ethanol

    Hydantoin

    Coumarin

weight gain have been parameters that led to the diagnosis of IUGR (Figure 17.2). The uterine fundus normally reaches to the umbilicus at approximately 20 weeks and continues to grow about 1 cm per week when measured from the top of the symphysis pubis to the top of the uterine fundus. Clearly, this measurement is a crude parameter and today is considered merely as a screen for possible IUGR. Nevertheless, it is a sign that should not be ignored. The ultrasound findings that are most commonly utilized in making the diagnosis of IUGR include placental grade, amniotic fluid volume, biparietal diameter, abdominal circumference, head circumference, and femur length.

CLINICAL CORRELATION

L. C. has an ultrasound done that afternoon. The amniotic fluid volume is low, with no single pocket being greater than 1 cm in diameter. The placenta shows some calcifications diffusely. The biparietal diameter, femur length, head circumference, and abdominal circumference are all consistent with 26 to 27 weeks gestational age. The ratio of head circumference to abdominal circumference is 1.1. Active fetal movement is seen. Sonographic examination of the fetus does not reveal any other signs of genetic or structural abnormalities. The estimated fetal weight is 1600 g, which is below the tenth percentile for 32 weeks gestational age.

The measurements obtained at ultrasound also give information about whether the growth restriction is symmetrical or asymmetrical. In asymmetrical growth restriction, one finds an increased ratio of the head circumference to the abdominal circumference (AC). The AC is felt to be relatively lowered by a smaller liver volume secondary to decreased glycogen storage. Asymmetrical IUGR is most commonly associated with maternal vascular disease, whereas most other etiologies of IUGR result in symmetrical IUGR.

Management of gestations diagnosed with IUGR is aimed at improving fetal outcome and diminishing factors responsible for the growth

tations. Placental factors include abnormal placental vasculature, abruption, or uteroplacental insufficiency secondary to early placental calcification and aging. Maternal factors include infection (most commonly rubella and cytomegalovirus), starvation, vascular disease, smoking, and drug ingestion.

Historically, fundal height and maternal

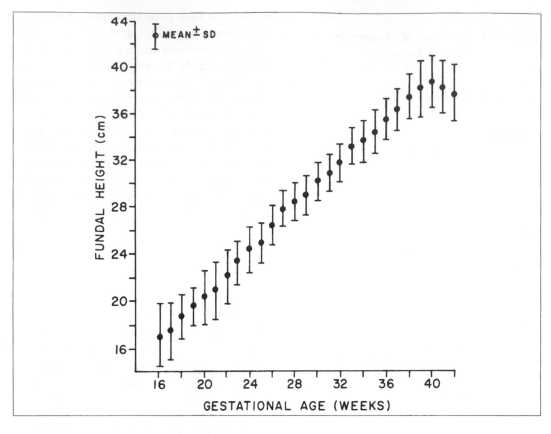

Figure 17.2 Fundal height over pregnancy

Source: Gabbe SG, Niebyl JR, Simpson JL, eds. Obstetrics: normal and problem pregnancies, 2nd ed. New York: Churchill Livingstone, 1991:227.

restriction. Antenatal testing may begin early and include nonstress testing, a biophysical profile, or contraction stress testing. Other sonographic measurements that may indicate the necessity for intervention include Doppler flow studies of the umbilical artery. Fetuses with absence of end-diastolic flow in the umbilical artery or fetal aorta are at high risk for hypoxia and poor outcomes. Maternal drug or alcohol ingestion should be curtailed if at all possible. If the mother has cyanotic heart disease, some suggest that supplemental oxygen may improve fetal oxygenation. Diagnosis of chromosomal abnormalities is important even in later gestation so as to plan modes of delivery and intervention based on the likelihood of survivability in the genetically damaged fetus.

Amniocentesis can also be valuable in predicting the likelihood of respiratory distress syndrome (RDS) occurring in the fetus if it is delivered. Gestations with IUGR are often sig-

nificantly stressed, which increases the maturation of the lungs. Therefore, if delivery is necessary, the IUGR-affected fetus of a particular gestational age may have a decreased likelihood of RDS relative to nonstressed gestations. Testing of amniotic fluid for the presence of phosphotidylglycerol or a mature lecithin/sphingomyelin ratio (L/S > 2.0) is indicative of pulmonary maturity.

Nonstress testing (NST) assessment with daily maternal assessment of fetal activity should be done twice per week in those patients for whom the physician plans to try to delay delivery once the diagnosis of IUGR is made (Figure 17.3). The NST is normally reactive after 32 weeks, nonreactive in approximately 15% of normal gestations between 28 and 32 weeks, and nonreactive in 50% of normal gestations between 24 and 28 weeks. Ultrasound should be performed every two to three weeks to assess interval growth. If the re-

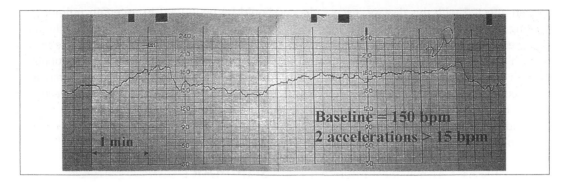

Figure 17.3   Reactive nonstress test (NST). The baseline of the fetal heart tones is approximately 150 beats per minute. Within the recording are two accelerations greater than 15 beats per minute and lasting longer than 15 seconds.

sults of NST are nonreassuring or continued declines in interval growth occur, strong consideration should be given to delivering the fetus.

CLINICAL CORRELATION

L. C. is admitted to labor and delivery after the ultrasound. Fetal heart rate tracings reveal a minimally reactive pattern. An amniocentesis is performed, and the L/S ratio is 1.9 with weakly positive phosphatidylglycerol. A maternal toxicology screen returns positive for cocaine, nicotine, and ethanol. When a contraction stress test is performed that evening, late decelerations are noted with every other contraction. On the basis of these findings, a cesarean delivery is performed that evening with delivery of a 1590 g male infant with Apgars of 5 at one minute and 7 at five minutes. The newborn quickly becomes hypoglycemic, a condition that is managed in the neonatal intensive care unit. The neonate recovers uneventfully and is discharged on day 7 when he is tolerating bottle feeds without difficulty. L. C. agrees to participate in outpatient rehabilitation for drug and alcohol abuse.

Table 17.2 lists the immediate neonatal morbidity associated with IUGR. Electrolyte disturbances are common. Hypoglycemia is very frequently observed secondary to inadequate glycogen stores and a gluconeogenic

pathway that may be poorly responsive to hypoglycemia. Hypothermia can occur due to decreased body fat stores. As noted earlier, RDS and intraventricular hemorrhage are decreased in the IUGR neonates compared to normal neonates born at the same gestational age, probably due to a protective effect of intrauterine stress.

MACROSOMIA

Macrosomia—the disorder of a fetus being too large for its gestational age—is usually a condition associated with maternal diabetes. In

Table 17.2   Immediate Neonatal Morbidity in IUGR

Birth asphyxia

Meconium aspiration

Hypoglycemia

Hypocalcemia

Hypothermia

Polycythemia, hyperviscosity

Thrombocytopenia

Pulmonary hemorrhage

Malformations

Sepsis

Source: Adapted from Gabbe SG, Niebyl JR, Simpson JL, ed. Obstetrics: normal and problem pregnancies, 2nd ed. New York: Churchill Livingstone, 1991:923.

women affected with this disease, excess circulating glucose is converted by the fetus to fat stores. Most clinicians define macrosomia as birth weight in excess of 4000 or 4500 g. As with small gestational size, excess size is screened for by noting increased uterine growth during pregnancy, which prompts ultrasound estimation of fetal weight. In maternal diabetes, macrosomia is found in muscles and fat but not in brain tissue. Such fetuses will typically have asymmetrical macrosomia —that is, an enlarged abdominal circumference but a normal head circumference. Estimated fetal weight exceeding the ninetieth percentile defines macrosomia.

The majority of complications associated with macrosomia are related to the birth process. Shoulder dystocia, birth trauma, and asphyxia are all increased in the macrosomic fetus. Meticulous maternal control of blood sugar can decrease but not eliminate the incidence of macrosomia associated with diabetes. In diabetic gestations, particularly if they are well controlled, delivery should be planned for after 38.5 weeks if antenatal testing gives reassuring results. Prior to this time, amniocentesis should be performed to ascertain pulmonary maturity if delivery is being considered. In diabetic patients, there is an increase in false-positive results with the L/S ratio; consequently, newborns need to be closely monitored for RDS. Judicious use of cesarean delivery can avoid most instances of birth trauma and shoulder dystocia in macrosomic neonates.

SUMMARY

Fetal growth abnormalities are indicators of serious problems with a gestation. Early detection of growth anomalies is possible with careful monitoring of the mother and changes in the fundal height. Although the ultimate determination of growth abnormalities is made with serial sonography, this assessment is begun in most cases only once an abnormal uterine growth is detected. Once the diagnosis of IUGR or macrosomia is made, investigation into the etiology of that abnormality and alterations in the management of the pregnancy are undertaken to achieve the best possible outcome.

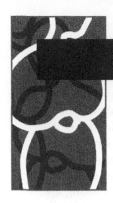

CHAPTER 18

Teratology

Alexander F. Burnett

Birth defects make a significant contribution to morbidity and mortality in the United States. In fact, congenital abnormalities account for more than 20% of infant deaths in that country. The etiology of birth defects is often multifactorial and, more often, unknown. Genetic abnormalities account for some 25% of developmental defects, with approximately one-fifth of these problems resulting from chromosomal aberrations and the rest from genetic transmission of defects. Environmental causes account for 7% to 10% of defects, with the remainder of defects being due to unknown or poorly understood factors. This chapter will discuss some of the commonly known factors associated with developmental defects, including genetic abnormalities and teratogenic agents.

CLINICAL CORRELATION

L. C. is a 34-year-old, G1P1 female who gave birth to a male child at term two months ago. She visits her obstetrician at her routine post-partum appointment. She comments that her baby has not gained much weight since birth (less than 1 lb), that he always appears fussy and is a poor sleeper, and that his face looks different than the faces on her friends' children. Although she is concerned, when you ask about her visits to the pediatrician, she states that she has yet to "get around to it." She does request oral contraceptives. The remainder of the history and physical are within normal limits, with the exception of a faint alcohol odor on her breath. You make a note of this fact as it is only 10:00 A.M., and have the office staff make an appointment with a pediatrician in your office building for the following morning.

TERATOGENIC AGENTS

A great many factors may contribute to the identification of a specific agent as causative in birth defects. Exposure to a particular compound, as measured in terms of amounts, time in gestation, route of administration, potency to induce defects, and offspring susceptibility, is important in determining the likelihood that the agent produced the perceived effect. Most teratogens have been identified through conducting animal studies and then extrapolating those data to humans. This method has limitations in that metabolism of an agent, sensitivity to that agent, and even transport of the agent to developing embryos may be vastly different between animals and humans. Consider the case of thalidomide, a potent human teratogen that produces such defects as phocomelia and cardiac malformations. Animal studies in the rat had revealed the drug to be relatively innocuous even at high doses, the drug was approved for marketing based on this information.

Today, the U.S. Food and Drug Administration requires extensive animal data to be collected and analyzed before it will approve any drug that could potentially be used in early pregnancy. On the basis of animal studies and observational data in humans, if available, drugs are classified into one of five categories (Table 18.1).

The other limitation of animal testing for teratogenicity is that typically very high doses of agents are used to better detect rare events in offspring. Agents that are harmful in very high doses to animals may not be harmful when given in the usual dose to humans. Nevertheless, "err on the side of caution" remains the prudent rule.

In addition to information gleaned from animal studies, data are collected from humans who have first trimester exposure to various agents, generally when they did not realize they were pregnant. The first trimester during organogenesis (up to 10 to 12 weeks) is the period when the fetus is most at risk for incurring significant structural damage from an offending agent. When exposure occurs later in pregnancy, the manifestations may include growth deficiencies or mental deficiencies, but would not show absence of particular organs.

When observational data are used, very long periods may pass before the risk of exposure is realized. For instance, diethylstilbestrol (DES) was a drug used in an effort to reduce spontaneous miscarriages. The drug was used for nearly 30 years in the United States before some researchers began to notice that women who had been exposed to the agent early in their fetal life had some common abnormalities of their genital tracts, including adenosis of the vagina, abnormal cervical formation, and abnormally shaped uteri. Occasionally, in about 1 woman per 1000 exposed, clear cell carcinoma of the vagina developed at a young age (otherwise an extremely rare cancer, generally affecting very elderly women).

This case demonstrates the difficulty in determining with complete accuracy the safety of any new drug for the developing fetus. Most physicians recommend that no drugs, unless absolutely necessary, be given during pregnancy or during the time when a woman may be attempting to conceive.

Legal and illegal substances of abuse may also play a role in birth defects, as discussed in Table 18.2. Cocaine use has been associated with bowel atresia; congenital malformations of the heart, limbs, face and genitourinary tract; microcephaly; growth restriction; and cerebral infarctions. In addition, hypertensive episodes related acutely to cocaine ingestion may lead to placental abruption or maternal death. Narcotic abuse presents the highest risk for the fetus if the mother should withdraw during pregnancy. As a result, the fetus suffer from with-

---

Table 18.1   FDA Risk Categories for Drugs

Category A	Studies fail to demonstrate a risk to the fetus in the first trimester and the possibility of fetal harm appears remote. Example: prenatal vitamins taken in normal doses.
Category B	Either animal reproduction studies have not demonstrated fetal risk but no controlled studies in pregnant women have been reported, or animal reproduction studies have shown an adverse effect that was not confirmed in controlled studies in women in the first trimester. Example: ampicilin.
Category C	Either studies in animals have revealed adverse effects on the fetus (teratogenic, embryocidal, or other) but no controlled studies in women have been reported, or studies in women and animals are not available. Drugs should be given only if the potential benefit justifies the potential risk to the fetus. Example: zidovudine used to decrease perinatal transmission of human immunodeficiency virus.
Category D	Positive evidence of human fetal risk exists, but the benefits from use in pregnant women may be acceptable despite the risk. Example: phenytoin.
Category X	Studies in animals or humans have demonstrated fetal abnormalities, or evidence exists of fetal risk based on human experience, or both, and the risk in pregnant women clearly outweighs any possible benefit. The drug is contraindicated in women who are or may become pregnant. Example: isotretinoin.

Source: ACOG educational bulletin: teratology, no. 236. Int J Gyn & Ob 1997;57:319.

Table 18.2   Drugs and Their Effects on the Fetus

Alcohol	Fetal alcohol syndrome (prenatal and postnatal growth deficiency, CNS abnormalities such as irritability and hyperactivity, and craniofacial abnormalities).
Tobacco	Low birth weight, increased perinatal mortality, increased preterm birth, increased placenta previa, abruption, and premature rupture of membranes.
Cocaine	Decreased birth weight, impaired fetal growth, increased preterm labor and delivery, increased placental abruption, increased cerebral infarctions, possible increase in genitourinary anomalies, SIDS, and premature rupture of membranes.
Amphetamines	Decreased birth weight and length, cerebral ischemia and infarctions possible, increase in intraventricular hemorrhage, possible increased anomalies.
Marijuana	Possible decrease in birth weight and length, although data are conflicting when controlling for other variables such as concurrent alcohol or tobacco use. No definite sequelae noted in neurodevelopment testing or postnatal growth.
Opiates	Intrauterine growth restriction, preterm delivery, fetal death, decreased head circumference, depressed Apgar scores, meconium staining of amniotic fluid, premature rupture of membranes, chorioamnionitis, neonatal withdrawal.
Caffeine	Most studies suggest an increased risk of fetal growth delay among women consuming more than 300 mg/day (3–4 cups of coffee/day).

Source: Adapted from Creasy RK, Resnick R, eds. Maternal—fetal medicine, 4th ed. Philadelphia: W. B. Saunders, 1999:146–158.

drawal as well, with the potential for death. Intrauterine growth restriction is also increased in narcotics abusers. Although marijuana has not been shown to be teratogenic, several studies have found diminished learning abilities in children of mothers who smoked marijuana during their pregnancy. Likewise, tobacco smoke has not been shown to be teratogenic; when mothers smoke, however, there is an increased risk of spontaneous abortions, intrauterine fetal death, neonatal death, and prematurity. Tobacco smoke exposure also reduces birth weight, birth length, and head circumference.

The most commonly abused agent during pregnancy is alcohol. Fetal alcohol syndrome (FAS) may affect 0.2% to 0.4% of infants born in the United States. The likelihood of having a child with FAS is related to the amount of alcohol ingested. Women who ingest six drinks per day during pregnancy have a 40% risk of having offspring with some manifestations of FAS. The most common findings include the following:

- Prenatal growth deficiency for weight, height, and head circumference
- Distinct craniofacial features including midfacial hypoplasia and microcephaly

- Mild to moderate mental retardation (Figure 18.1).

The average IQ among affected offspring is 65 but may range from 16 to 105. Hypotonia and poor motor coordination are often present. Diagnosis is based on the presence of some of these findings when high alcohol ingestion is documented in the mother.

CLINICAL CORRELATION

L. C. is asked the TACE questions (see Chapter 7). She answers that it requires at least two highball drinks to make her feel high (tolerance). She also admits to being annoyed by her husband's criticism of her drinking, has felt that at times she should cut down on her drinking (but has been unable to do so), and rarely requires a morning drink (eye-opener) to calm her nerves. She relates that both of her parents are alcoholics and that her husband is also a heavy drinker. It is explained to her that some of the problems with her child may be related to alcohol consumption during pregnancy, and the pediatrician is alerted to examine the infant carefully for sequelae of FAS.

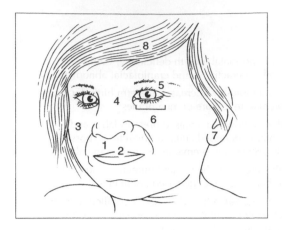

Figure 18.1 Facial features associated with fetal alcohol syndrome include: 1) absent philtrum, 2) thinned upper vermilion, 3) hypoplastic midface, 4) low nasal bridge, 5) epicanthal fold, 6) shortened palpebral fissure, 7) low-set ears, and 8) microcephaly.

Source: Coles CD. Impact of prenatal alcohol exposure on the newborn and the child. Clin Obstet Gynecol 1993;36:255.

Environmental exposure to several compounds has been associated with birth defects. For example, exposure to lead may affect fetal central nervous system development. Exposure to organic mercury can lead to cerebral atrophy, microcephaly, mental retardation, spasticity, seizures, or blindness. Contact with organic solvents and polychlorinated biphenyls may also cause specific defects and increase spontaneous abortions and cognitive impairment. Table 18.3 lists other agents associated with birth defects.

Infectious agents that can lead to birth defects include any of the TORCH infections (toxoplasmosis, rubella, cytomegalovirus, herpes virus). Exposure to syphilis and varicella is also associated with specific defects. These infections are discussed in detail in Chapter 28. Table 18.4 details common manifestations of prenatal infection with these agents.

Exposure to ionizing radiation can lead to infant microcephaly and mental retardation

Table 18.3 Additional Teratogens

COMPOUND	EFFECTS	COMMENTS
Androgens	Virilization of females, advanced genital development of males	Effects are dose-dependent and also depend on stage of development when exposure occurs
Angiotensin-converting enzyme inhibitors	Fetal renal tubular dysplasia, oligohydramnios, lack of cranial ossification, IUGR	Fetal morbidity of 30%
Coumarin	Nasal hypoplasia and stippled bond epiphyses, IUGR, CNS anomalies	Risk of seriously affected offspring 15%–25% when used in first trimester
Carbamazepine	Neural tube defects, microcephaly, IUGR	Increased risk when used with other antiseizure medications
Methotrexate	Increased spontaneous abortions and various anomalies	
Lithium	Congenital heart disease (Ebstein anomaly)	Risk is low
Phenytoin	IUGR, mental retardation, microcephaly, cardiac defects, hypoplastic nails, dysmorphic faces	Full syndrome occurs in less than 10%; 30% with some manifestations
Tetracycline	Hypoplasia of tooth enamel, permanent discoloration of deciduous teeth	
Valproic acid	Neural tube defects, spina bifida	
Vitamin A derivatives (isotretinoin)	Increased abortions, microtia, CNS defects, thymic agenesis, cardiovascular anomalies	

Table 18.4 TORCH, Syphilis, and Varicella Infection Manifestations

Toxoplasmosis	Microcephaly, hydrocephaly, cerebral calcifications. Chorioretinitis is common. Initial maternal infection must occur during pregnancy to place the fetus at risk.
Rubella	Microcephaly, mental retardation, cataracts, deafness, congenital heart disease. Malformation rate is 50% if the mother is infected during the first trimester.
Cytomegalovirus	Hydrocephaly, microcephaly, chorioretinitis, cerebral calcifications, IUGR, microphthalmos, brain damage, mental retardation, hearing loss. The most common congenital infection. The congenital infection rate is 40% after primary infection.
Syphilis	Fetal demise with hydrops. Mild infections result in abnormalities of the skin, teeth, and bones. Penicillin is effective therapy. The worst damage occurs when the infection persists for longer than 20 weeks.
Varicella	Skin scarring, chorioretinitis, cataracts, microcephaly, hypoplasia of hands and feet, muscle atrophy. The risk of congenital varicella is low.

(Table 18.5). Higher doses, particularly early in pregnancy, are associated with increased spontaneous miscarriage and fetal death. Studies of the Japanese atomic bomb survivors show the highest incidence of mental retarda-tion among those exposed between 8 and 15 weeks gestation. Microcephaly and mental re-tardation was almost nonexistent in those who were exposed to this radiation during the third trimester. Prior to any radiographic study in a reproductive-age woman, her pregnancy sta-tus should be ascertained. Where appropriate, the abdomen may be shielded to minimize ex-posure to the fetus. For abdominal evaluations during pregnancy, ultrasound and MRI avoid the exposure to ionizing radiation.

Table 18.5 Fetal Dose for Radiographic Tests

EXAMINATION	FETAL DOSE RANGE (gGY)
CXR	0.00006
Abdominal X ray	0.024–1.416
Lumbar spine	0.002–2.901
Pelvic X ray	0.008–1.587
IVP	0.024–3.069
Upper GI	<0.001–1.228
BE	0.005–9.218
Bone scan	0.13–0.33
CT chest	0.006–0.05
CT abdomen	0.8–4.9
CT pelvis	2.5–7.9
V/Q scan	0.002–0.04
Mammogram	Undetectable

Sources: Mossman KL, Hill LT. Ob Gyn 1982;60:237; Fattibene P, Mazzei F, Nuccetelli C, Resica S. Acta Pediatrica 1999;88:693.

GENETIC ABNORMALITIES

Chromosomal and genetic alterations may give rise to specific physical manifestations in the offspring.

The most frequent autosomal chromo-somal syndrome is Down syndrome (trisomy 21). Common anomalies associated with this syndrome include facial anomalies (such as brachycephaly, epicanthal folds, and low-set ears), cardiac anomalies, duodenal atresia, and single palmar crease (Figure 18.2). These in-fants generally have lower birth weights and exhibit moderate to severe mental retardation.

Trisomy 18 occurs much less frequently. Common facial anomalies in this syndrome include microcephaly, micrognathia, and low-set, pointed ears. Rocker-bottom feet with pro-trusion of the calcaneum may be present. Car-

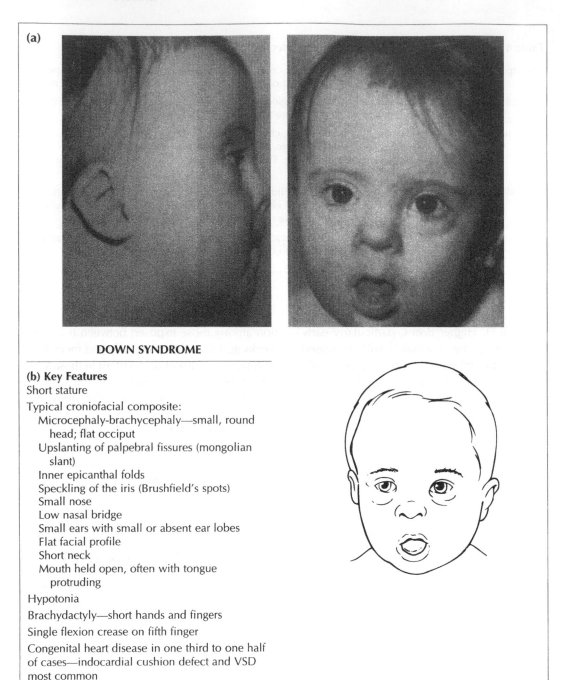

(a)

DOWN SYNDROME

(b) Key Features

Short stature

Typical croniofacial composite:
  Microcephaly-brachycephaly—small, round
    head; flat occiput
  Upslanting of palpebral fissures (mongolian
    slant)
  Inner epicanthal folds
  Speckling of the iris (Brushfield's spots)
  Small nose
  Low nasal bridge
  Small ears with small or absent ear lobes
  Flat facial profile
  Short neck
  Mouth held open, often with tongue
    protruding

Hypotonia

Brachydactyly—short hands and fingers

Single flexion crease on fifth finger

Congenital heart disease in one third to one half
of cases—indocardial cushion defect and VSD
most common

Figure 18.2   (a) A child with Down syndrome (trisomy 21). (b) Key features of Down syndrome.

Sources: (a) Cunningham FG, MacDonald PC, Gant NF, Leveno KJ, Gilstrap LG III, eds. Williams obstetrics, 19th ed. Norwalk, CT: Appleton & Lange, 1993:921. (b) Oski FA, DeAngelis CD, McMillan JA, Feigin RD, Warsaw JB, eds. Principles and practice of pediatrics, 2nd ed. Philadelphia: J. B. Lippincott, 1994:2184.

Table 18.6 Sex Chromosomal Abnormalities

ABNORMALITY	CHROMOSOMAL DEFECT	MANIFESTATIONS
Turner's syndrome Monosomy X	45,XO	Gonadal dysgenesis (streak ovaries) Shield chest, renal and cardiac anomalies, cubitus valgus, rarely fertile
Klinefelter syndrome Males with two or more X chromosomes	47,XXY, 48,XXXY 49,XXXXY	Small testes, azoospermia, elevated FSH and LH, decreased testosterone
Polysomy X in females	47,XXX	Increased mental retardation
Polysomy Y in males	47,XYY 48,XXYY	More likely tall and more likely to display sociopathic behavior

diac anomalies and renal anomalies are common. Most infants with trisomy 18 die within the first few months; those who survive exhibit severe retardation.

Trisomy 13 is very rare. If the infant affected with this syndrome survives to term, he or she will often have severe anomalies including holoprosencephaly, cleft lip and palate, polydactyly, cardiac defects, and eye anomalies.

Sex chromosomal abnormalities are less common than Down syndrome, but most are compatible with a normal life span. Table 18.6 lists the major features of the most common sex chromosomal abnormalities.

SUMMARY

Birth defects are most commonly multifactorial in origin. There are some well-recognized syndromes associated with specific chromosomal abnormalities and some defects associated with a limited number of external agents. The risk of defects from an exposure to a particular teratogen depends on the timing of exposure, the strength of the exposure, and the susceptibility of the developing fetus. Because of their potential for harm, medications should be used only when absolutely necessary during pregnancy.

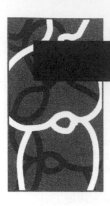

CHAPTER 19

Preterm Labor

Alexander F. Burnett

Labor is defined as regular uterine contractions resulting in progressive effacement and dilation of the cervix. Preterm (premature) labor is that which occurs prior to 37 weeks gestational age. In practical terms, intervention is begun prior to dilation of the cervix, if at all possible, in an effort to prevent preterm delivery. In general, women from lower socioeconomic classes tend to have a higher incidence of preterm labor and low-birth-weight deliveries, as do women who are at the extremes of reproductive age and women who smoke. Similarly, women who do not receive adequate prenatal care are at risk for preterm labor and delivery.

Preterm birth is defined as delivery prior to 37 weeks gestational age. The incidence of premature delivery is approximately 9%. Prematurity is responsible for 75% of neonatal deaths (excluding congenital malformations). The incidence of preterm delivery has not changed significantly since 1950. Low birth weight (LBW) is not identical to prematurity, as some other causes of low birth weight exist. LBW is an important determinant of neonatal morbidity and mortality. By definition, LBW is defined as a neonate weighing less than 2500 g at birth. Its incidence varies with variable populations and various altitudes. Very low birth weight (VLBW) is less than 1500 g. Incidences of LBW and VLBW are reported as 7% and 1.2% of all deliveries, respectively. Both the degree of prematurity and the birth weight are closely correlated with neonatal morbidity and mortality (Table 19.1).

CLINICAL CORRELATION

L. B. is a 16-year-old primigravida at 28 weeks since her last menstrual period. She is brought into labor and delivery by ambulance, complaining of regular uterine contractions for several hours. She has had only one prenatal visit, eight weeks ago. An ultrasound was arranged at the first prenatal visit, but she failed to keep that appointment. L. B. states that she has felt regular, hard uterine "cramps" for about six hours. She feels the baby move quite well and denies any leakage of fluid or bleeding from her vagina. She has not had any fevers or chills. She denies recent intercourse and illicit drug use.

L. B. is placed on a monitor in the labor and delivery department. The fetal heart tones are in the 150s. Uterine contractions are detected every four to five minutes. The contractions last about 30 seconds and are felt to be moderate by the labor and delivery nurse. L. B. is afebrile, but has a blood pressure of 140/90 with a normal pulse and respirations.

ETIOLOGY OF PRETERM LABOR

In roughly one-third of all preterm labor cases, the etiology involves maternal or fetal compli-

Table 19.1 Approximate Neonatal Survival to Discharge of Preterm Infants Born in a Tertiary-Care Center

GESTATIONAL AGE (WEEKS)	BIRTH WEIGHT (G)	SURVIVORS (%)
24–25	500–750	55
26–27	751–1000	80
28–29	100–1250	93
30–31	1251–1500	96
32–33	150–1750	99
≥34	1751–2000	99+

cations (Table 19.2). Examples of these complications include maternal hypertensive disorders, placental abruption, placenta previa, multiple fetal pregnancy, polyhydramnios, and congenital anomalies. Maternal uterine anomalies include large myomas, septations, bicornuate uterus, or other malformations that may restrict normal uterine expansion over the course of the pregnancy. Women who were themselves exposed to diethylstilbestrol (DES) in utero may fall into this category. Fetal malformations resulting in oligohydramnios, such as abnormal kidney formation or urethral strictures, also increase the likelihood of preterm labor and birth. Likewise, maternal infections outside of the uterus—such as pneumonia, pyelonephritis, or viral syndromes—are associated with preterm labor. Cervical incompetence due to prior surgical procedures, congenital anomalies, or idiopathic reasons typically results in and is defined by painless dilation and effacement of the cervix, which can initiate labor or premature rupture of membranes.

Another one-third of cases of preterm labor and delivery can be traced to premature rupture of membranes (discussed in Chapter 20). The remaining one-third of preterm labor cases are considered "idiopathic," as these women have intact membranes and no identifiable explanation for the preterm labor. Many feel that subclinical infections are responsible for the majority of these cases—perhaps ascending infections from the lower genital tract to the uterus.

Table 19.2 Risk Factors in the Prediction of Spontaneous Preterm Labor

MAJOR	MINOR
Multiple gestation	Febrile illness
Diethylstilbestrol exposure	Bleeding after 12 weeks
Hydramnios	History of pyelonephritis
Uterine anomaly	Cigarettes—more than 10/day
Cervix dilated >1 cm at 32 weeks	Second-trimester abortion >1
More than two second-trimester abortions	More than two first-trimester abortions
Previous preterm delivery	
Previous preterm labor—term delivery	
Abdominal surgery during pregnancy	
History of cone biopsy	
Cervical shortening <1 cm at 32 weeks	
Uterine irritability	

The presence of one or more major factors and/or two or more minor factors places the patient in the high-risk group.

CLINICAL CORRELATION

L. B. undergoes an ultrasound evaluation, which reveals a singleton gestation in vertex presentation. Measurements of the head circumference, biparietal diameter, abdominal circumference, and femur length are all consistent with 27 to 29 weeks gestational age. The fetus is active and adequate amniotic fluid is present. The placenta shows calcifications consistent with grade 2 (Figure 19.1), which are more pronounced than those anticipated for this stage of gestation. The placenta is anterior fundal in location. Upon examination, the cervix is noted to be soft, 50% effaced, and nondilated. Cultures for group B streptococcus, gonorrhea, and Chlamydia are taken from the cervix. Laboratory tests are undertaken, including complete blood count, toxicology screen, type and screen, electrolytes and blood glucose, and urinalysis with urine and blood cultures. An intravenous line is begun, and L. B. is given a rapid infusion of 1 L of balanced salt solution, followed by a maintenance rate of 125 cm³/hr.

MANAGEMENT OF PRETERM LABOR

Once the diagnosis is established by the presence of regular uterine contractions and physical changes in the cervix, the decision is made about whether to place the mother on tocolytic therapy. If the ultrasound reveals anomalies in the fetus that are incompatible with life, then one should not heroically intervene to try to prolong the gestation. Tocolytic therapy should be given at a time in gestation where a delay in birth will have a positive benefit for the neonate. Generally, tocolytics are used between 24 and 34 weeks gestation.

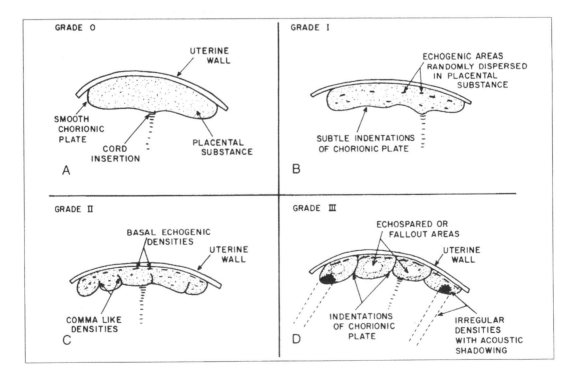

Figure 19.1   Placental grading

Source: Gabbe SG, Niebyl JR, Simpson JL, eds. Obstetrics: normal and problem pregnancies, 2nd ed. New York: Churchill Livingstone, 1991:414.

Table 19.3 Approximate Neonatal Morbidity Rates (percent) by Gestational Age at Birth

| | GESTATIONAL AGE (WEEKS) | | | | | | |
	24–25	26–27	28–29	30–31	32–33	34	35
RDS	85	81	65	30	30	20	3
PDA	80	50	50	21	17	13	—
Sepsis	25	25	20	10	7	5	5
NEC	8	6	5	5	3	—	—
IVH grades III and IV	30	9	7	5	3	—	—

RDS: Respiratory distress syndrome: PDA; patent ductus arteriosus; NEC: necrotizing enterocolitis; IVH: intraventricular hemorrhage (Papille's classification).

Cases must be decided on an individual basis when preterm labor occurs outside of this time frame. Table 19.3 describes the common neonatal morbidity associated with prematurity. Frequently occurring, serious sequelae of prematurity include respiratory distress syndrome (RDS), patent ductus arteriosus (PDA), necrotizing enterocolitis (NEC), sepsis, and intraventricular hemorrhage (IVH).

Tocolytic agents are intended to reduce or eliminate uterine contractions. Ritodrine is the only drug with FDA approval as a tocolytic agent, although similar agents, such as terbutaline, and alternative agents, such as magnesium sulfate, are also commonly used. Other agents, such as prostaglandin inhibitors (indomethacin) and calcium-channel blockers (nifedipine), are occasionally utilized in tocolytic regimens.

Beta-mimetics (ritodrine and terbutaline) function by simulating beta-receptors, which results in smooth muscle relaxation in vascular, gastrointestinal, and uterine sites. Side effects from beta-mimetics include tachycardia with rare dysrhythmias, pulmonary edema, hypokalemia, hypotension, hyperglycemia, chest pain, and shortness of breath. Pulmonary edema is the most frequent serious complication of beta-mimetic therapy and requires careful attention to fluid balance in these patients. Maternal cardiac disorders are a contraindication to beta-mimetic therapy.

Alternatively, magnesium sulfate may be given to provide tocolysis. Its mechanism of action is likely competition with calcium in the uterine smooth muscle, which reduces the excitability of the muscle. Magnesium sulfate has an efficacy as a tocolytic similar to that of beta-mimetics, but offers reduced incidence of pulmonary edema and chest pain. Consequently, many institutions prefer to use magnesium sulfate as first-line therapy for tocolysis. Serum magnesium levels should be monitored and maintained between 5 and 8 mg/dL. Higher serum concentrations may result in respiratory compromise and even arrest. Immediate reversal of magnesium toxicity may be achieved by administering an ampule of calcium gluconate, which should always be at the bedside of a patient on magnesium sulfate.

Contraindications to tocolysis may be maternal or fetal in nature and represent situations in which it is deemed unsafe or unwise to prolong the gestation. Maternal contraindications include significant hypertension (such as eclampsia), antepartum hemorrhage, significant cardiac disease, and hypersensitivity to a specific tocolytic agent. Some of these contraindications may be relative—for example, in the mildly bleeding premature gestation with placenta previa, tocolysis may be indicated to prevent further hemorrhage. Fetal contraindications to tocolysis include gestational age greater than 36 weeks, advanced dilation/effacement of the cervix, birth weight greater than 2500 g, fetal death or lethal anomaly, chorioamnionitis, and evidence of in utero fetal distress.

Antibiotic use in preterm labor remains controversial. Reports conflict regarding the effects of prolongation of pregnancy with antibiotic use alone. If the patient has an identified infection, such as the urinary tract or cervical group B streptococcus, it should be actively treated.

Glucocorticoids have long been recognized to accelerate fetal lung maturation. Commonly employed glucocorticoids are betamethasone and dexamethasone. Studies have shown that use of these agents in the patient between 28 and 32 weeks gestation significantly reduces the incidence of RDS, IVH, PDA, NEC, and neurologic abnormalities in prematurely born infants. To realize the greatest benefits, the agents must be given at least 24 hours but no more than 7 days prior to birth. Therefore, these agents are given weekly between 28 and 32 weeks as long as the gestation continues. After 32 to 34 weeks, the benefit of glucocorticoids is not as clear.

CLINICAL CORRELATION

L. B. is begun on magnesium sulfate therapy with an intravenous bolus of 4 g followed by an infusion of 2 g/hr. Her magnesium levels are checked on a regular basis. The urine culture returns with greater than 100,000 E. coli; this infection is treated with ampicillin given intravenously. Her cervical cultures are negative. A toxicology screen is positive for cocaine and nicotine. L. B.'s contractions abate after 8 hours of magnesium therapy and antibiotics. Her blood pressure 8 hours after admission is 130/82. She is maintained on magnesium sulfate for 24 hours, at which time the cervical examination is unchanged and uterine contractions are no longer detectable. L. B. is transferred to the antepartum floor after the magnesium therapy is discontinued and does well for 48 hours. At that point, contractions begin again. She returns to labor and delivery. Her cervix is now completely effaced and 2 cm dilated. L. B. is administered magnesium sulfate

again as well as betamethasone. Once again, her contractions stop. Nevertheless, she is maintained in labor and delivery on magnesium for the next four weeks, receiving weekly betamethasone.

At 32 weeks gestational age, L.B. begins contracting while on magnesium sulfate. A trial of ritodrine is attempted but fails to stop the progressive dilation of her cervix. The fetus is in cephalic presentation, and she delivers a male infant via spontaneous vaginal delivery who weighs 1500 g. The Apgar scores are 5 at one minute and 7 at five minutes. Supplemental oxygen is given to the neonate, but he does not require intubation. He is sent home one month later without obvious neurologic sequelae.

Delivery of the premature infant depends on the position of the fetus. Nonvertex presentations (transverse, breech) should be delivered via cesarean delivery when they are premature. Vertex presentations can safely deliver vaginally, with most researchers recommending a generous episiotomy to reduce forces on the small, soft head.

Prevention of preterm labor in future pregnancies focuses on meticulous prenatal care, including regular examinations of the cervix. For those women with cervical incompetence, a cerclage stitch may be placed in the cervix to help prevent silent dilation (Figure 19.2). Typically, it will be emplaced between 12 and 16 weeks after a viable pregnancy has been established.

Another controversial issue related to the prevention of preterm birth is the use of home monitors, which transmit information on uterine activity via phone lines to the physician. Data gathered so far are not clear regarding the efficacy of this technique.

In any event, it is clear that frequent contact with medical personnel and education on signs and symptoms of preterm labor are beneficial in detecting preterm labor at an earlier stage. Prophylactic use of tocolytics when a woman has had a prior preterm delivery, in the absence of contractions during the present gestation, has not been proven to be beneficial.

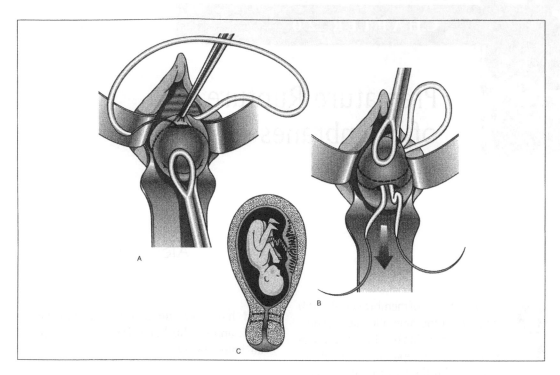

Figure 19.2 Cerclage of the cervix

Source: Callahan TL, Caughey AB, Heffner LJ. Blueprints in obstetrics and gynecology. Malden, MA: Blackwell Science, 1998:13.

SUMMARY

Prematurity continues to be the major factor in neonatal morbidity and mortality. Prevention of premature birth involves early recognition of preterm labor, when intervention is most likely to be successful in tocolysis, and treatment of infections contributing to preterm labor. When possible, delivery of the preterm infant should be performed under controlled conditions with access to neonatal resuscitation and specialized personnel.

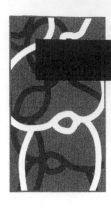

CHAPTER 20

Premature Rupture of Membranes

Alexander F. Burnett

Premature rupture of membranes (PROM) occurs when the amniotic sac ruptures prior to the initiation of labor. This problem occurs with approximately 15% of all pregnancies, with the vast majority occurring in term gestations. When rupture of membranes occurs in a preterm gestation (prior to 37 weeks), the condition is called preterm PROM (PPROM). Approximately 3% to 4% of all gestations are affected by PPROM. The majority of patients who have PROM will undergo spontaneous labor within 48 hours. Consequently, complications are most frequently related to the gestational time at which PROM occurs.

PROM has a significant effect on maternal and neonatal morbidity and mortality. Approximately 10% of perinatal deaths are associated with this condition.

CLINICAL CORRELATION

P. T. is a 28-year-old, G1 female who is at 22 weeks gestational age when she feels a sudden gush of fluid from her vagina as she is going into bed at night. She calls her obstetrician immediately. She denies any passage of blood from her vagina, uterine cramping or pain, or fevers or chills. P. T. began to feel the baby move (quickening) about two weeks prior to this episode and states that she has felt the baby move this evening. Her prenatal care began at eight weeks gestational age and has been uncomplicated thus far. P. T. and her husband drive to the hospital immediately.

The common presenting symptom for premature rupture of membranes is the passage of fluid from the vagina that is neither associated with uterine contractions nor felt to be urine by the patient. Rarely, rupture of membranes is detected in an asymptomatic patient based on oligohydramnios (diminished amniotic fluid) and subsequent documentation of passage of amniotic fluid.

The diagnosis of PROM is not always easily confirmed. Several tests are available to evaluate fluid in the vagina to determine whether it is amniotic fluid. Nevertheless, other fluids may be normally present in the vagina—for example, urine, cervical mucus, bath water, vaginal discharge, blood, meconium, or semen. Alternatively, the patient may report sudden vaginal fluid loss but on evaluation be found to have no fluid in the vagina. The initial evaluation of the patient with this history is to perform a sterile speculum examination, looking for pooling of fluid in the posterior vagina and visualizing the cervix for evidence of dilation. A sterile swab is then used to sample the fluid (Figure 20.1).

After its collection, the fluid is evaluated for pH. The pH of the vagina is typically fairly acidic, ranging between 5.2 and 6.0. The amniotic fluid pH is more basic, ranging be-

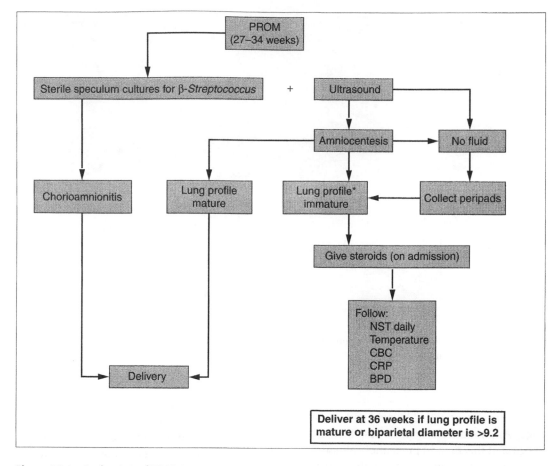

Figure 20.1 Evaluation of PROM

Source: Mishell DR, Brenner PF, eds. Management of common problems in obstetrics and gynecology, 3rd ed. Boston: Blackwell Scientific Publications, 1994:110.

tween 7.0 and 7.7. Nitrazine paper (sodium dinitrophenylazonaphthol) changes color from orange to blue at a pH of 6.4 to 6.8. This color change is nearly 90% accurate in predicting rupture of membranes. False-positive results may occur when the sample contains blood, semen, soap, or antiseptics, or occasionally when the patient has a vaginal infection involving *Trichomonas* or bacterial vaginosis. Urine, if infected with *Proteus,* may also undergo alkalization and lead to a false-positive result.

In addition to being evaluated in terms of its pH, the fluid is spread over a microscope slide and allowed to air-dry. When amniotic fluid dries, it becomes crystallized and forms a pattern resembling a fern when viewed under the microscope. This process is referred to as ferning and reflects the presence of salts within amniotic fluid (Figure 20.2). Ferning evaluation is between 85% and 98% accurate in diagnosing amniotic fluid.

CLINICAL CORRELATION

When P. T. undergoes a sterile speculum examination, a pool of clear fluid is noted in the posterior vagina. The fluid turns the nitrazine paper blue and ferns on a microscope slide as it dries. A culture is taken of the cervix, which appears long and closed. P. T. is placed on the monitor, which does not detect any uterine contractions. She is afebrile. Routine admission laboratory tests are sent and an ultrasound is performed. There is a single intrauterine gestation with

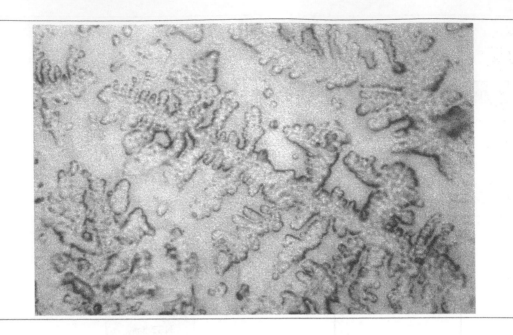

Figure 20.2   The ferning pattern seen when amniotic fluid is allowed to dry on a glass slide after removal of a sample from the vaginal pool

a size consistent with 22 weeks gestational age. Amniotic fluid appears less than expected at this time in pregnancy, although some pockets measure 7 cm in their greatest dimension. Gross examination does not reveal any obvious abnormalities of the fetus.

ETIOLOGY OF PROM

Multiple factors may contribute to the occurrence of premature rupture of membranes. Whatever the etiology, the event involves a weakening of the collagen within the amniotic sac. Some studies have demonstrated that pregnancies complicated with PROM have a diminished collagen content within the amnion (Table 20.1).

Infection is felt to be a major cause of PROM. Organisms that have been implicated in PROM include group B streptococcus, *Neisseria gonorrhea, Bacteroides* species, *Trichomonas vaginalis, Chlamydia trachomatis,* and possibly *Mycoplasma.* Women who are colonized with group B streptococcus (GBS) have a higher incidence of PROM than those who are not. For all patients, cultures

should be taken of the cervix at the time of evaluation for PROM.

Vaginal pH may be related to the onset of PROM. Infection with several of the previously mentioned infections (GBS, *N. gonorrhea,* anaerobes) causes the vaginal pH to be raised.

Table 20.1   Factors Associated with PROM

1. Cervical incompetence

2. Overdistended uterus (multiple gestations, polyhydramnios)

3. Inherited membrane defect (genetic conditions, low maternal serum copper, vitamin C deficiency)

4. Exogenous effects on the membranes (by proteolytic enzymes produced by mycoplasma, *E. coli, Streptococcus* B and D, and by the release of collagenase-like enzymes present in seminal fluid)

5. Unknown

Source: Mishell DR, Brenner PF, eds. Management of common problems in obstetrics and gynecology, 3rd ed. Boston: Blackwell Scientific Publications, 1994:109.

Studies have shown that women at risk for PROM who had a vaginal pH greater than 4.5 had an increased chance of PROM compared with women with a pH less than 4.5.

Vitamin and mineral deficiencies that have been associated with PROM include lack of vitamin C, zinc, and copper. Smoking during pregnancy is also associated with an increased risk of PROM. Anatomical defects of the cervix—particularly cervical incompetence—is associated with PROM, most likely due to increased exposure of the amniotic membranes to the flora of the vagina. Intercourse during pregnancy has also been theorized to increase the likelihood of rupture of membranes; as yet, no studies have confirmed this theory.

CLINICAL CORRELATION

The cervical culture taken at the time of P. T.'s evaluation for PROM returns positive for group B streptococcus. P. T. is given antibiotic therapy with ampicillin. She does not exhibit any signs of contractions while being monitored in labor and delivery, nor does she show clinical signs of infection (such as fever, elevated white blood cell count, or elevated C-reactive protein).

MANAGEMENT OF PROM

The management of PROM depends on several factors. Most important is the point during the gestation at which the rupture of membranes occurs. For this reason, accurate dating of the gestation is essential. When PROM occurs at term, the question becomes one of expectant versus active management (intervention with induction of labor). Approximately 90% of women at term who rupture their membranes will have spontaneous labor within 24 hours. The trade-offs between expectant versus active management include a higher rate of chorioamnionitis the longer the membranes remain ruptured without delivery versus a higher cesarean birth rate if women are induced with an unfavorable cervix. Certainly delivery should be expedited in a situation where infection is present or fetal distress occurs; however, one cannot easily predict who is at risk for these complications.

A woman who is approaching term at 35 to 36 weeks gestation may have labor induced with a low expected rate of neonatal pulmonary complications. Between 32 and 35 weeks, some clinicians advocate waiting 16 hours before initiating induction, as this delay has been associated with less pulmonary sequelae in the neonate. If the fetus is estimated to weigh more than 2000 g, delay is probably not necessary. If, at 32 to 35 weeks, labor has not begun within 16 hours, it should probably be induced, as the longer a woman remains with ruptured membranes, the higher is the likelihood of infection occurring.

Bimanual examinations of the cervix in a patient with PROM are discouraged because they tend to introduce vaginal flora into the cervix and lower uterine segment, increasing the likelihood of infection. At the initial evaluation, if a vaginal pool of fluid is observed, some should be collected in a sterile fashion and analyzed for the presence of phosphotidylglycerol (PG) as an indicator of pulmonary maturity. If the PG test is negative and the patient is neither infected nor in active labor, she should be placed on bedrest, preferably in slight Trendelenberg position to allow amniotic fluid to reaccumulate. If the mother has an infection, labor should be induced and antibiotics should be given during labor. If the pathogen is known, the antibiotic administered should be specific for that organism. More likely the pathogen will be unknown, so a reasonable choice of antibiotics would be a combination of ampicillin and gentamicin during labor.

When PROM occurs between 28 and 32 weeks gestation, the choice of whether to administer corticosteroids to hasten pulmonary maturity is a controversial one. Clearly, in nonruptured women, steroids decrease neonatal RDS between 28 and 32 weeks (see Chapter 19). In the face of ruptured membranes, however, steroids may increase the incidence of amnionitis. Another controversial topic is the role of tocolytic therapy in the patient with ruptured membranes. This debate is related to the potential for an infectious agent to serve as the etiology for membrane rupture and the choice of prolonging a pregnancy when amnionitis is present. Generally, in patients with PROM, expectant management (bedrest, fetal monitoring intermittently, daily observation of mother and fetus) appears to be the most reasonable approach. If clinical chorioamnionitis develops, the fetus should be delivered.

In the previable gestation with PROM, the patient may be allowed to stay home on bedrest as much as possible, if no signs of infection are present. If the pregnancy continues to the time of viability, admission to the hospital may be reasonable so as to monitor both mother and fetus more closely. In the previable PROM, the mother should be given the option of terminating the pregnancy.

COMPLICATIONS OF PROM

Other than prematurity, the major complications associated with PROM include infection (as previously stated) and consequences of oligohydramnios (lack of amniotic fluid). In oligohydramnios, a tetrad of consequences have been described. The most serious is pulmonary hypoplasia, most likely caused by abnormal fluid dynamics. Other sequelae include a typical facial deformity with low-set, flattened ears, extremity deformities from compression and immobility, and fetal growth restriction (Table 20.2).

CLINICAL CORRELATION

P. T. is given the options of terminating the pregnancy or attempting to maintain the pregnancy to viability. She elects to maintain the pregnancy and is placed on maximum bedrest at home. Weekly examinations are performed by her obstetrician that document adequate fundal growth and no evidence of infection. When an ultrasound

---

is performed with a portable ultrasound machine at 25 weeks, it reveals an adequate amount of amniotic fluid and good interval growth of the fetus.

P. T. is transferred to the antepartum ward at the hospital at 26 weeks and maintained on bedrest with daily monitoring of fetal heart rate. She continues to leak small amounts of fluid from her vagina while on bedrest. P. T. begins contracting at 31 weeks and proceeds to deliver a viable male infant via spontaneous vaginal delivery. The infant has Apgars of 5 at one minute and 8 at five minutes. He requires supplemental oxygen but does not need to be intubated. Morphologically, the infant appears completely normal.

FETAL SURVEILLANCE WITH PROM

Once the gestation reaches viability, surveillance is done via ultrasound and fetal heart rate monitoring as a biophysical profile (see Chapter 33). Fetal heart rate monitoring looks for signs of cord compression, such as deep variable decelerations that occur because of lack of amniotic fluid. In addition, an elevated fetal heart rate may indicate a fetal infection. Fetal measurements intended to identify interval growth should also be made. Fetal movements, breathing movements, and reactive fetal heart tones are all indicators of fetal well-being.

If the pregnancy should develop signs of uterine infection or fetal compromise, the decision will usually made to proceed with active induction and delivery. Cesarean delivery is undertaken for obstetrical indications and

---

Table 20.2   Complications of PROM

- Infections: chorioamnionitis, neonatal sepsis, maternal sepsis
- Premature labor and delivery: respiratory distress syndrome, intraventricular hemorrhage, necrotizing enterocolitis
- Hypoxia and asphyxia secondary to umbilical cord compression: cord prolapse
- Increased rates of cesarean delivery
- Fetal deformations secondary to oligohydramnios: pulmonary hypoplasia, compression deformities of the face and/or limbs

not on the basis of PROM per se. The outcome will depend on the extent of prematurity and the presence of any sequelae of oligohydramnios.

SUMMARY

PROM occurs when the membranes rupture prior to the onset of labor. When this condition arises in a preterm gestation, the morbidity and mortality can be high, mostly due to prematurity (the majority of patients with PROM will spontaneously enter labor). The underlying cause of PROM should be investigated, particularly if it is anticipated that the pregnancy will continue. Prematurity versus infectious complications must often be weighed in the decision to try to prolong a pregnancy with premature rupture of membranes.

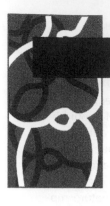

CHAPTER 21

Third Trimester Bleeding

Shaun G. Lencki

The obstetrical patient may understandably become anxious at the sight of vaginal bleeding, particularly during the third trimester of pregnancy. Its implications can be serious for both the fetus and the expectant mother. A rapid and appropriate obstetrical response can tremendously improve the neonatal outcome. Conversely, an unsuitable response by the obstetrician can have disastrous consequences for the newborn and mother. Because third trimester bleeding is not unusual, the physician must carefully evaluate each episode reported by the patient. Once the source of bleeding is determined, a conservative route of therapy may be taken or a more drastic action (such as prompt delivery) may be required.

CLINICAL CORRELATION

H. P. is a 34-year-old female, G4P2012, with a fetus at 36 weeks gestational age, who presents to labor and delivery by ambulance. Her chief complaint is vaginal bleeding that began two hours earlier. She denies any abdominal pain. Extensive vaginal bleeding soiled the patient's undergarments, socks, and shoes. Her prenatal care was uncomplicated. She had a cesarean delivery three years earlier because of arrested dilation at term. Five years ago, she had an elective abortion at 11 weeks gestation.

DIFFERENTIAL DIAGNOSIS

Vaginal bleeding is considered abnormal in pregnancy with the exception of bloody show. Although the differential diagnosis is not complicated, a thorough investigation is mandatory. Traumatic injury to the cervicovaginal epithelium, cervicitis, and intraepithelial neoplasia must be excluded in the pregnant patient with third trimester bleeding. Occasionally, the anxious patient may confuse bleeding from rectal fissures or hemorrhoids with vaginal bleeding. Preterm labor may cause vaginal bleeding related to cervical dilation. Similarly, patients close to their estimated date of confinement (EDC) may report vaginal mucus tinged with blood. This condition, known as bloody show, is not problematic.

The obstetrician must exclude three possibilities (Table 21.1):

- Placenta previa
- Abruptio placentae
- Vasa previa

Each of these diagnoses can pose an immediate threat to the survival of the fetus, mother, or both if it goes unrecognized or neglected.

PLACENTA PREVIA

The incidence of placenta previa is 1 per 250 births. If the placenta becomes implanted in he lower uterine segment, its edge may lie ad-jacent to the internal os (marginal previa), incompletely occlude the internal os (partial

Table 21.1   The Differences Between Placenta Previa, Abruptio Placentae, and Vasa Previa

	PLACENTA PREVIA	ABRUPTIO PLACENTAE	VASA PREVIA
Condition	Placenta over the cervical os	Separation of placenta from uterine wall	Umbilical vessels over os without support of placenta
Incidence	1/200 pregnancies	1/120 pregnancies	1/2500 pregnancies
Risk factors	Prior previa	Hypertension	Velamentous insertion
	Prior cesarean scar	Advanced maternal age	Bilobed, low placenta
	Large placenta	Cocaine abuse	
	Maternal smoking	Maternal smoking	
		Multiparity	
		Poor nutrition	
Symptoms	Painless vaginal bleeding	Painful bleeding, although 30% have small, asymptomatic bleeds	Very profuse bleeding
Diagnosis	Ultrasound of placenta	Clinical inspection of placenta postpartum; ultrasound diagnosis is rare	Ultrasound
Treatment	Stabilization if hemodynamically stable; otherwise, emergency delivery	Emergency delivery	Emergency delivery
Fetal complications	Prematurity	15%–20% mortality	30%–100% mortality
Maternal complications	Depends on amount of bleeding	May lead to DIC, shock, death	Usually mild, bleeding is fetal

previa), or completely cover the os (complete previa) (Figure 21.1). Placenta previa accounts for approximately 20% of third trimester bleeding. Risk factors for this condition include a prior pregnancy complicated by previa, multiparity, previous cesarean delivery, prior elective abortion, and uterine surgery with endometrial cavity entry such as with certain myomectomies.

Bleeding from a placenta previa can range from a scant spot to a torrential flow of blood. Such bleeding can cause severe maternal hypotension and fetal decompensation. The neonate may be hypotensive due to hypovolemia. The complete previa usually becomes symptomatic earlier than the partial or marginal variety. Approximately one-third of previa patients experience symptomatic bleeding before 28 weeks gestation, one-third between 28 and 34 weeks, and the remainder after 34 weeks. Approximately 90% of all pa-

tients develop vaginal bleeding by their due dates.

ABRUPTIO PLACENTAE

Abruptio placentae is more common than placenta previa. Its incidence is 1 per 150 births, although it may occur more commonly when marginal sinus separation is included. Abruptio placentae accounts for 30% of all third trimester bleeding (Figure 21.2); marginal sinus separation and idiopathic causes account for the remainder.

The major difference between placenta previa and abruption relates to the presence of abdominal pain. Placental abruption is invariably associated with uterine contractions that range from mild contractions, to regular contractions every minute, to tetanic contractions without uterine relaxation. Vaginal bleeding may be absent, light, or massive associated with maternal hemodynamic instability. Eighty

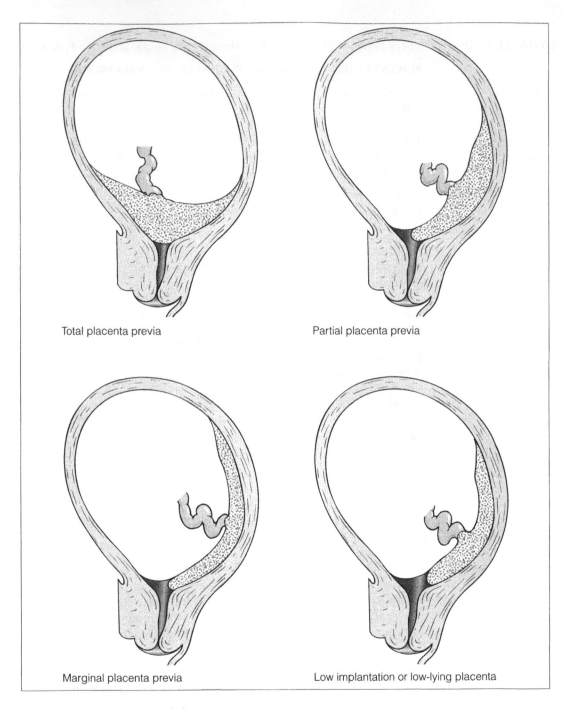

Total placenta previa

Partial placenta previa

Marginal placenta previa

Low implantation or low-lying placenta

Figure 21.1   Classifications of placenta previa

Source: Callahan TL, Caughey AB, Heffner LJ. Blueprints in obstetrics and gynecology. Malden, MA: Blackwell Science, 1998:35.

percent of patients with placental abruption will exhibit vaginal bleeding. Those who do not are considered to harbor a "concealed" abruption. A concealed abruption can contain a large portion of the patient's intravascular volume in a retroplacental hemorrhage. In this instance, the patient will have unexplained hypotension, shock, and/or disseminated intravascular coagulopathy (DIC). Similar to the situation with placenta previa, the fetus can de-

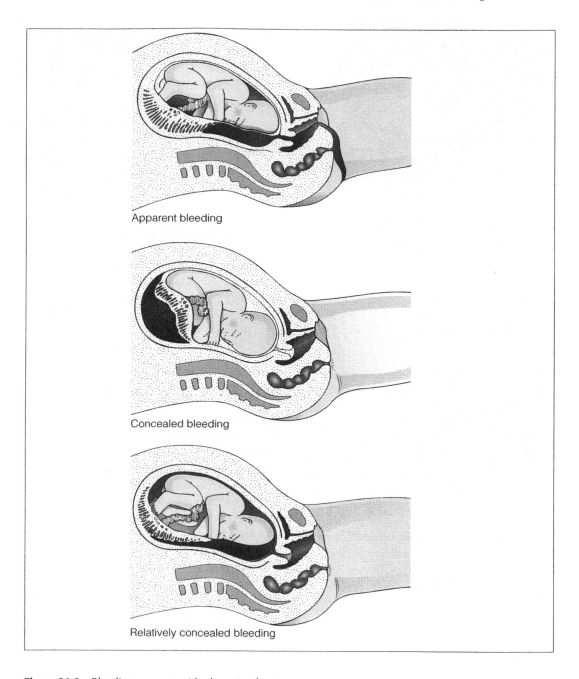

Apparent bleeding

Concealed bleeding

Relatively concealed bleeding

Figure 21.2   Bleeding patterns with abruptio placentae

Source: Callahan TL, Caughey AB, Heffner LJ. Blueprints in obstetrics and gynecology. Malden, MA: Blackwell Science, 1998:35.

velop severe anemia due to hemorrhage. Fetal–maternal hemorrhage may also occur.

Risk factors for abruptio placentae include a prior pregnancy with an abruption, severe maternal hypertension, blunt abdominal trauma, cocaine intoxication, antiphospholipid syn-

drome, polyhydramnios, and chorioamnionitis.

Vasa Previa

A rare problem usually recognized after delivery is vasa previa (Figure 21.3). It is classically

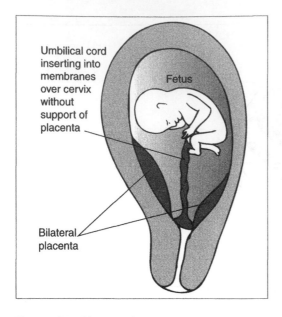

Figure 21.3   Vasa previa

155 with absent variability. Uterine contractions occur every 5 minutes. Shortly after maternal intravenous hydration, H. P.'s vital signs improve, with her blood pressure reaching 100/60 and her pulse 95.

Ultrasound is performed using the portable machine available in labor and delivery. The patient is found to have a complete posterior placenta previa. The fetal measurements are consistent with the gestational dates and the amniotic fluid volume is normal. Blood work is sent stat to obtain a complete blood count, type and cross, and coagulation profile. Four units of packed RBCs are ordered from the blood bank. A brief history and physical examination are completed, but the sterile speculum examination is avoided. The neonatologist is notified.

described as velamentous insertion of the umbilical cord into the amnion and chorion laeve (membranes) instead of the chorion frondosum. Velamentous insertion has been found in less than 1% of placentas studied after birth. Another scenario for vasa previa involves a satellite placental lobe (succenturiate placenta), which communicates with the primary placenta by small vessels. In either circumstance, if the vessels course over the internal os of the cervix, a vasa previa occurs. The most dangerous time related to this condition is when labor starts and the membranes rupture spontaneously or artificially. These vessels can become torn with the membranes, leading to fetal exsanguination and death.

CLINICAL CORRELATION

H. P. is immediately evaluated by the labor and delivery staff. The maternal pulse is 120, blood pressure is 80/30, respiratory rate is 20, and the temperature is 98.6 °F. No jugulovenous distention is present. A peripheral 18-gauge intravenous catheter is emplaced, and 1.5 L of normal saline is quickly infused. Concomitantly, the fetal heart rate is monitored by continuous external Doppler. The baseline fetal heart rate is

---

DIAGNOSTIC EVALUATION

The history and physical examination may provide important hints as to the etiology of third trimester bleeding. Upon inspection, the patient with an abruption is usually in discomfort because of the frequent uterine contractions. Fundal height measurements may acutely increase in the face of a large retroplacental hemorrhage. On palpation, the uterus appears firm during contractions and may not relax between contractions, indicating uterine tetany. Abdominal pain may also occur due to extravasation of blood into the myometrium, resulting in a couvelaire uterus. Compared with placental abruption, the patient with placenta previa does not experience pain unless she goes into preterm labor concurrently. The presenting part of the fetus may lie well above the maternal symphysis pubis during palpation. Auscultation with a stethoscope over the pubic symphysis can reveal sounds of the placental soufflé, or blood flow. The quantity of blood loss does not differentiate the patient with placenta previa versus abruption.

Ultrasound is the diagnostic cornerstone for identifying third trimester bleeding. An obstetrical ultrasound should precede the pelvic examination. This procedure is easily done in most instances by using the abdominal ultrasound technique with a full maternal urinary bladder. Occasionally, a transvaginal or translabial approach is required. The latter approaches are most helpful with posteriorly positioned placentas near the cervix. Although both are helpful and safe, vigorous movements of the transvaginal transducer may incite more bleeding.

Placental tissue between the cervical internal os and the fetus is required for the diagnosis of placenta previa. The interface between the internal os and fetal compartment is normally separated by a thin amniotic membrane. In contrast, placenta previa creates a much thicker and more echogenic interface. "Placental migration" refers to the resolution of placenta previa diagnosed earlier in pregnancy. Placenta previa is noted on 5% of sonograms performed in the second trimester for genetic amniocentesis. Fortunately, 90% of these tissue developments migrate away from the cervical os as the lower uterine segment develops throughout the remainder of the pregnancy.

In the absence of a placenta previa documented by ultrasound, placental abruption becomes a strong possibility. Although placental separation as small as 60 cm³ may be seen on sonogram, the diagnosis is made on a clinical basis. The separation may occur in any of three sites:

- Retroplacental
- Between the amnion and chorion along the chorionic plate
- In the space between the decidua and the chorion laeve

Vasa previa is usually diagnosed in retrospect when either spontaneous or artificial rupture of membranes is followed by a large gush of vaginal bleeding. Antenatal diagnosis has been noted with ultrasound by demonstration of fetal vessels inserted into the membranes near the internal os.

CLINICAL CORRELATION

H. P. undergoes emergency cesarean delivery under general anesthesia. A transverse incision is performed over the lower uterine segment. The infant is delivered with Apgar scores of 8 at one minute and 9 at five minutes. The placenta is removed in multiple fragments, whereupon brisk bleeding from the placental bed is seen. The uterine tone is firm after intravenous pitocin. Placenta accreta is suspected. The anesthesiologist orders a CBC, prothrombin time, partial thromboplastin time, fibrin split products, and fibrinogen tests. Although the bilateral hypogastric artery ligation is complete, the bleeding remains heavy. The patient does not have a coagulopathy or thrombocytopenia. A hysterectomy is required to stop the blood loss. Three units of packed RBCs, intravenous antibiotics, and crystalloid fluids are administered. The patient's post-operative course remains uncomplicated, and she is discharged on post-operative day 5.

MANAGEMENT

The proper management of third trimester bleeding is primarily dependent on the gestational age, fetal well-being, and maternal hemodynamic status and secondarily dependent on the cause of the bleeding. The initial management requires rapid maternal and fetal assessment. Peripheral venous access with large catheters and administration of isotonic fluids to maintain maternal perfusion is mandatory. Laboratory tests for CBC, type and cross match, PT, PTT, FSP, and fibrinogen must be ordered as stat requests. In addition, external fetal monitoring is absolutely necessary to exclude nonreassuring fetal heart rate changes. An obstetrical ultrasound should be performed in labor and delivery for the hemodynamically unstable patient. A history should be obtained from the patient, spouse, or emergency transport team. Although a complete physical examination is essential, a vaginal examination should not be performed until a placenta previa has been excluded by ultrasound.

If the patient is Rh-negative, Rh-immune globulin therapy is indicated. Because vaginal bleeding is associated with fetal–maternal hemorrhage, a KB stain should precede Rh-immune globulin administration. After the fetal cells in the maternal circulation are quantified, the appropriate amount of Rh-immune globulin can be ordered (20 μg/mL fetal red blood cells).

The patient who presents with symptomatic placenta previa beyond 34 weeks gestation is best managed by cesarean delivery. Nevertheless, the premature fetus at 26 weeks will derive great benefit if conservative therapy is kept as an option. Its use requires the mother to have a stable hemodynamic profile and external fetal monitoring to be reassuring. Conservative management would include maternal beta-methasone steroid treatment to induce fetal lung maturation. At extremely premature gestational ages, maternal blood transfusion may be considered if maternal anemia develops.

Because preterm labor can exacerbate vaginal bleeding, tocolytic therapy should be given if preterm labor occurs. Intravenous magnesium sulfate is preferred over beta-mimetics such as ritodrine, as the latter agents may induce maternal tachycardia and hypotension. Perinatal morbidity and mortality are decreased in selected premature gestations complicated by placenta previa who are treated with tocolytic therapy.

In the symptomatic patient, the presence of maternal tachycardia suggests a 15% to 20% intravascular loss; the presence of hypotension suggests an even greater loss. Nonreassuring fetal heart rate patterns such as late decelerations suggest uteroplacental compromise due to maternal intravascular hypovolemia. Either maternal hemodynamic disturbances or fetal decompensation are indications for emergency delivery.

The asymptomatic patient with a complete placenta previa should have an amniocentesis for fetal lung maturity at 36 weeks and undergo cesarean delivery as soon as fetal maturity is documented. The delivery route for complete or partial placenta previa is cesarean section, although the marginal placenta previa may occasionally be delivered vaginally. Marginal placenta previa or an equivocal ultrasound for placenta previa may require a "double setup" vaginal examination when delivery is indicated. This examination is conducted in the operating room with a surgical team prepared for emergency cesarean delivery. The vaginal fornices are examined for fullness due to placental tissue. Eventually, an examining finger is placed in the external os. If the placenta is palpated, a cesarean section is performed.

The uterine incision must be carefully determined with a cesarean delivery. If the placenta is located posteriorly, then a low segment transverse incision of Kerr can be attempted in the well-developed lower uterine segment. The anterior previa often requires a classical uterine incision to avoid the placenta. Maternal and fetal anemia is more likely if the placenta is traversed during delivery. Intraoperative ultrasound can map the anterior placenta prior to uterine incision to help avoid placental entry.

Every patient with placenta previa must be counseled regarding the risk of placenta accreta. Placenta accreta refers to abnormal trophoblastic invasion into the myometrial layer. This problem is increased with placenta previa (5%) and particularly likely to occur with a prior cesarean delivery and placenta previa (10% to 15%).

Placenta increta (deep myometrial invasion) and placenta percreta (invasion through the myometrium to urinary bladder or surrounding structures) may also occur (Figure 21.4). Treatment of placenta accreta may include endometrial bed sutures, bilateral ascending uterine artery ligation, bilateral hypogastric artery ligation, utero-ovarian ligation, bilateral uterine artery radiographic embolization, or cesarean hysterectomy.

If a sonogram excludes a placenta previa and the patient presents with painful vaginal bleeding in the third trimester, a placental abruption must be suspected. Abruptio placentae is a clinical diagnosis. The physical examination may reveal a firm uterus due to uterine tetany. This finding represents a sustained contraction of the myometrium that may occur in response to the examiner's palpation of the abdomen. The persistent uterine contraction leads to fetal hypoxia because utero-placental exchange cannot occur.

Fetal heart rate monitoring and maternal evaluation must be done simultaneously. Once

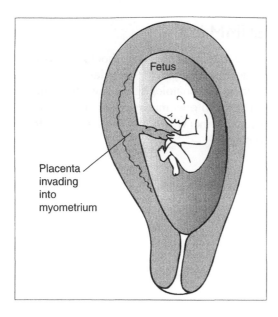

Figure 21.4 Placenta percreta

an acute abruption is diagnosed, delivery is usually indicated. Occasionally, however, chronic abruptions can be managed conservatively. The severity of placental separation is determined by identifying the presence of maternal hemodynamic instability, the fetal status, and the presence of coagulopathy (Table 21.2). The most severe form of abruptio placentae (grade 3) is associated with fetal death in utero, disseminated intravascular coagulopathy, and maternal hemorrhagic shock. More commonly, placental abruption is mild and occurs without fetal heart rate changes, DIC, or maternal hemodynamic changes (grades 0 to 1). The de-

livery method is dependent upon the findings of the cervical examination, fetal heart rate monitoring, and maternal status. The gestation at 30 weeks with a long, closed cervix requires a cesarean delivery. On the other hand, the patient who presents completely effaced and dilated with the presenting part at a +3 station can presumably deliver vaginally.

The irritation of the uterus by a placental abruption may greatly speed up the labor process, even in a primiparous woman. Therefore, an examination of the cervix should be done prior to performing a cesarean delivery. Forceps or vacuum may be needed to expedite delivery.

Because patients with placental abruption usually present with uterine contractions, it is important to distinguish this problem from the entity of preterm labor. It must be stressed that the patient suspected to have an acute abruption should not be managed with tocolytic therapy. Most patients diagnosed with preterm labor do not develop vaginal bleeding. Conversely, the majority of placental abruptions do exhibit vaginal bleeding. In addition, a small subset of preterm labor patients may have a concealed abruption.

If vaginal bleeding follows spontaneous or artificial rupture of membranes with initially clear amniotic fluid, a vasa previa must be suspected. Fetal bradycardia occurs shortly thereafter and emergency delivery is required. Again, the route of delivery is based on the results of the cervical examination.

The neonatal outcome for placenta

Table 21.2	Grades of Placental Abruption
Grade 1	Slight vaginal bleeding and uterine irritability. Maternal blood pressure unaffected. Maternal fibrinogen level normal. Fetal heart rate pattern normal.
Grade 2	External uterine bleeding mild to moderate. Uterus is irritable and may have tetanic contractions. Maternal blood pressure maintained. Maternal pulse elevated. Fibrinogen usually reduced to 150 to 250 mg %. Fetal heart rate often shows signs of fetal distress.
Grade 3	Bleeding is moderate to severe but may be concealed. Uterus is tetanic and painful. Maternal hypotension frequently present. Fetal death has occurred. Fibrinogen often less than 150 mg % with other coagulation abnormalities present (thrombocytopenia, factor depletion).

Source: Adapted from Gabbe SG. Obstetrics: normal and problem pregnancies, 2nd ed. New York: Churchill Livingstone, 1991: 579–580.

previa, abruptio placenta, and vasa previa is dependent on the appropriate diagnosis, obstetrical management, and neonatal staff preparation. Because the neonate may present in hypovolemic shock, the forewarned neonatology team can have the appropriate resuscitation medications and fluids immediately available.

SUMMARY

Third trimester bleeding should provoke concern on the part of the patient, obstetrician, and neonatologist. A complete evaluation and proper management in a coordinated manner will result in the best possible outcome.

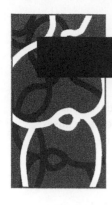

CHAPTER 22

Pre-eclampsia and Eclampsia

Gary D. Helmbrecht

Despite the remarkable advances in medicine during the twentieth century, pre-eclampsia and eclampsia continue to represent a major obstetric health problem worldwide. Overall, hypertensive disorders of pregnancy are responsible for 17% of all maternal deaths in the United States. Indeed, perinatal mortality rates (stillbirths plus neonatal deaths) as high as 182 per 1000 have been reported. Although eclampsia has been recognized for centuries, pre-eclampsia went unrecognized until the early 1800s, when it was discovered that proteinuria preceded the seizures. By 1896, the sphygmomanometer was developed, which led to recognition of the classic triad of pre-eclampsia: hypertension, proteinuria, and edema. Maternal and neonatal mortality remained quite high until the 1960s, however, when the combination of anticonvulsant and antihypertensive therapy was introduced to treat this condition. The exact cause of pre-eclampsia remains unknown.

DEFINITIONS AND CLASSIFICATIONS

Hypertensive disorders of pregnancy encompass all forms of hypertension occurring during gestation and are seen with an overall frequency of approximately 7%. Pre-eclampsia is the most common hypertensive condition, accounting for 70% of all cases. The clinical significance of the disease varies according to the gestational age at onset, the severity of the disease, and the organ systems involved. For example, mild transient hypertension developing at 37 weeks gestation will have few effects on maternal or neonatal morbidity, whereas severe pre-eclampsia with liver and renal failure at 26 weeks gestation conveys a significant risk for serious maternal and fetal complications.

Proper management of hypertensive disorders during pregnancy depends on their rapid and correct recognition and classification, as treatments vary according to the specific disease process. As outlined by the Committee on Terminology of the American College of Obstetricians and Gynecologists, hypertensive disorders of pregnancy are divided into four subgroups (Table 22.1): (1) pre-eclampsia/eclampsia; (2) chronic hypertension; (3) chronic hypertension with superimposed pre-eclampsia; and (4) transient hypertension.

PRE-ECLAMPSIA/ECLAMPSIA

The diagnosis of pre-eclampsia rests on the classic triad of hypertension, proteinuria, and edema.

- Hypertension is defined as a blood pressure increase of at least 30 mm Hg systolic or 15 mm Hg diastolic over previously recorded values. If prior blood pressures are unknown, a reading of at least 140/90 mm Hg after 20 weeks gestation is sufficient to make the diagnosis. In either case, the elevation in blood pressure must be documented on two measurements taken at least six hours apart. The Committee on

Terminology of the American College of Obstetricians and Gynecologists further defines hypertension in terms of mean arterial pressure (one-third the pulse pressure plus the diastolic pressure). An increase in mean arterial pressure of 20 mm Hg or more or, if prior pressures are unknown, a mean arterial pressure of 105 mm Hg or more after 20 weeks gestation is considered diagnostic of hypertension.

- Proteinuria is defined as at least 0.1 g/L on two random specimens collected 3 hours apart or 0.3 g in a 24-hour urine collection.

- Edema, defined as an accumulation of extravascular fluid, develops as a result of vascular endothelial cell injury. Generally, it is clinically manifested as swelling in dependent portions of the body such as the lower extremities. In its most severe form, known as anasarca, edema occurs in non-dependent areas—particularly the hands and face. Rapid fluid retention may occur without clinically recognizable edema; in those patients, sudden weight gain may be the only clue.

Pre-eclampsia may be categorized as either mild or severe, as noted in Table 22.1. It is more frequently associated with primigravidas on the extremes of reproductive age groups (the young and the older primigravida), multi-ple gestations, and chronic hypertension, although none may be present in a patient with pre-eclampsia.

Eclampsia is diagnosed when a seizure occurs that is not attributed to other causes such as epilepsy, cocaine toxicity, or head trauma.

CHRONIC HYPERTENSION

A patient is thought to have chronic hypertension if a blood pressure greater than 140/90 is documented prior to the onset of pregnancy or before the twentieth week of gestation. Likewise, chronic hypertension is diagnosed if the elevation in blood pressure persists beyond 6 weeks post-partum. Another clue to the diagnosis of chronic hypertension comes from the absence of the midtrimester nadir in blood pressure.

The form of chronic hypertension most commonly observed is primary essential hypertension. Many other causes exist as well, including renal (diabetic nephropathy, lupus nephritis, chronic and acute glomerulonephritis), endocrine (Cushing's, pheochromocytoma, thyrotoxicosis), neurologic (quadriplegia), and autoimmune (antiphospholipid syndrome) etiologies. These causes of secondary hypertension should be evaluated because treatment directed at the specific etiology may be life-saving for the patient and her fetus.

Table 22.1 Criteria for Classification of Pre-eclampsia and Eclampsia

DISORDER	BLOOD PRESSURE	PROTEINURIA	EDEMA	OTHER SIGNS OR SYMPTOMS
Pre-eclampsia				
Mild	140–160/90–110 or > 30 mm Hg increase in SBP or > 15 mm Hg increase in DBP	> 300 mg, < 5 g/24 hours or 1–2 plus dipstick	Hands or face	
Severe	>160/110	> 5 g/24 hours or 3–4 plus dipstick	Hands or face	Mild pre-eclampsia with: oliguria, pulmonary edema, headache, scotoma, right upper quadrant pain, elevated liver functions, thrombocytopenia, IUGR
Eclampsia				Pre-eclampsia with seizures not due to other causes

SBP: systolic blood pressure; DBP: diastolic blood pressure; IUGR: intrauterine growth restriction.

Chronic Hypertension with Superimposed Pre-eclampsia

Women with chronic hypertension tend to develop signs and symptoms of pre-eclampsia with increased frequency and at an earlier gestational age compared to normotensive gravidas. The Committee on Terminology recommends that this diagnosis be made based on elevation of blood pressure, as outlined earlier for chronic hypertension, in association with the appearance of proteinuria and/or generalized edema.

Transient Hypertension

Transient hypertension can occur at any time in gestation or within 24 hours post-partum. It is not accompanied by any other signs or symptoms of pre-eclampsia and resolves within 10 days post-partum. This benign condition does not require treatment.

HISTORY AND PHYSICAL

Sources for a complete history should include the patient, the medical record, and family members, if necessary. Because the clinical manifestations of pre-eclampsia can develop insidiously over several days to weeks, careful attention should be paid to subtle changes in blood pressure, weight gain, and symptoms such as headache, upper-right-quadrant abdominal pain (suggesting hepatic swelling against the liver capsule), or visual disturbances. Any abnormal laboratory test values obtained should be acted on quickly—once the disease process becomes overtly apparent, progression to seizures (eclampsia) may be rapid and cause severe morbidity or mortality. A patient with mild pre-eclampsia is just as likely to have a seizure as one with severe pre-eclampsia.

CLINICAL CORRELATION

E. S. is a 24-year-old African American female, G1P0, with a fetus at 27 weeks estimated gestational age. She is brought to labor and delivery by ambulance after having a seizure at home. She received Valium in the field and is currently heavily sedated. On arrival at the hospital, her blood pressure is 189/115, pulse 112, respirations 18, and temperature 36.9 °C. Fetal heart tones are auscultated at 160 beats per minute. The seizure was witnessed by her husband, who stated that she began to complain of a severe frontal headache and difficulty focusing her vision about an hour earlier. E. S. then fell to the floor with violent tonic-clonic movements of all extremities lasting approximately 60 seconds. She was incontinent of stool and urine and began bleeding from a laceration of her tongue. When the paramedics arrived, she developed a second seizure. This one lasted several minutes and finally stopped after 5 mg of Valium was administered through an intravenous line.

Review of E. S.'s prenatal record revealed a first trimester blood pressure of 160/96. Pressures remained in the 140–160/84–96 range throughout her visits and did not decline in the midtrimester. Uterine size at 10 weeks and a first trimester sonogram were consistent with the estimated gestational age based on her last menstrual period. Her last office visit was one week ago. At that time, her blood pressure was 168/98, urine was 2+ for protein on semiquantitative analysis, and her weight had increased 12 lb over the past four weeks. A 24-hour urine and some blood work were ordered, but her husband states that she was very busy at her job and had not yet completed these tests. E. S. has no prior history of seizure disorder and is not taking any medications other than prenatal vitamins. Her family history is remarkable for essential hypertension in both parents and two other siblings. Her mother suffers from systemic lupus erythematosis (SLE).

E. S. clearly has chronic hypertension. The historical finding of lupus in her mother raises the possibility that she may have SLE as well. When she went to her obstetrician's office during the previous week for her prenatal visit, she was showing signs of superimposed pre-eclampsia characterized by new-onset proteinuria and sudden weight gain. Hospital admission at that time would have been appropriate and may have prevented the seizures. Nevertheless, E. S. now presents as an obstetric emergency that must be rapidly evaluated and treated to prevent further harm.

The physical examination of this patient should incorporate a detailed neurologic assessment of the mother, including a magnetic resonance imaging scan of her brain. The fetus should be evaluated by ultrasound to assess its growth and immediate well-being. Intrauterine growth restriction occurs in approximately 50% of such pre-eclampsia cases, and placental abruption is seen in 10%. In addition, immediate steps must also be taken to control E. S.'s blood pressure and prevent further seizures. Laboratory data should be obtained to rule out HELLP (Hemolysis, Elevated Liver enzymes, Low Platelets) syndrome and disseminated intravascular coagulopathy, both of which frequently accompany severe pre-eclampsia/eclampsia. Finally, if delivery can be delayed, consideration should be given to accelerating fetal lung maturation with corticosteroids.

CLINICAL CORRELATION

Upon completion of the history, E. S. is started on an intravenous infusion of magnesium sulfate for seizure prophylaxis. The drug is given as an initial bolus of 4 g over 20 minutes followed by a continuous infusion of 2 g/hr. Her blood pressure stabilizes at 168/110; the other vital signs remain unchanged. On the external fetal monitor, the fetal heart rate is 170 beats per minute with little or no variability. E. S. is conscious, oriented to person, place, and time, and continues to complain of a severe frontal headache. Her extraocular eye movements are sluggish and incoordinate. Her pupils are equal and reactive to light. Her face, hands, abdomen, and feet are markedly edematous with 3+ pitting. The chest is clear to auscultation and percussion, and the cardiac examination reveals a regular rate with an S3 gallop. The abdomen is gravid and tight. The uterine fundus extends 22 cm above the symphysis pubis. The liver is percussed 10 cm below the right costal margin and is exquisitely tender. A fluid wave is elicited in the upper abdomen. Deep tendon reflexes are symmet-

ric and brisk, with clonus evoked in both lower extremities. The Babinski reflexes are normal. The remainder of the physical examination is unremarkable.

A sonogram of the uterus reveals a singleton fetus in a vertex presentation. The fetal measurements are consistent with a 24-week pregnancy, and the amniotic fluid volume is low. The anterior placenta is heavily calcified, with approximately one-third of its lower edge being separated from its uterine wall implantation site.

The Foley catheter previously placed has drained only 10 cm³ of urine in the past hour. The urine dipstick is 4+ for protein. CBC shows a WBC of $12,000/cm^3$, hemoglobin and hematocrit are 8 g/dL and 22% respectively, and a platelet count is $28,000/cm^3$. Remarkable serum chemistries include SGOT (AST) 585, SGPT (ALT) 490, LDH 600, creatinine 2.6, and uric acid 8.6. Clotting studies show a prolonged PT and PTT. The serum fibrinogen is 60 and the fibrin split products are elevated (more than 480).

MANAGEMENT AND TREATMENT

Management of E. S. should initially focus on stabilization of the mother, after which attention will be directed toward the fetus. Her blood pressure must be rapidly controlled, and invasive monitoring should be initiated using central venous pressure and arterial lines. The coagulopathy should be corrected with fresh frozen plasma and platelets to avoid excessive bleeding during surgery.

Magnesium sulfate is most commonly prescribed to prevent the onset of seizures in a pre-eclamptic patient or repeated seizures in an eclamptic patient. When the magnesium level in the blood stream is therapeutic (4 to 6 mEq/L), neuromuscular conduction and depression of central nervous system irritability slow, thereby preventing seizures. If the levels become too high (greater than 12 mg/dL), the patient is at risk for muscular paralysis and respiratory difficulties; in addition, very high levels have been associated with cardiac arrest. If levels become toxic, reversal of toxicity will occur following treatment with calcium gluconate. The magnesium is given for at least 24 hours after delivery, as this time is the most likely period in which a seizure may be encountered. Magnesium sulfate has a long history of use during pregnancy and appears to be safe for the fetus.

The patient needs careful volume replacement with crystalloids and packed RBCs preoperatively in the event that hemorrhage is encountered. Such patients are at risk for pulmonary edema, and excessive volume replacement may precipitate this development. Delivery of the fetus is the cure for pre-eclampsia or eclampsia. Once stabilized, the fetus should be delivered and transported to a high-risk, intensive care nursery. Although vaginal delivery can be attempted for the stabilized patient, cesarean delivery is performed for obstetric or fetal indications. The neonatologist should be informed of the growth retardation and placental abruption detected by sonography in this case, so that the labor and delivery staff will be prepared to provide appropriate volume resuscitation to the infant at delivery.

CLINICAL CORRELATION

Following stabilization, E. S. undergoes emergency cesarean delivery. The infant weighs 960 g and has Apgar scores of 3 at one minute and 5 at five minutes. The mother remains in labor and delivery on a continuous infusion of magnesium sulfate for the next 24 hours. During this time, the MRI shows no intracranial hemorrhage, her liver and renal function improve, her blood pressure stabilizes at 140/85, and her coagulation parameters normalize spontaneously. She requires three more units of PRBC as her vascular space reexpands during this recovery phase. E. S. is discharged on the fourth post-operative day in satisfactory condition. She continues to require antihypertensive medication to keep her diastolic blood pressures below 100 mm Hg. Her infant is discharged 82 days later with bronchopulmonary dysplasia as a consequence of chronic mechanical ventilation.

E. S. and her infant suffered from the complications of pre-eclampsia/eclampsia and prematurity that may have been prevented by taking a more careful history and paying greater attention to the physical findings. Many preventive strategies have been tested in the recent past. Based on several promising reports, chemoprophylaxis with low-dose aspirin gained widespread use in the United States and Europe. Pre-eclampsia is characterized by vasospasm and activation of the coagulation systems. Platelet activation with production of increased amounts of thromboxane, a potent vasoconstrictor, seems to play a central role. Aspirin irreversibly binds to cyclo-oxygenase and inhibits prostaglandin production. Its effect was thought to be more pronounced on platelet production of thromboxane than it is on endothelial cell production of prostacyclin, a vasodilator. Several studies had demonstrated a reduction in the incidence of pre-eclampsia in women at risk who received low-dose aspirin during their pregnancies. Finally, a large, multicentered clinical trial sponsored by the NICHD failed to identify any benefit from this therapy. Supplementation with other agents (such as zinc, calcium, magnesium, and protein) have not proved beneficial, either.

Like the E and I series prostaglandins, nitric oxide is a potent endothelial cell-derived vasodilator. Alterations in its metabolism are thought to play a role in the pathogenesis of pre-eclampsia. Recent data suggest that increasing the bioavailability of this compound in pregnancies at risk for pre-eclampsia may prove protective. Although this agent seems promising, further study is needed before it can be safely used.

Prompt hospital admission for bedrest, blood pressure control, and fetal testing would also have helped E. S. Such conservative management can extend pregnancies by an average of two or more weeks. This delay permits administration of corticosteroids to stimulate fetal lung maturity and further in utero fetal maturation. Improved fetal outcomes have been documented when such a delay has occurred safely, as opposed to immediate delivery at the time of diagnosis. The most favorable results occur when pre-eclampsia is detected in its mild forms, as opposed to a history of eclampsia.

For the woman with chronic hypertension, it is generally recommended that she continue with her antihypertensive regimen when she becomes pregnant. Agents that have been used in pregnancy include methyldopa, hydralazine, beta blockers, labetalol (alpha and beta blockers), and calcium-channel blockers. For acute therapy of hypertension, labetalol appears to be a safe option and is more effective than hydralazine. Beta blockers have been associated with increased risk of intrauterine growth restriction. Diuretics are generally avoided, as one does not wish to diminish intravascular volume and therefore blood flow to the uterus; they may be necessary in the patient with congestive heart failure, however. Angiotensin-converting enzyme (ACE) inhibitors have been associated with oligohydramnios, neonatal anuria, cranial defects, and stillbirths; their use should therefore be avoided in pregnancy.

REPRODUCTIVE COUNSELING FOR WOMEN WHO HAVE HAD PRE-ECLAMPSIA/ECLAMPSIA

Any woman affected with severe pre-eclampsia warrants close observation in subsequent pregnancies. The overall recurrence risk is 25% in the next pregnancy, falling to 12% in any subsequent pregnancy. If pre-eclampsia developed in midtrimester in the index pregnancy, the recurrence risk increases to 60% with the woman's next pregnancy, with roughly half of these patients again developing pre-eclampsia in midtrimester. The likelihood of developing chronic hypertension is also increased in women who have experienced severe pre-eclampsia complicating pregnancy. Approximately half of these women can be expected to require treatment for hypertension within 10 years of the pregnancy. Siblings and daughters of women who have had severe pre-eclampsia are also at increased risk for the disease. Based on this information, a woman may decide to limit the size of her family. If she does conceive again, she will require close attention from her obstetric care professionals.

SUMMARY

Hypertensive disorders in pregnancy are serious contributors to neonatal morbidity and mortality, and they can also severely affect the mother. Early detection of pre-eclampsia and aggressive management of this condition are critical for improving maternal and fetal outcomes. In previously unscreened women, pregnancy may be the first opportunity to detect chronic hypertension and to begin patients on regimens that will affect their overall survival.

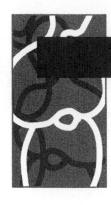

CHAPTER 23

Medical and Surgical Complications of Pregnancy

Marc H. Incerpi and Alexander F. Burnett

The reproductive-age woman is generally a healthy patient. Because of the sheer numbers of women who become pregnant, however, the obstetrician will undoubtedly come into contact with various medical conditions that may complicate or be complicated by pregnancy on a frequent basis. At times, the best management for the patient would include referral to a specialist in high-risk gestations. Not all areas of the country have such clinicians readily available, however, so a thorough understanding of some medical conditions commonly encountered during pregnancy is warranted. The intensive screening of a woman early in her pregnancy may also present an opportunity to diagnose underlying conditions previously not recognized.

ANEMIA

During pregnancy, the maternal plasma volume undergoes an expansion, with a less significant increase in red blood cell mass occurring as well. This difference often leads to a physiologic anemia during pregnancy. Approximately half of all pregnant women will have a hematocrit lower than 32% in the third trimester.

The majority of cases of anemia are due to iron deficiency. Iron stores are used up by the increase in red blood cell mass and go to the developing fetus and placenta. Consequently, prophylactic iron supplementation is advised in pregnancy. Daily supplementation with 300 mg of ferrous sulfate will usually satisfy preg-

nancy requirements and, therefore, prevent the development of iron deficiency anemia. During pregnancy, the intestine increases its iron absorption capacity from 1.3 to 2.6 mg of elemental iron per day. Except in the cases of extreme hemorrhage associated with birth, most women with pregnancy-induced iron deficiency anemia have returned to a normal hematocrit by six weeks post-partum. For this reason, iron supplementation should be continued during the post-partum period.

Folate deficiency is a less common cause of anemia in pregnancy, although it is the most common cause of megaloblastic anemia during pregnancy. Women at risk are those with poor eating habits, who fail to consume adequate amounts of green vegetables and nuts in their diets. Folate deficiency is a common complication seen in alcoholics. Most prenatal vitamins contain 1 mg of folic acid; this amount, if taken daily, is more than adequate to overcome a deficiency. Recent studies have indicated that folic acid may play a key role in helping to prevent neural tube defects in the fetus.

Various hemoglobinopathies may also be encountered in the pregnant population. Sickle cell anemia occurs in approximately 1 of every 708 adult African Americans in the United States. Sickle cell trait is identified in 1 per every 12 adult African Americans. Screening for this disease should be advised in the African American population. The patients should be advised that if both parents have the trait, there is a 50% chance that their offspring will also have the trait and a 25% chance that their offspring will have the disease. Women with sickle cell anemia often have difficulty with their pregnancies, with spontaneous abortions occurring in as many as 25% of such pregnancies. The incidence of infectious complications is increased in the pregnant woman with sickle cell anemia, and all infections must be recognized promptly before fever and dehydration develop, as these problems will increase the severity of a sickling crisis. Pneumonia and pregnancy-induced hypertension are also common findings in sickle cell patients. The role of prophylactic blood transfusions to correct the anemia remains controversial in pregnancy.

DIABETES MELLITUS

Patients with diabetes mellitus require extremely close monitoring throughout pregnancy, with observation ideally beginning prior to conception. Before the discovery of insulin, the fetal and neonatal mortality rate for pregnant diabetics was approximately 65%. Today, that rate is only 2% to 5%, although the potential for major complications persists. Human placental lactogen is a polypeptide produced normally by the placenta. It has actions that serve to reduce the body's sensitivity to insulin, which in turn contributes to a physiologic diabetogenic state during pregnancy. In nondiabetics, the pancreas will increase its production of insulin to counteract this effect. In the diabetic patient, such compensation is not possible. As a consequence, insulin requirements will rise throughout pregnancy.

Congenital malformations occur two to four times more often in children born to diabetics relative to children born to nondiabetic mothers. The measurement of glycosylated hemoglobin (Hb A1C) at the time of conception reflects the degree of glucose control. Levels greater than 7.5 have been associated with a higher incidence of congenital anomalies (Table 23.1). Table 23.2 lists the major malformations associated with these patients. Because malformations occur at the time of organogenesis (which is completed by seven weeks of gestation), tight glucose control prior to conception is a major priority in diabetic

Table 23.1   Fetal Complications of Diabetes Mellitus

Macrosomia with traumatic delivery
Delayed organ maturity
    Pulmonary
    Hepatic
    Neurologic
    Pituitary-thyroid axis
Congenital abnormalities
    Cardiovascular
    Neural tube defect
    Caudal regression syndrome
Intrauterine growth restriction
    Intrauterine death
    Abnormal fetal heart rate patterns
    Small-for-date babies

women. The role of preconception counseling and teaching cannot be overemphasized.

Macrosomia (excessive fetal growth) can occur as a result of elevated circulating sugar levels, which easily pass to the developing fetus. In this condition, there is increased growth of the shoulders and trunk compared to the head, which increases the likelihood of fetal injury with a vaginal delivery. Conversely, intrauterine growth restriction (IUGR) can occur when diabetes is accompanied by underlying vascular disease.

GESTATIONAL DIABETES

The rise in human placental lactogen decreases sensitivity to insulin to a point in some women that they will experience difficulty with glucose regulation, even though they were not diabetic prior to gestation. Diagnosis of gestational diabetes is accomplished by using a 50 g oral glucose tolerance test, which is routinely administered at 24 to 28 weeks gestation in all pregnant women, or earlier if there is a strong suspicion of this condition (Table 23.3). The cut-off value most commonly used for this screen is a plasma glucose of 140 mg/dL measured one hour after administration of the glucose cola. If the value exceeds 140 mg/dL, the patient should undergo

Table 23.2   Congenital Anomalies Associated with Diabetes Mellitus

CARDIOVASCULAR

Transposition of the great vessels

Ventricular septal defect

Atrial septal defect

Hypoplastic left ventricle

Situs inversus

CENTRAL NERVOUS SYSTEM

Anencephaly

Encephalocele

Meningomyelocele

Holoprosencephaly

Microcephaly

SKELETAL

Caudal regression syndrome

Spina bifida

GENITOURINARY

Absent kidneys (Potter syndrome)

Polycystic kidneys

Double ureter

GASTROINTESTINAL

Tracheoesophageal fistula

Bowel atresia

Imperforate anus

Source: London MB. Diabetes mellitus and other endocrine deseases. In: Gabbe SG, Niebyl JR, Simpson JL, ed. Obstetrics: normal and problem pregnancies. New York: Churchill Livingstone, 1991:1101.

Table 23.3   Glucose Screening Tests During Pregnancy

TEST	NORMAL GLUCOSE LEVEL (mg/dL)
Fasting	<100
1 hr after a 50 g glucose load	<140
2 hr after a 100 g glucose load	<165

tributed over three meals and two snacks during the day. Goals for glucose monitoring are fasting blood sugar measurements of less than 100 to 105 mg/dL and two-hour post-prandial sugar measurements of less than 120 mg/dL. If adequate glucose control is not achieved through diet alone, patients should be started on insulin. Oral hypoglycemics are not used in pregnancy because of the paucity of data available regarding their teratogenic potential and because of these agents' lack of efficacy for controlling blood sugars during gestation.

In women with good glucose control over pregnancy, antepartum testing can begin at 36 weeks gestation. Most centers recommend weekly or biweekly nonstress testing; some recommend frequent biophysical profiles as well. With gestational diabetes complicated by other problems such as hypertension or previous stillbirth, testing should begin earlier and will often occur twice per week. Ultrasound examination is important as the woman gets closer to term so as to estimate fetal weight with greater accuracy.

Although the presence of gestational diabetes is not an indication for early delivery, most physicians prefer to not allow diabetic women to go much beyond their due date. In the past, it was taught that elective induction or cesarean delivery should be undertaken only after amniocentesis was performed to document pulmonary maturity. Today, it is recommended that amniocentesis need not be performed if the patient has a well-dated pregnancy at term with good glucose control. Complications of gestational diabetes such as hypertension, macrosomia, and oligohydram-

a standard 100 g, three-hour glucose tolerance test. The values accepted with a three-hour test (Table 23.4) are as follows: fasting blood sugar, 105 mg/dL or less; one hour, 190 mg/dL; two hours, 165 mg/dL; and three hours, 145 mg/dL. Gestational diabetes is diagnosed when two or more of the patient's measured values meet or exceed these standards.

Initial management of patients with abnormal glucose metabolism should include nutrition counseling. Generally, diets should include 30 to 35 kcal/kg ideal body weight dis-

Table 23.4   Three-Hour Glucose Tolerance Test: Venous and Plasma Criteria for GDM

TIMING OF GLUCOSE MEASUREMENT	NORMAL WHOLE VENOUS BLOOD GLUCOSE (mg/dL)	NORMAL PLASMA GLUCOSE
Fasting	90	105
1 hr	165	190
2 hr	145	165
3 hr	125	145

nios or abnormal antepartum testing may be indications for early delivery.

INFECTIOUS DISEASES IN PREGNANCY

HERPES SIMPLEX VIRUS

Genital herpes infection has the potential of being transmitted to the neonate with devastating results. The neonate may acquire infection via passage through an infected birth canal, ascending infections, or passage through the placenta. Approximately half of all infants born vaginally to mothers with primary genital herpes infection will develop disseminated herpes infection, with a mortality of about 60%. The transmission rate in mothers with recurrent herpes simplex virus (HSV) infection is only 4%. It should be noted on the first prenatal visit if the mother or father has a history of genital herpes.

If a lesion is present or prodromal herpes infection symptoms are present at the onset of labor or membrane rupture, the fetus should be delivered via cesarean section to diminish the likelihood of viral transmission to the neonate. This tactic does not guarantee that the newborn will avoid infection, but it does decrease the likelihood of infection and lead to a smaller viral load should infection occur. Acyclovir has been used extensively during pregnancy without reported harm to the fetus. The U.S. Food and Drug Administration has not approved its use during pregnancy, however, and it should therefore be used only in severe maternal infections. The use of acyclovir in late pregnancy to prevent herpes outbreaks has been shown to reduce clinical recurrences without harming the fetus.

RUBELLA

Maternal rubella infection begins with prodromal symptoms of low-grade fever, malaise, and lymphadenopathy, followed by a characteristic macular rash that begins on the face and spreads rapidly to the trunk and extremities. Infection in the first trimester may result in a wide range of consequences to the fetus—from no fetal infection to severe, multiorgan damage. Approximately 20% of infants born to mothers infected during the first trimester of pregnancy will show signs of congenital rubella at birth (Table 23.5). The most common abnormalities are cataracts, patent ductus arteriosus, and deafness. Rubella defects are not found in those neonates infected after the twentieth week of gestation. All pregnant patients should be screened for rubella immunity at the first prenatal visit. If a mother is found to be seronegative, rubella vaccine is indicated after delivery and before discharge from the hospital.

For a woman concerned about contracting rubella infection, a hemagglutination inhibition serologic test should be performed as soon after the suspected exposure as possible. The presence of antibodies within a few days of exposure is indicative of prior infection and current immunity. Similarly, an antibody titer of 1:16 or higher is generally conclusive for immunity. A titer of 1:8 may represent an early rise in antibody levels from recent exposure. A second blood specimen should be drawn 10 days later and the two specimens run at the same time. If there is a fourfold or greater increase in titer, the diagnosis of rubella is confirmed. A woman with current or recent rubella infection will have elevated levels of IgM. IgM antibody specific for rubella should

Table 23.5 Congenital Anomalies Associated with Rubella Infection

COMMON	LESS FREQUENT
Patent ductus arteriosus	CNS defects
Pulmonary artery hypoplasia	Coarctation of the aorta
Deafness or hearing impairment	Diabetes
Eye lesions	Interstitial pneumonitis
Cataracts	Jaundice
Retinopathy	Meningoencephalitis
Growth retardation	Micrognathia
Hepatosplenomegaly	Microphthalmia
	Myocardial necrosis
	Psychomotor retardation
	Radiolucencies of long bones
	Thrombocytopenic purpura

Source: Reproduced with permission. Horstmann DM. Rubella. In: Qeenan JT, ed. Management of high-risk pregnancy, 3rd ed. Boston: Blackwell Scientific Publications, 1994:310.

disappear within 5 to 10 weeks after exposure. Therefore, if the titer is elevated and all of the antibody found is of the IgG class, then the patient can be considered immune.

The rubella vaccine currently available in the United States is a live, attenuated virus grown in human diploid cells. This virus has been detected in the placenta and fetal tissue of abortions when the mother had been recently vaccinated. Due to this finding, the rubella vaccine is contraindicated in pregnancy. Nevertheless, when the Centers for Disease Control (CDC) set up a registry from 1971 to 1989 of women who had been vaccinated for rubella between three months prior to conception to three months after conception, there were no reported cases of fetal rubella sequelae. Therefore, it is not recommended to terminate a pregnancy if a woman has been given the rubella vaccine accidentally during pregnancy.

Women who have not been immunized against rubella will usually be vaccinated after giving birth and prior to leaving the hospital. Breast-feeding is not a contraindication to vaccination.

The number of cases of rubella in the United States declined from 50,000 in 1969 to an all-time low of 225 in 1988. Since then, the number of rubella cases has been rising as vaccination has been utilized less. In 1991, there were 1401 cases of rubella in the United States, with 11 cases of congenital rubella syndrome reported.

GROUP B STREPTOCOCCUS

Group B streptococcus (GBS) sepsis in the newborn has been recognized for approximately 35 years. Maternal colonization of the cervix and vagina generally remains asymptomatic, and routine surveillance for this organism has unclear value. The diseases that GBS can cause in the mother include urinary tract infection, intra-amniotic infection, post-partum endometritis, and maternal bacteremia. It is in the neonate, however, that the most significant sequelae may be found. Neonatal sepsis with this organism is associated with a mortality rate of approximately 4%, with that rate rising several-fold in preterm infants. Risk factors for neonatal development of GBS sepsis include heavy maternal colonization with GBS, prolonged rupture of membranes, prolonged labor, maternal fever or endometritis during labor, and prematurity.

Prenatal treatment of pregnant women who have cultures positive for GBS has not been effective in reducing neonatal sepsis. As a result, treatment is directed at the woman in labor or with ruptured membranes in an effort to diminish the vertical transmission to the neonate. The American College of Obstetricians and Gynecologists currently recommends prophylaxis for GBS in women with preterm labor or premature rupture of membranes, prolonged rupture of membranes (for more than 18 hours), birth of a prior child with symptomatic GBS infection, prior colonization or infection with GBS, or maternal fever during labor. Ampicillin remains the treatment of choice. In patients without maternal infection, the antibiotic is stopped immediately after delivery.

HEPATITIS B

The most common form of viral hepatitis seen in the United States is hepatitis B. Immunization for this infection is now available, and the CDC recommends routine vaccination of all infants. All pregnant mothers should be tested for hepatitis B; the testing is designed to detect hepatitis B surface (Hep B s) antigen, which is indicative of active infection. The likelihood of a fulminant course for the disease is greater during pregnancy. Untreated neonates have a 20% to 50% of dying of cirrhosis or hepatocellular carcinoma. Those born to mothers who test positive for Hep B s antigen should also be treated with hepatitis B immunoglobulin at birth. The combination of immunoglobulin and vaccine prevents infection in approximately 95% of infants born to Hep B s antigen-positive mothers.

Vertical transmission of hepatitis B occurs 80% to 100% of the time when the mother is both Hep B e antigen-positive and Hep B s antigen-positive, as opposed to 25% of the time when she is only Hep B s antigen-positive. Neonatal infection generally is manifested postpartum rather than at birth. Maternal immunization and treatment with hepatitis B immunoglobulin are effective in preventing perinatal transmission in 90% of high-risk cases. The mode of delivery does not seem to influence likelihood of neonatal infection.

HUMAN IMMUNODEFICIENCY VIRUS INFECTION

Human immunodeficiency virus (HIV) counseling and testing should be offered to all pregnant women, preferably prior to conception so that women may make informed decisions about contraception. Women remain one of the fastest-growing cohorts of HIV-seropositive patients in the United States, with the majority becoming infected through heterosexual contact. Pregnancy does not appear to have an adverse effect on the course of HIV infection. HIV-infected pregnant women should receive vaccinations against influenza, hepatitis, and *Streptococcus pneumoniae*. Because they are at high risk, these mothers should be screened for sexually transmitted diseases and tuberculosis.

The rate of HIV transmission to neonates is estimated at 25% to 35%, although recent studies have shown a marked decrease—to 8%—when mothers were treated with zidovidine (AZT) during the pregnancy. It is now recommended that AZT be offered to all HIV-infected pregnant women. There does not appear to be a difference in the transmission rates for the various modes of delivery (cesarean section versus vaginal). Invasive procedures on the fetus, such as placement of a fetal scalp electrode, should be avoided, if possible, in the HIV-infected mother. Breastfeeding also should be avoided, some reports of post-natal transmission of HIV by breast milk have surfaced. Those infants who develop HIV disease have a very poor outcome, with most dying within the first few years of life.

Universal precautions should be exercised by all members of the health care team in dealing with all women, not just those identified as HIV-positive.

OTHER SEXUALLY TRANSMITTED DISEASES

Gonorrhea and Chlamydia

Routine testing for gonorrhea and Chlamydia are frequently performed during the first prenatal visit. Both of these infections may play a role in premature rupture of membranes and preterm labor. The course of these diseases in the pregnant woman may range from asymptomatic infection to fulminant sepsis. Antibiotics should be used to treat women who have positive cervical cultures for gonorrhea or Chlamydia. Neonatal complications include gonococcal ophthalmia (a leading cause of blindness in the preantibiotic era), neonatal sepsis, conjunctivitis, and pneumonia. Ophthalmic ointment is routinely placed in newborns' eyes in the delivery room to prevent the possible ocular complications.

Syphilis

Infection with *Treponema pallidum* (syphilis) can have devastating results on the developing fetus. Congenital syphilis may be manifested as stillbirth, nonimmune hydrops, IUGR, or premature labor during pregnancy. The neonate may exhibit hepatosplenomegaly, rhinitis, and mucocutaneous pemphigus eruptions. In many cases, the placenta is enlarged and edematous. Late-onset congenital syphilis may appear with minimal symptoms at birth; as the disease progresses, however, the sequelae may come to include characteristic dental malformations, bone deformities, neurosyphilis, interstitial keratitis of the eye, and cardiovascular abnormalities.

Diagnosis of syphilis is made most commonly by nonspecific serologic tests that measure host antibodies to cardiolipin, which is present in elevated levels in syphilis infections. All pregnant women should be screened for this condition at the initial prenatal visit. An elevated titer may also occur when the mother has a connective tissue disorder, such as systemic lupus erythematosis. More specific tests are available that measure antibody directed against the treponemal antigens, such as FTA-ABS (florescent treponemal antibody-absorbed test) and MHA-TP (microhemagglutination assay for *T. pallidum*). If the nonspecific test gives a positive result, one of these other tests should be performed to confirm the diagnosis of syphilis.

Treatment of syphilis in pregnancy consists of penicillin antibiotics given for an extended course. If the patient has a history of penicillin allergy, skin testing to confirm this reaction is performed, followed by penicillin desensitization.

CYTOMEGALOVIRUS AND VARICELLA

CYTOMEGALOVIRUS

Cytomegalovirus (CMV) is the most common congenital viral infection, affecting approximately 1% of all births. The majority of neonates with congenital CMV are unaffected at birth (90%). Approximately 10% will exhibit sequelae of CMV at birth; of the initially asymptomatic patients, approximately 10% will exhibit sequelae later in life, such as mental retardation and deafness. Major effects of CMV infection are listed in Table 23.6.

Diagnosis may be difficult in the mother because CMV infections are often asymptomatic or minimally symptomatic. In the fetus, some sonographic findings are suggestive of infection, including hydrops, IUGR, polyhydramnios, fetal ascites, and brain ventriculomegaly. Definitive diagnosis is made on the basis of elevated levels of IgM antibodies specific for CMV and viral cultures. Culturing the virus from amniotic fluid may offer the best diagnostic test.

Treatment for both mother and child is generally intended to eliminate the symptoms. Treatment of severe cases of neonatal infection may include antiviral agents such as acyclovir.

VARICELLA

Varicella infection during pregnancy can have severe consequences for the mother. In particular, varicella pneumonia can be life-threatening. If the developing fetus is exposed to varicella during the first four months of pregnancy, approximately 3% will go on to develop defects, such as low birth weight, neurologic and ocular anomalies, limb defects, skin scars, and Horner's syndrome. Babies who are born within five days of the mother's acquisition of varicella or who are exposed to the organism during the first three to four weeks of life are also at high risk for becoming infected, without having the benefit of passage of maternal varicella antibodies.

Varicella-zoster immunoglobulin (VZIG) can be used as prophylaxis in patients prone to developing severe infections as well as in the newborn when either is exposed to this pathogen. Acyclovir is recommended therapy during pregnancy if severe varicella infection is present.

CARDIAC DISEASE AND PREGNANCY

The alterations of hemodynamics associated with pregnancy may significantly affect the patient with cardiac disease. Increases in heart rate and stroke volume translate into increases in cardiac output during gestation. In patients who have undergone prior curative cardiac

Table 23.6   Characteristics of CMV Infection in the Newborn

EARLY FINDINGS

COMMON	LESS COMMON
Hepatosplenomegaly	Chorioretinitis
Purpura/petechiae	Microphthalmia
Microcephaly	Cerebral calcifications
Jaundice	Seizures
Hemolytic anemia	Brain atrophy
Hepatitis	Interstitial pneumonitis
Thrombocytopenia	Dental anomalies
	Hernias
	Prenatal findings:
	IUGR
	Small for gestational age
	Fetal death in utero

LATE-ONSET FINDINGS

COMMON	LESS COMMON
Mental retardation	Optic atrophy
Hearing loss	Spasticity
	Dental defects
	Neuromuscular defects
	Learning disability
	Psychomotor retardation

Source: Sison AV, Sever JL. Cytomegalovirus Infections in Pregnancy and the Neonate. In: Queenan JT, ed. Management of high-risk pregnancy, 3rd ed. Boston: Blackwell Scientific Publications, 1994:318.

surgery, such as repair of atrial septal defect, pregnancy may place them at no increased risk. In contrast, in mothers with significant valvular disease or other anatomical lesions, mortality may be greatly increased by pregnancy (Table 23.7). Such patients should be counseled prior to conception about the potential risks and treatments that may be used. In the most severe circumstances in which pregnancy may be life-threatening (for example, patients with pulmonary hypertension), a therapeutic abortion may be considered.

The use of cardiac drugs may need to be altered during pregnancy. Oral anticoagulants (coumadin) are potentially teratogenic and cross the placenta. In patients requiring anticoagulation for risk of thromboembolism, subcutaneous heparin should be administered—this large molecule does not cross the placenta. Beta blockers have the potential to stimulate the uterus and cause preterm labor. In addition, these agents have been associated with neonatal hypoglycemia, bradycardia, and respiratory depression. Digitalis appears to be safe to the fetus, but may stimulate preterm labor. Thiazide diuretics may cause electrolyte disturbances in the newborn. As with all medications used during pregnancy, the absolute necessity of the drugs and possible alternatives should be scrutinized carefully.

In the severe cardiac patient who has managed to survive to term, one needs to con-

Table 23.7 Maternal Mortality Rates for High-Risk Cardiovascular Disease

CARDIOVASCULAR LESION	MATERNAL MORTALITY (%)
Coarctation of the aorta	9
Marfan's syndrome	50
Tetralogy of Fallot	12
Eisenmenger syndrome	33
Primary pulmonary hypertension	53
Mitral stenosis	
All classes	1
Classes III, IV	4–5
With atrial fibrillation	14–17
Closed valvotomy	4–6
Peripartum cardiomyopathy	15–60
Prosthetic heart valves (all)	2

Source: Ueland K. The Cardiac Patient. In: Queenan JT, ed. Management of high-risk pregnancy, 3rd ed. Boston: Blackwell Scientific Publications, 1994:225.

sider the effects of the stress of labor and delivery on the mother. Occasionally, it will be safer to deliver the patient electively by cesarean section. At other times, one will wish to limit the pushing performed by the mother in the second stage of labor and therefore will elect to undertake an operative vaginal delivery. Cardiac monitoring and careful fluid management both intrapartum and immediately post-partum are essential in the cardiac patient. Collaboration with the mother's internist or cardiologist will help to assure the best outcome for mother and child.

ASTHMA

Most studies have found that, of women with asthma who become pregnant, approximately one-third experience an improvement of their asthma, one-third have no change in their asthma, and one-third have worsening of their

asthma. The physiologic changes to the lungs that occur during pregnancy include an increase in the tidal volume and decrease in airway resistance. Overall, in most situations where the mother is carefully monitored during pregnancy, the outcome is good, even for asthmatics who are steroid-dependent.

The major goal of treating the asthmatic during pregnancy is avoidance of status asthmaticus and its accompanying hypoxia. When the pO_2 falls below 70 mm Hg, the fetus will also become hypoxic, with potentially devastating results. Treatment during an acute attack should include oxygen therapy, hydration, bronchodilators, steroids if required, antibiotics if an infectious component is suspected, and intubation if the pCO_2 should rise above 60 mm Hg or the pO_2 should fall below 60 mm Hg. On a chronic basis, prednisone and theophylline appear to be safe in pregnancy. In general, the management of asthma in pregnancy is similar to that in a nonpregnant individual.

SURGERY DURING PREGNANCY

Abdominal masses are reported at rates varying from 1 of every 81 births to 1 of every 2500 live births. Given the trend toward more widespread screening by obstetrical ultrasound and the increased age at which women are becoming pregnant, the incidence of this condition is likely to rise in the future. An acute abdomen during pregnancy is most commonly due to appendicitis, which has an incidence of roughly 1 per 2000 pregnancies. Clinically, appendicitis may present with confusing symptoms during pregnancy, as the point of maximum tenderness will shift from the classic McBurney's point to higher up along the right abdominal wall as the uterus enlarges and elevates the appendix (Figure 23.1). Once a presumptive diagnosis is made, surgery should be performed by making an incision directly over the area of maximal pain. In the case of unruptured appendicitis, removal of the appendix is a safe procedure that does not require antibiotics or tocolytic therapy. If the appendix is ruptured and generalized peritonitis ensues, broad-spectrum antibiotic coverage should be begun

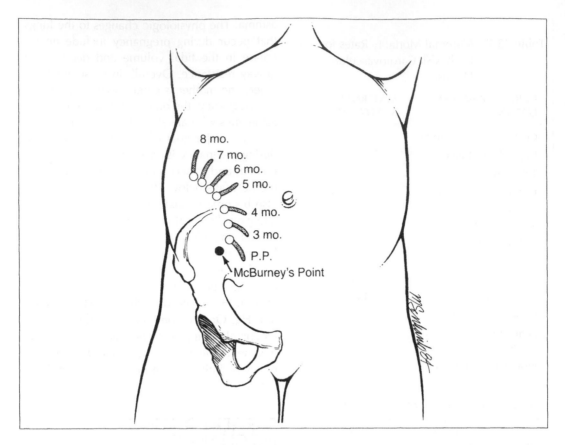

Figure 23.1 Location of appendix over the course of pregnancy

Source: Gabbe SG, Niebyl JR, Simpson JL, eds. Obstetrics: normal and problem pregnancies, 2nd ed. New York: Churchill Livingstone, 1991:685.

and drainage may be required. Peritonitis will increase uterine irritability and greatly increase the risk of preterm labor.

The majority of adnexal masses during pregnancy are benign. Most series report that between 2% and 10% of pelvic masses in pregnancy represent cancer. In addition to the possibility of cancer, other concerns of a pelvic mass include the possibility of torsion of the mass (particularly as it is elevated out of the pelvis by the expanding uterus), rupture of the mass and subsequent hemoperitoneum, and the possibility of the mass obstructing the birth canal. Common functional tumors of the ovary that may occur during pregnancy include corpus luteum cysts, hyperreactio gestationalis, and follicular cysts. Hyperreactio luteinalis is a condition of multiple, theca lutein cysts leading to bilateral ovarian enlargement

during pregnancy. The enlargement is due to either increased gonadotropin production or increased ovarian sensitivity to gonadotropins. The treatment is conservative, as the enlargement will regress spontaneously after the pregnancy. Corpus luteum cysts are produced by either maintenance of or hemorrhage into the corpus luteum of pregnancy with enlargement of the cyst. The luteoma of pregnancy is a rare disorder of a benign, hyperplastic reaction of ovarian theca cells to the pregnancy. Approximately one-third of these cases are bilateral, and they have an increased prevalence in multiparous African American women. Roughly one-third may be hormone-producing and lead to masculinization of the mother or female fetus. These problems will regress spontaneously after the pregnancy.

Characteristics of a mass that raise concerns about malignancy include size greater than 6 cm, complex architecture as revealed by ultrasound, bilaterality, ascites, and elevated levels of CA-125. CA-125 is a serum tumor marker for epithelial ovarian cancers (see Chapter 54), which is normally mildly elevated in pregnancy. Nevertheless, values exceeding 95 μg/mL should raise the suspicion of malignancy.

Recently, magnetic resonance imaging (MRI) has been utilized during pregnancy with excellent results in characterizing pelvic masses. MRI has an advantage in that it does not involve radiation and has been safely used in pregnancy. At times, the diagnosis by MRI may be accurate enough to allow cancellation of surgery for benign conditions such as uterine myomata (shown in Figure 23.2).

Surgery should be avoided if at all possible during pregnancy. If laparotomy becomes necessary, however, this procedure appears to be safe for the mother and fetus at almost any time during gestation. Most would avoid operating during the first trimester for three reasons:

- It is preferable to avoid the teratogenic potential of drugs during organogenesis.

- Often, functional cysts will resolve spontaneously by the second trimester.

- If the patient should miscarry, it would be unclear whether that event followed from the surgery or would have occurred spontaneously anyway.

If the ovary with the corpus luteum is removed during early pregnancy, the pregnancy will need to be supported with exogenous progesterone until the placenta makes sufficient hCG to continue the gestation. The highest likelihood of pregnancy loss will occur if the patient has generalized peritonitis associated with the indication for laparotomy. In later pregnancy, tocolytic therapy may be beneficial to avoid preterm delivery.

When an ovarian carcinoma is discovered during pregnancy, the general approach is to perform the minimal amount of surgery needed to obtain a diagnosis. Chemotherapy has been used during pregnancy. When it is administered in the second and third trimesters, the fetus often suffers some growth deficits, though these are generally transient. Delivery should be coordinated when the patient is not in a blood-count nadir from the chemotherapy. Chemotherapy during the period of

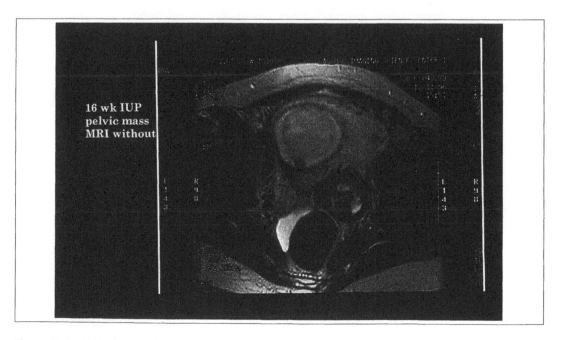

16 wk IUP
pelvic mass
MRI without

Figure 23.2 MRI of 16-week intrauterine pregnancy with a mass in the uterus. This examination is without gadolinium contrast.

organogenesis is associated with a high incidence of fetal death and anomalies. Radiation therapy does not appear to be safe for the fetus at any time during pregnancy.

SUMMARY

Pregnancy is often complicated by pre-existing medical conditions and occasionally by conditions that are initially diag-nosed during this time. Consultation with experts in other areas will help to devise plans that will provide the best care for the mother and fetus. In life-threatening ill-nesses, the mother should be counseled on the potential risks of continuing the preg-nancy. The neonatologist or pediatrician should be appraised of all the mother's medical conditions and treatments so that they may best serve the newborn.

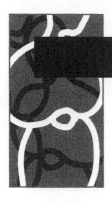

CHAPTER 24

Post-term Pregnancy

Alexander F. Burnett

Post-term pregnancy is one of the more common complications of pregnancy. "Post-term" describes a pregnancy that goes 42 weeks or beyond (294 days or more from the first day of the last menstrual period). Although inaccurate dating of the pregnancy is often the culprit in post-term pregnancy, legitimate extended gestations pose a high risk for perinatal morbidity and mortality and must be aggressively monitored for signs of fetal decompensation. This chapter focuses on the problems associated with post-term pregnancies, the correct diagnosis of this condition, and management strategies in post-term gestations.

CLINICAL CORRELATION

M. N. is a 34-year-old female, gravida 2, para 1, who is 41 3/7 weeks by her last menstrual period and a first trimester sonogram. She complains of being pregnant past her due date and feels generally miserable without any focal complaints. She states that the baby moves a little less than it did about two to three weeks ago.

The diagnosis of post-term or post-dates pregnancy requires knowledge of the expected date of confinement (EDC) or due date. Dating of a pregnancy is therefore critical in managing these patients. The earlier in pregnancy that dates are determined, the more accurate that those dates will be. Crown-rump length in the early first trimester (prior to 12 weeks) is considered accurate within plus/minus three to five days, whereas sonographic findings in the third trimester are accurate only within plus/minus three weeks. If the patient has been evaluated during the first trimester and her dates, as estimated by examination and sonogram, are consistent at that time, then those values can accurately be used to diagnose post-dates if the pregnancy should go more than two weeks beyond the EDC.

The cause of prolongation of pregnancy usually remains unknown. Rare conditions such as fetal anencephaly and placental sulfatase deficiency are associated with failure to enter into spontaneous labor by term.

The complications to the mother and baby increase exponentially as the pregnancy passes beyond the forty-second week. The incidence of cesarean delivery at more than 42 weeks gestation is double that in gestations of 38 to 40 weeks, due mostly to the greater fetal size. Larger babies also increase vaginal birth complications due to vaginal trauma or uterine atony and hemorrhage.

Neonatal complications due to postmaturity include placental insufficiency, macrosomia, and meconium aspiration. Perinatal mortality doubles by the time the gestation reaches 42 weeks. As the placenta ages, it becomes less able to provide sufficient exchange of oxygen and nutrients. The post-term fetus will typically begin to lose weight and is often born hypoglycemic. As oxygenation decreases, the likelihood of hypoxic events increases.

Hypoxia stimulates the parasympathetic system, thereby increasing the likelihood of passage of meconium. Approximately 25% to 30% of post-term babies have meconium staining at delivery, about double the rate for term gestations. In many cases, there is decreased amniotic fluid volume as the fetal plasma volume is reduced. As a result, if meconium is in the amniotic fluid, it will tend to be thicker and can create more risk of respiratory compromise.

CLINICAL CORRELATION

Evaluation of M. N. reveals the fundal height to be 41 cm. The fetus is in cephalic presentation with a left longitudinal lie. Fetal heart tones are heard and are approximately 150 beats per minute. During the examination, the fetus is felt to kick against the abdominal wall once strongly. The cervix is long, thick, and closed. A biophysical profile is ordered to assess fetal well-being.

Evaluation of the fetus in an otherwise normal pregnancy will alter once the gestation reaches 41 weeks. The cervix should be examined to assess induceability. A decision is then made to either induce cervical ripening and labor or to observe with antenatal testing. The agents used to ripen the cervix are discussed in detail in Chapter 26.

Antenatal testing includes several different procedures. The easiest and least expensive testing is termed the nonstress test (NST). It involves monitoring the fetal heart rate with continuous external monitor for a period of time while the mother marks on the monitor those times when she feels the fetus actively kick or move. The test is termed "reactive" if at least two episodes of fetal heart rate acceleration of at least 15 beats per minute over baseline and lasting at least 15 seconds occur during a 20-minute observation period. There are no contraindications to performing an NST. This test's ability to predict when a fetus is in trouble improves when it is used twice per week as opposed to once per week. Spontaneous decelerations of fetal heart tones on NST may signal significant trouble for the fetus.

A contraction stress test (CST) observes the fetal heart tones as the uterus is stimulated to contract at least three times in a 10-minute period. This test has been shown to have a low false-negative rate (defined as a stillbirth within seven days of a negative test) and is predictive of fetal survival for the next week. The CST needs to be performed only once per week. Decelerations—particularly late decelerations after a contraction—may signal uteroplacental insufficiency and indicate that the fetus is at risk for hypoxia. If the NST is reactive but the CST is positive (late decelerations with contractions), induction should begin immediately. In such circumstances, approximately two-thirds of women will have a successful vaginal delivery. If the NST is nonreactive and the CST is positive, then an immediate cesarean delivery should be considered.

Ultrasound is used to assess parameters of fetal well-being in the biophysical profile (BPP). Sonographic examination over a 30-minute observation period looks for fetal breathing movements, gross body movements, fetal tone as defined by extension/flexion of the limbs or trunk, and amniotic fluid volume as determined by the greatest measurable pocket. The results of the test are then graded for each component as 0 or 2, with the highest total possible score being 8. Some clinicians also include the NST in the profile, giving a total possible score of 10 (Table 24.1). Often the amniotic fluid index (AFI) is used to assess the amniotic fluid volume. The AFI is determined by measuring the largest pocket in each of the four quadrants of the amniotic sac and adding these measurements together. A value less than or equal to 5 cm receives 0 points; a value greater than 5 cm receives 2 points. If the total score of the BPP is less than 6, most physicians would commence with delivery. If the score is equal to 6, some obstetricians would repeat the BPP the following day, whereas others would proceed with delivery at that time.

CLINICAL CORRELATION

M. N. has a reactive NST. When BPP is performed, her AFI is 7 cm. The fetus has several episodes of more than 30 seconds of fetal breathing movements. Four discrete, gross body movements are observed

Table 24.1 The Biophysical Profile

BIOPHYSICAL PARAMETER	NORMAL (SCORE = 2)	ABNORMAL (SCORE = 0)
Fetal breathing movements	At least one episode > 30 seconds in 30-minute observation period	No episode of > 30 seconds' duration in 30 minutes
Gross body movement	At least 3 discrete body/limb movements in 30 minutes	Up to 2 episodes of body/limb movements in 30 minutes
Fetal tone	At least 1 episode of active extension with return to flexion of fetal limbs or trunk	Either slow extension with return to partial flexion or movement of limb in full extension or absent fetal movement
Reactive fetal heart rate	At least 2 episodes of acceleration of greater than or equal to 15 bpm and 15 seconds' duration associated with fetal movement in 30 minutes	Less than 2 accelerations or acceleration < 15 bpm in 30 minutes
Amniotic fluid volume	At least one pocket of amniotic fluid measuring 2 cm in two perpendicular planes or AFI > 5 cm	No pocket greater than or equal to 2 cm AFI less than or equal to 5 cm

bpm: beats per minute.

during the test. The fetus shows slow extension with return to partial flexion. The total score of the BPP is 8/10. On the basis of M. N.'s dates and the BPP findings, cervical ripening is initiated, with prostaglandin E_2 gel being placed into the cervix. M. N. is observed for two hours with normal fetal heart tones and returns the following morning for labor induction. On admission to labor and delivery, the cervix is 2 cm dilated and completely effaced, and uterine contractions are noted every five to six minutes. Effective labor begins after artificial rupture of membranes with lightly meconium-stained amniotic fluid. M. N. delivers a female infant after six hours of active labor, by spontaneous vaginal delivery. The baby weighs 8 lb, 8 oz. The Apgar scores are 6 at one minute and 7 at five minutes. The newborn is observed and shows no evidence of meconium aspiration.

SUMMARY

Post-term gestation is one of the more common complications of pregnancy. When a pregnancy goes to 42 weeks, the incidence of cesarean delivery and neonatal morbidity and mortality rise significantly. Intervention is warranted to prevent fetal death once the gestation has reached 42 weeks. The earlier in pregnancy that prenatal care begins, the more accurate is the assessment of fetal age. Surveillance in the post-term gestation includes ultrasound with biophysical profile, contraction stress testing, and cervical assessment to predict ease of labor induction.

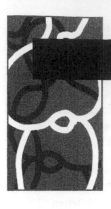

CHAPTER 25

Intrapartum Care: Management of Labor and Delivery

Alexander F. Burnett

L abor can be defined as the progressive dilation and effacement of the cervix caused by painful, regular uterine contractions. Uterine contractions associated with labor become gradually more intense and more frequent as time progresses. True labor must be differentiated from false labor, in which the contractions tend to occur at irregular intervals and do not increase in intensity or frequency with the passage of time. The discomfort of false labor is generally felt only in the lower abdomen; in true labor, the pain is felt in the back and abdomen. By definition, false labor does not lead to cervical dilation. Braxton-Hicks contractions are irregular uterine contractions that occur throughout pregnancy starting in the first trimester. Generally only mild discomfort, if any, is associated with these contractions. Some physicians use the term "Braxton-Hicks contractions" as a synonym for "false labor."

Labor is commonly divided into four stages:

1. The first stage of labor begins with the onset of labor and ends with full cervical dilation.

2. The second stage begins with the full dilation of the cervix and ends with delivery of the infant.

3. The third stage begins after delivery of the infant and ends with delivery of the placenta.

4. The fourth stage of labor refers to the immediate post-partum period—that is, the first one to two hours after delivery of the placenta, when most post-delivery complications will occur.

Each stage of labor lasts a characteristic amount of time. When substantial deviation from these normal time limits occurs, labor is considered either precipitous or protracted.

The first stage of labor (Figure 25.1) can further be subdivided into a latent phase and an active phase. During the *latent phase,* uterine contractions may remain somewhat irregular. This period of labor is characterized by the softening of the cervix, resulting in effacement, or thinning, of the cervix; it is followed by the early dilation of the cervix up to about 4 cm. The latent phase also involves changes to the collagen and other connective tissue components of the cervix. The *active phase* begins when the cervical dilation occurs more rapidly, generally when the cervix is dilated about 4 to 5 cm. This phase is also characterized by descent of the fetus.

As defined by *Friedman,* the normal duration of the latent phase in a primiparous woman is a maximum of 20 hours and in a multiparous woman a maximum of 14 hours. Prolonged latent phases are uncommon, affecting only some 3% to 4% of all gravidas. The mean duration of the active phase is approximately 4.9 hours for primiparous women and 3.0 hours for multiparous women. For primiparous patients, the minimum rate of cervical dilation in the active phase is 1.2 cm/hr; multiparous patients tend to progress at a mini-

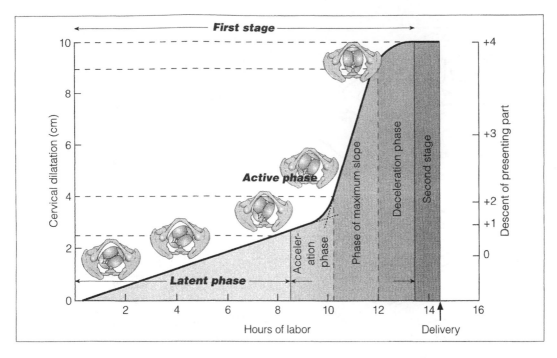

Figure 25.1   First stage of labor

Source: Callahan TL, Caughey AB, Heffner LJ. Blueprints in obstetrics and gynecology. Malden, MA: Blackwell Science, 1998:26.

mum rate of 1.5 cm/hr. Active-phase disorders—either protraction (slower than normal) or arrest (cessation of progress)—are the most common abnormalities of labor, occurring in 26% of nulliparous patients and 16% of multiparous patients.

Friedman's analysis of the active phase also takes into account fetal descent, which occurs simultaneously with dilation. In primigravidas, descent usually commences when the cervix is dilated about 7 to 8 cm and occurs most rapidly after 8 cm. In some multiparous patients, significant descent may not occur until the second stage of labor, when active pushing begins. Descent is described as the relationship between the presenting part and the ischial spines. If the presenting part is 1 or 2 cm above the ischial spines, it is designated as −1 or −2 station, respectively. If the presenting part is at the ischial spines, it is at 0 station. If it is below the ischial spines, it is a +1, +2, or +3 station depending on whether it is 1, 2, or 3 cm below the ischial spines, respectively.

The second stage of labor—the pushing stage—concludes with the delivery of the in-

fant. It has a median duration of 50 minutes in nulliparous women and 20 minutes in multiparous women. Many of the cardinal movements of the fetus take place at this time. The cardinal movements of labor refer to the changes in the fetal head position as the head passes through the birth canal. Because the vertex (fetal occiput) presents first to the pelvis in 95% of term deliveries, the cardinal movements are defined relative to this presentation.

The cardinal movements (Figure 25.2) are as follows: engagement, descent, flexion, internal rotation, extension, external rotation, and expulsion.

Engagement is the descent of the biparietal diameter of the fetal head below the pelvic inlet. It can be diagnosed clinically by palpating the presenting part below 0 station (that is, below the level of the ischial spines of the maternal pelvis). In nulliparous patients, the fetal head is commonly engaged in the pelvis at the onset of labor, which suggests that the maternal bony pelvis is adequate for fetal head descent. Many primiparous patients will feel the fetus "drop" into the pelvis prior to the onset of labor.

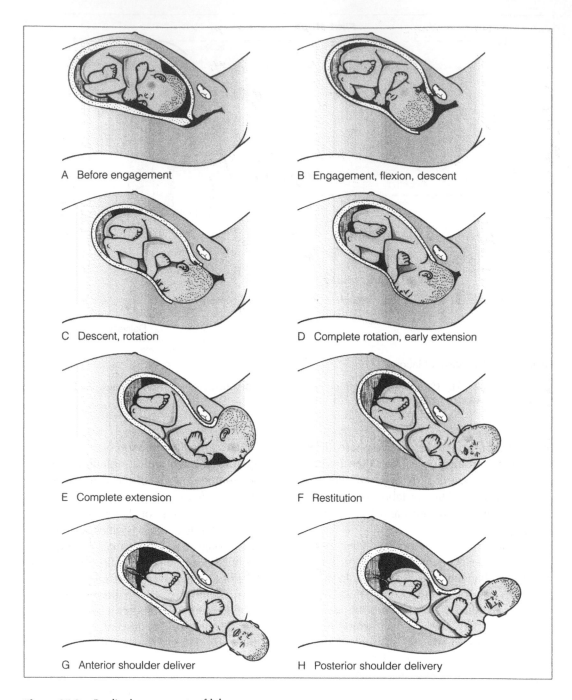

Figure 25.2   Cardinal movements of labor

Source: Callahan TL, Caughey AB, Heffner LJ. Blueprints in obstetrics and gynecology. Malden, MA: Blackwell Science, 1998:25.

Descent is the point at which the greatest rate of movement occurs during the latter part of the first stage and during the second stage.

Flexion is the point at which the fetal chin reaches its chest, which allows for the smaller diameter of the fetal head to present to the maternal pelvis. This transition will aid in descent.

Internal rotation also facilitates presentation of the optimal diameters of the fetal head to the bony pelvis.

Extension of the neck occurs at the introitus to accommodate the upward curve of the birth canal.

External rotation occurs after delivery of the fetal head.

Expulsion is the final delivery of the fetus from the birth canal.

These movements typically occur simultaneously to achieve delivery of the infant.

CLINICAL CORRELATION

Mrs. Jones is a 32-year-old, G1P0 female who presents to labor and delivery suite at 39 4/7 weeks gestational age at 10 A.M. on December 24, complaining that she thinks she is in labor. She reports that she has been experiencing tightening of the abdomen every 5 to 8 minutes for the last 4 hours. The tightening episodes last 20 to 30 seconds, and she can breathe and talk through them. Mrs. Jones reports good fetal movement. She denies any vaginal bleeding. She thinks she may have leaked a little bit of fluid from her vagina, but she is not sure whether the fluid may have come from her bladder. The resident is called to evaluate the patient.

In general, patients are instructed to come to the hospital for evaluation if they are experiencing regular painful uterine contractions that occur every five minutes or less for longer than one hour, if there is a question of spontaneous rupture of membranes suggested by a sudden gush or persistent leakage of fluid from the vagina, or if fetal movement decreases significantly. When the patient arrives in labor and delivery, the nurse will place her on an external fetal monitor to document the fetal heart rate reactivity and the frequency and length of uterine contractions. The patient's prenatal records are reviewed to verify the gestational age and identify any medical complications or other high risk factors in the prenatal course. The uterine contractions are palpated abdominally to document their intensity.

Leopold maneuvers (Figure 25.3) are performed to determine the fetal lie, presentation, and position. The fetal lie is the relationship of the long axis of the fetus to the long axis of the

mother. In 99% of cases, the fetal lie is longitudinal. Alternatively, the lie can be transverse or oblique. If a question arises about the fetal lie, sonography should be performed to confirm the position. The presentation refers to the portion of the fetus lowest in the birth canal—that is, breech or cephalic. The position refers to the relationship of the fetal presenting part to the right or left side of the maternal pelvis. For example, a right occiput anterior presentation (ROA) of the fetal vertex means that the fetal occiput is the presenting part and is positioned such that the occiput is oriented toward the mother's right side and occupies an anterior position (toward the symphysis pubis).

A sterile speculum examination should be performed to document spontaneous rupture of membranes in selected cases based on patient history. A nitrazine and fern test can then be done on any fluid that may pool in the posterior vaginal fornix. Next, a digital examination is performed to document the cervical status and fetal station. The extent of cervical thinning or effacement is described as a percentage of normal fetal length and the amount of cervical dilation is described in centimeters. The location of the fetal presenting part is noted with respect to the ischial spines. This position is referred to as the station and, as noted earlier, is reported as the number of centimeters above or below the spines (−3 to +3). The cervical position in the vagina is described as posterior, midposition, or anterior. The cervical consistency is referred to as firm or soft.

CLINICAL CORRELATION

The nurses place Mrs. Jones on an external fetal monitor. The resident physician reviews her prenatal records. The reports from her early examinations and the availability of a reliable last menstrual period confirm the patient's gestational age. She has experienced an uncomplicated prenatal course and has not developed any other medical problems. The external monitor reveals the presence of irregular uterine contractions every 5 to 10 minutes. They palpate as mild and last approximately 30 seconds. The fetal heart rate tracing is reactive. Leopold maneuvers reveal a fetus

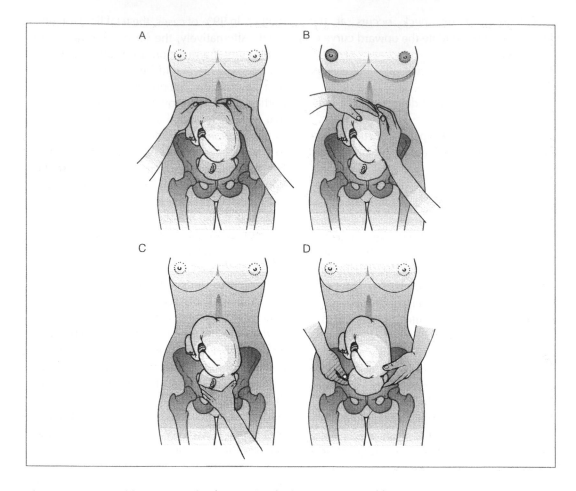

Figure 25.3 Leopold maneuvers for determining fetal presentation and lie

Source: Callahan TL, Caughey AB, Heffner LJ. Blueprints in obstetrics and gynecology. Malden, MA: Blackwell Science, 1998:17

with longitudinal lie and vertex presentation. A sterile speculum examination reveals a small amount of secretions in the vagina but no pooled fluid. The results of both the nitrazine and fern tests are negative. Digital examination reveals a soft cervix, in the midposition with 50% effacement and 1 cm dilation. The vertex is at 0 station. The assessment is false labor, and the patient is discharged home with labor precautions.

By 6 P.M., Mrs. Jones's contractions are occurring every 4 to 5 minutes and last approximately 1 minute. She reports good fetal movement and no leakage of fluid per vagina. She stays at home until 3 A.M., when the contractions become quite strong. Mrs.

Jones then returns to labor and delivery. Examination by the same resident reveals no significant change in the cervix, but the contractions are now palpably strong, lasting 1 minute and occurring every 4 minutes.

Mrs. Jones has now been reporting painful uterine contractions for approximately 12 hours. As the contractions are now more intense, more frequent, and of longer duration, she is likely in true labor, but is still in the latent phase as no significant cervical change has occurred. She is now exhausted from the contractions. A trial of therapeutic rest is a reasonable way to allow a patient to rest in early labor. In response to 10 to 15 mg of IM morphine, approximately 10% of patients will wake from sleeping and no longer be contracting; these patients can be discharged to their homes until true active labor begins. About 85% of patients will awaken with significant cervical change and will have entered active labor. The remaining 5% of patients will persist with ineffective uterine contractions and will require labor stimulation via artificial rupture of membranes or administration of oxytocics. The majority of patients who respond to therapeutic rest by entering active labor will eventually deliver vaginally. This one-time dose of narcotic given early in labor will not harm the fetus.

CLINICAL CORRELATION

The attending physician asks the resident to administer 15 mg of morphine IM to Mrs. Jones. She sleeps for six hours. At 10 A.M. on December 25, her cervix is rechecked. It is found to be completely effaced, 4 cm dilated, and at 0 station. Her uterine contractions are now palpating as moderate to strong in intensity and occur about every three minutes. The fetal heart rate demonstrates good variability. Mrs. Jones is now admitted and permitted to ambulate.

Mrs. Jones has now entered the active phase of labor. Admission laboratory tests include a urinalysis, CBC, and a type and screen. While they are in labor, patients are usually restricted to sips of clear liquids, ice chips, and hard candies. Maternal vital signs are recorded every 30 minutes, and fetal heart rate auscultation is performed at least every 15 minutes. The patient does not have to have continuous infusion of intravenous fluids unless she is dehydrated, but venous access via a 16- to 18-guage heplock is desirable in the event that intravenous drugs, large doses of fluids, or blood needs to be administered.

CLINICAL CORRELATION

At 12 noon, Mrs. Jones becomes very uncomfortable and wishes to discuss her options for analgesia. The resident checks her cervix. She is now completely effaced, 6 cm dilated, and the presenting part is at 0 station.

The use of anesthesia in obstetrics is complicated by the facts that a fetus is present and that pregnancy brings on maternal physiologic changes. All analgesic/anesthetic agents cross the placenta to some degree. The type of anesthesia used may depend on the type of delivery performed, the stage of labor, and the parity of the patient. A thorough review of anesthesia in obstetrics is presented in Chapter 5.

CLINICAL CORRELATION

Mrs. Jones elects to have an epidural placed. Continuous external monitors are placed so as to observe fetal heart rate tracing and the frequency of uterine contractions. Uterine contractions continued every two to three minutes after the epidural catheter was emplaced. At 2 P.M., the cervix was examined again and found to be unchanged from 12 noon.

Mrs. Jones should be progressing at about 1.2 cm/hr in the active phase of labor. A protraction disorder occurs when there is an abnormally slow rate of cervical dilation or fetal descent. Arrest disorders occur when no cervical change or fetal descent occurs over a two-hour period in the active phase. The obstetrician must assess three key components of the delivery process: the powers (the uterine contractions), the passages (the maternal soft tissues and bony pelvis), and the passenger (the fetal size and position).

The uterine contractions cannot be adequately assessed by an external monitor. Quantification of the strength and duration of the contractions requires an intrauterine pressure catheter—that is, a soft catheter introduced into the uterine cavity around the fetus. Contractions of less than 25 mm Hg rarely result in cervical dilation. Generally, if uterine contractions are less than 50 mm Hg and occur less often than every 3 minutes and labor is progressing abnormally, then one would augment labor with oxytocin.

Assessment of the passenger involves estimating the fetal weight, position, and attitude (flexion). Abnormalities of fetal head position or size may result in the head presenting in an abnormally broad diameter as it negotiates the pelvis. This problem may occur in cases of asynclitism (lateral flexion of the fetal head), posterior presentation, or an extended attitude. Certain less common abnormalities, such as hydrocephalus or encephalocele, may also obstruct labor. A simple test that can evaluate whether the fetal presenting part is too large for the pelvis is the Miller-Hillus maneuver. To perform this technique, gentle fundal pressure is applied while a hand is placed vaginally; the hand will receive the impression of easy downward movement of the presenting part if the fetus is not too large for the pelvis.

The maternal bony pelvis is rarely the limiting factor in a vaginal delivery. Clinical pelvimetry will identify the rare instance of a grossly misshapen pelvis and identify architectural anomalies of the pelvis.

Assisted or artificial rupture of membranes (AROM) should be performed in cases of protracted or arrested labor. This technique is accomplished with a plastic hook that gently tears the membranes. Rupturing the amniotic sac will improve labor in two ways. First, AROM results in greater pressure of the head on the lower uterine segment. Second, it releases arachidonic acid from the membranes, which will be converted to prostaglandins and enhance uterine activity. Rupture of the membranes allows placement of intrauterine catheters to quantify the powers of labor. Membrane rupture should be performed only if the head is well applied to the cervix so as to avoid prolapse of the umbilical cord. A fetal scalp electrode can also be placed to better document fetal heart rate variability.

The most common cause of arrest disorders of labor is inadequate uterine contractions. Pitocin (oxytocin) is given initially at 1 mU/min and can be increased by 1 to 2 mU/min every 20 to 40 minutes until an adequate labor pattern is achieved. Ninety-five percent of women will require less than 10 mU/min of Pitocin to achieve adequate labor.

CLINICAL CORRELATION

The resident re-examines Mrs. Jones and estimates a fetal weight of 7½ lb. The vertex is in a LOT (left occiput transverse) position. After the Miller-Hillus maneuver is performed, the head easily descends to the +1 station with gentle fundal pressure. The resident then performs assisted rupture of membranes with clear amniotic fluid. An internal pressure catheter and fetal scalp electrode are emplaced. The uterine contractions are occurring every three to four minutes with a strength of 40 mm Hg. Pitocin augmentation is begun, and an adequate labor pattern is achieved at a Pitocin level of 5 mU/min.

At 4 P.M., the patient complains of rectal pressure. The cervix is now completely effaced and completely dilated (10 cm), and the vertex is at the +2 station in the LOA position (left occiput anterior). The patient is instructed on how to push.

In the second stage of labor, voluntary maternal effort enhances the involuntary uterine contractions to effect delivery of the fetus. During the pushing phase, the fetal head may undergo some changes as a result of negotiating the birth canal (Figure 25.4). Molding is the partial overlap of the bones of the fetal cranium. Caput succedaneum is edema of the portion of the fetal scalp immediately over the cervical os. This edema may prevent differentiation of the skull sutures and fontanelles of the fetus by the examiner. Crowning occurs when the fetal head is encircled by the vulvar ring at the time of delivery.

Episiotomies are midline or mediolateral incisions made by the obstetrician in the vaginal outlet to facilitate delivery of the fetal head in cases requiring vacuum or forceps use, delivery of a macrosomatic infant, or expedited delivery when the fetal heart rate is nonreassuring. Prophylactic episiotomy remains controversial: Proponents claim it leads to less blood loss, greater ease of repair, and greater pelvic support in later life; opponents claim a greater risk of laceration extension into the rectum and suggest that the procedure is unnecessary.

As the fetal head crowns, it delivers by extension to allow the smallest diameter of the head to pass over the perineum. During spontaneous delivery, the obstetrician may cover the patient's anus with a towel and perform the Ritgen maneuver (Figure 25.5), in which one hand controls the egress of the head by gentle pressure on the occiput and the other hand ex-

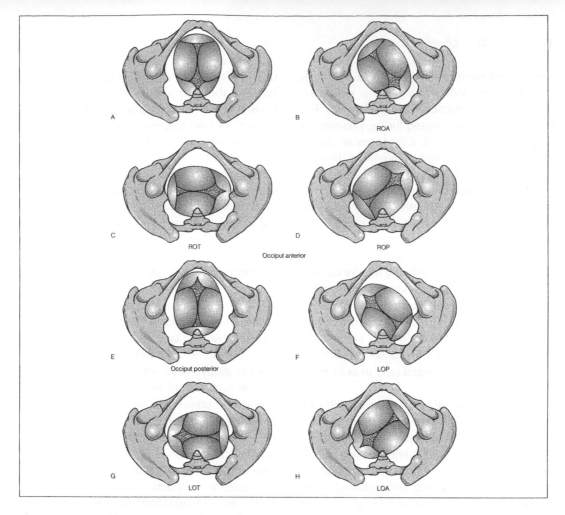

Figure 25.4 Fetal head position at delivery

Source: Callahan TL, Caughey AB, Heffner LJ. Blueprints in obstetrics and gynecology. Malden, MA: Blackwell Science, 1998:19.

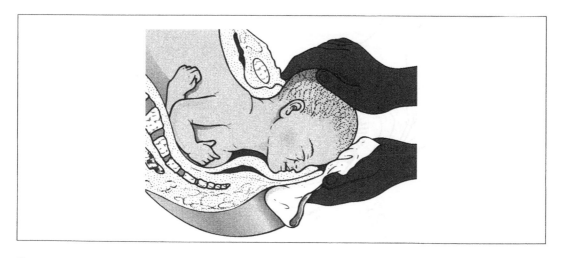

Figure 25.5 Ritgen maneuver for delivery of the fetal head

Source: Callahan TL, Caughey AB, Heffner LJ. Blueprints in obstetrics and gynecology. Malden, MA: Blackwell Science, 1998:26.

erts upward pressure on the fetal chin through the perineum. When the head is delivered, nasal and oral suctioning is performed. The fetal neck is then assessed for the presence of loops of umbilical cord. If the loops are loose, they should be reduced manually; if they are tight, they should be clamped and cut. At this point, the fetal shoulders should be located in the anteroposterior diameter of the pelvis. Gentle downward traction is then applied to the fetal head to release the anterior shoulder, followed by upward traction to deliver the posterior shoulder. The infant should then be cradled in the attendant's arms below the level of the placenta to allow transfusion of the placental blood to the infant. The umbilical cord is then clamped and cut if not done so earlier. The newborn should not be exposed to ambient temperatures for prolonged time so as to avoid heat loss.

The third stage of labor begins with the delivery of the infant and involves the separation and expulsion of the placenta. Placental expulsion is largely a result of uterine activity. A sudden gush of blood accompanied by lengthening of the umbilical cord and a change in the shape of the uterus from discoid to globular are signs of imminent placental separation. After expulsion of the placenta, uterine bleeding is usually limited by occlusion of blood vessels brought about by continued uterine contractions. After delivery, the placenta should be examined for completeness. It should be verified that the umbilical cord contains two arteries and one vein.

During this stage of labor, the vulva and birth canal should be explored for any lacerations requiring repair. Uterine tone and maternal vital signs should be monitored frequently for the next two to three hours. On average, blood loss at the time of delivery and during the immediate post-partum period is no more than 500 cm^3. Blood loss in excess of this amount would occur with post-partum hemorrhage. Causes of post-partum hemorrhage include unrealized lacerations, retained placental fragments in the uterus, coagulopathy, or uterine atony. Risks for uterine atony (poor uterine contraction) include excessive distention of the uterus with multiple gestations or polyhydramnios, precipitous labor, or uterine myoma that anatomically prevent adequate uterine contraction. Aggressive uterine massage and administration of agents that encourage uterine contraction (such as oxytocin, Methergine, or prostaglandins) will often alleviate this problem.

The placenta should be manually removed

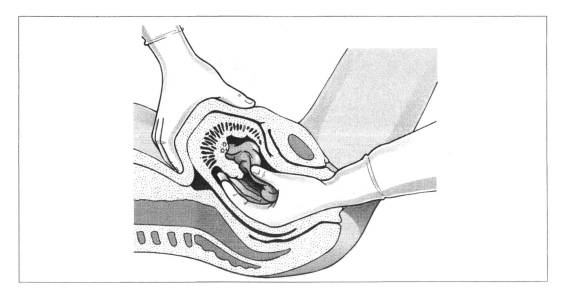

Figure 25.6   Manual removal of the placenta

Source: Callahan TL, Caughey AB, Heffner LJ. Blueprints in obstetrics and gynecology. Malden, MA: Blackwell Science, 1998:30.

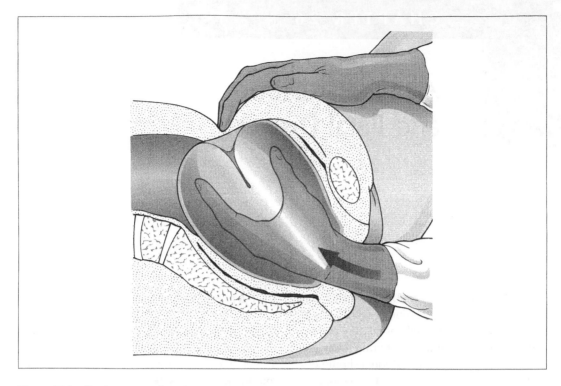

Figure 25.7   Replacement of uterine inversion

Source: Callahan TL, Caughey AB, Heffner LJ. Blueprints in obstetrics and gynecology. Malden, MA: Blackwell Science, 1998:79.

if excessive uterine bleeding occurs or the third stage of labor is prolonged (lasting more than 30 minutes) (Figure 25.6). Overzealous traction on the umbilical cord may result in uterine inversion, which can quickly lead to hemorrhage and shock. Correction of uterine inversion often requires relaxation with general anesthesia and manual replacement of the uterus (Figure 25.7).

The fourth stage of labor encompasses the immediate post-partum period—that is, approximately the first two hours after delivery of the placenta. The likelihood of serious post-partum complications is greatest during this time. The uterus should be frequently palpated to document firmness. Maternal vital signs should be closely monitored and the amount of bleeding recorded to ascertain at the earliest time possible whether post-partum hemorrhage

is occurring. All women should be checked in the post-partum period for their Rh status, and Rh-immune globulin given prior to their discharge if warranted.

SUMMARY

The management of women during labor demands close attention to the process of labor, the progressive dilation and effacement of the cervix with descent of the fetus, and the fetal well-being over this event. Management decisions will affect the outcomes for both the mother and the newborn. Only with a thorough understanding of the normal process of labor and delivery can one expect to detect those labors that are abnormal and may require intervention.

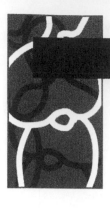

CHAPTER 26

Abnormal Labor and Fetal Distress

Alexander F. Burnett

C areful monitoring of the mother and fetus is essential during labor so as to detect abnormalities at the earliest possible time and permit intervention when appropriate. The student should understand the basics of fetal heart rate monitoring and those patterns that are cause for concern, uterine contraction monitoring, and the indications of abnormal labor. Indications and contraindications to labor augmentation are covered in this chapter. The physician must identify those cases that require emergency intervention and cesarean delivery. Also covered in this chapter is a rational approach to vaginal birth following cesarean delivery.

CLINICAL CORRELATION

T. S. is a 27-year-old female, gravida 1, para 0, whose fetus is at 38 weeks gestational age when she calls to complain of spontaneous rupture of membranes at 10:30 P.M. She has felt some uterine contractions occurring every 5 to 7 minutes and lasting 30 seconds. She was seen in the clinic two days prior to her current complaint, when an examination of the cervix revealed it to be soft, long, and closed. Her station was −1, and she had reported feeling the baby "drop" into her pelvis about a week ago. T. S. has no bleeding, and she reports good fetal movement. She is instructed to stay at home until the contractions begin to occur every 4 to 5 minutes or last 1 minute in duration.

FETAL MONITORING

Continuous monitoring of fetal heart tones during labor first became possible in the late 1960s. Prior to this time, fetal heart tones were intermittently measured during labor, with a relatively high incidence of fetal demise during labor and at the time of delivery. It was postulated that continuous monitoring might detect abnormalities indicative of fetal distress prior to death or significant neurologic injury. In the past few decades, basic patterns of fetal heart tones have been elucidated and correlated with outcome.

The fetal heart rate tracing can reveal evidence of perinatal asphyxia, cord compression, or severe anemia. The monitoring of the fetal heart rate is usually performed with an external monitor, which involves an ultrasound transducer that records movement of the fetal heart valves. A more accurate recording of the fetal heart rate becomes possible with placement of an electrode into the scalp of the fetus, as illustrated in Figure 26.1. Obviously, this technique requires rupture of the fetal membranes, which is not always a safe or desirable situation. Beat-to-beat variability is best shown with an internal monitor. This type of monitoring detects the rapid and constant changes of the fetal heart rate as the fetus responds to its environment. Long-term variability is the cyclic trends in the fetal heartbeat seen perhaps three to five times per minute as the heart rate trends toward deceleration and acceleration. It can be appreciated with the external monitor as well.

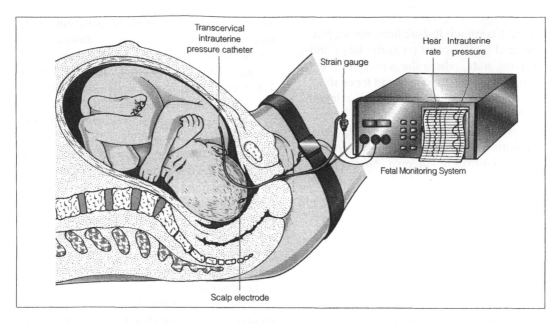

Transcervical intrauterine pressure catheter

Strain gauge

Hear rate   Intrauterine pressure

Fetal Monitoring System

Scalp electrode

Figure 26.1 Invasive monitoring of the fetus in labor

Source: Callahan TL, Caughey AB, Heffner LJ. Blueprints in obstetrics and gynecology. Malden, MA: Blackwell Science, 1998:24.

External monitoring of uterine contractions can be performed with a tocodynamometer, which records pressure differences over the uterus. Although they cannot provide accurate measurements of the strength of the contractions, these devices can reflect the duration of contractions and have been used to analyze fetal heart tones in relation to contractions. More accurate measuring of uterine pressure is obtained with internal monitors, which involve placement of a fluid-filled plastic sleeve into the uterine cavity that records pressure changes on the fluid within as wrought by the uterine contractions. This type of monitoring is more accurate in determining the strength and duration of contractions.

In certain low-risk pregnancies at term, intermittent external monitoring is adequate, particularly in early labor. Generally, fetal heart tones are auscultated for at least 30 seconds following a uterine contraction, with the auscultations taking place every 30 to 60 minutes in early labor. If all is well, the mother can continue walking, which may help in promoting the onset of active labor. For women who are in active labor, continuous monitoring may be recommended; indeed, it is often rec-

ommended in high-risk situations. Once continuous monitoring begins, the mother remains on bedrest but may interrupt monitoring on occasion to use the rest room or for other reasons if there is no contraindication to ambulation. Continuous monitoring gives more extensive information about the fetal reaction to contractions. Perinatal death rate is reduced with continuous monitoring. It is less clear, however, whether overall neonatal morbidity is decreased over intermittent monitoring. In fact, many studies have documented an increase in the cesarean delivery rate with continuous monitoring. Currently, controversy continues to swirl around the benefits of continuous versus intermittent fetal monitoring during labor.

CLINICAL CORRELATION

T. S. calls three hours later. Her contractions are now occurring every 4 to 5 minutes and last between 45 and 60 seconds. She states that they have become quite strong and she has difficulty talking during the contractions. She feels the baby move on occasion. Intermittently, small amounts of fluid continue to leak from her vagina. She and her husband go to the labor and delivery suite, where she is placed on external monitors. The fetal heart tones show a baseline of about 140 beats per minute, with occasional decelerations to 100 beats per minute lasting 10 to 15 seconds. Contractions occur every 4 minutes and endure for approximately 1 minute. An examination reveals the cervix to be completely effaced and 3 cm dilated.

Variability in the fetal heart rate is to be expected. Beat-to-beat variability is caused by the influences of the cardioinhibitory and cardioaccelerator centers in the fetal brain. Loss of beat-to-beat variability may indicate fetal anoxia, or it may reflect other processes such as fetal sleep, drug effects on the fetus (such as narcotics used for labor pain), fetal tachycardia, or other anomalies of the fetal heart or central nervous system. The presence of good beat-to-beat variability is a reassuring sign of fetal well-being.

The normal fetal heart rate pattern is considered to have a baseline between 110 and 160 beats per minute with accelerations, normal variability, and an absence of decelerations. Various problems may cause bradycardia or tachycardia, as indicated in Table 26.1. Fetal heart rate accelerations are considered normal and are definitive proof of a reactive pattern on a nonstress test (see Chapter 33).

Decelerations are classified as early, variable, and late, depending on when they occur in relation to the contraction. Early decelerations (Figure 26.2) begin when the contraction begins, have a uniform bowl-shaped configuration, and resolve at the end of the contraction. They rarely dip below 100 beats per minute. Such variations are felt to be due to head compression.

Late decelerations also have a uniform appearance and are repetitive. The slopes of the deceleration and return to baseline are less steep than those associated with the early decelerations. Typically, the return to baseline occurs some time after the contraction has completed. The deceleration may begin 30 seconds or more after the onset of the contraction. Such decelerations represent uteroplacental insufficiency and are a sign of de-

Table 26.1 Causes of Bradycardia and Tachycardia

BRADYCARDIA	TACHYCARDIA
Maternal medication	Maternal fever
Maternal hypotension or shock	Chorioamnionitis
Maternal convulsions	Maternal anxiety
Maternal hypothermia	Fetal anemia
Premature amniotomy	Fetal infection
Cord compression	Fetal hypoxia
Placental abruption	Following prolonged contractions
Excessive uterine activity	Paroxysmal atrial origin
Post-maturity	Atrial flutter
Fetal cardiac arrhythmia	"Doubling" of FHR
Complete A-V block	
Recording of maternal heart rate	
"Halving" of FHR	

Source: van Geijn HP. Developments in CTG analysis. Bailliere's Clin Ob Gyn 1996;10:185–209.

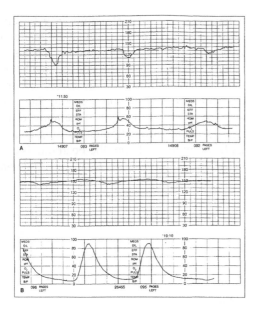

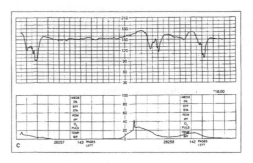

Figure 26.2 Various fetal heart rate tracing patterns

Source: Callahan TL, Caughey AB, Heffner LJ. Blueprints in obstetrics and gynecology. Malden, MA: Blackwell Science, 1998:23.

creased cerebral oxygenation. In many cases, poor variability is associated with late decelerations. When late decelerations occur, prompt intervention is required.

Variable decelerations do not have a uniform appearance and may occur during or apart from a contraction. Typically the heart rate falls quickly and returns quickly to baseline. Most variable decelerations are suspected to be due to umbilical cord compression, which may occur when the cord becomes wrapped around the fetus's neck or is compressed between the fetal body and the wall of the uterus. Prior to rupture of membranes, such decelerations may be an indicator of oligo-

hydramnios. Variable and late decelerations may be classified as mild, moderate, or severe (Table 26.2).

CLINICAL CORRELATION

T. S. continues to have regular contractions for the next two hours. After two and a half hours in labor and delivery, the fetus begins to exhibit variable decelerations that rapidly become moderate in nature. T. S.'s cervix is now 5 cm dilated. To better characterize the fetal heart rate pattern, an electrode is placed on the fetal scalp and an intrauterine pressure catheter is intro-

Table 26.2 Classification of Variable and Late Decelerations

GRADING CRITERIA	MILD	MODERATE	SEVERE
Variable decelerations			
Level of drop of FHR	<30 s, any FHR	<70 bpm, 30–60 s	<70 bpm, >60 s
Duration of drop	>80 bpm, any duration	70–80 bpm, > 60 s	
	70–80 bpm, < 60 s		
Late decelerations			
Level of drop in FHR	< 15 bpm	15–45 bpm	> 45 bpm

bpm: beats per minute.

duced. The fetal heart rate is 150 beats per minute with diminished beat-to-beat variability. Uterine contractions occur every 3 to 4 minutes with a duration of 60 seconds and an amplitude of 50 mm Hg.

Management of moderate or severe variable decelerations includes interventions to try to eliminate these decelerations. When the heart rate falls below 80 beats per minute during a variable deceleration, the risk of fetal acidosis increases, indicating either the presence of excess carbon dioxide or hypoxia. A sampling of the fetal blood from the scalp for a capillary pH determination may be done (Figure 26.3). The fetal capillary pH during labor is normally between 7.25 and 7.40. Some clinicians consider values between 7.20 and 7.24 to be in a pre-acidotic range. Values lower than 7.20—particularly if measured on two collections 5 to 10 minutes apart—are indicative of fetal acidosis and are considered sufficient to warrant termination of labor. These patients should be prepared for emergency delivery.

When a patient develops severe variable decelerations or if the fetal heart tone falls below 80 beats per minute and does not return to baseline, several techniques may be employed to try to remedy the situation. Maternal oxygen should be administered. Changes in maternal position from one side to the other or on to knee-chest position may successfully relieve positional cord compression. Stopping labor requires the use of stimulating drugs such as oxytocin. A stimulation drug should not be administered until the heart rate is corrected. If the variable decelerations are severe but do return to baseline levels, consideration of amnioinfusion to increase the fluid volume and thereby decrease cord compression may be considered. Finally, if the fetal heart tones fail to return to a normal range despite performance of all of the previously mentioned techniques, emergency cesarean delivery is indicated.

CLINICAL CORRELATION

The fetal heart rate tracing begins to show severe variable decelerations despite the infusion of saline into the uterine cavity through the pressure catheter. Analysis of a fetal scalp blood sample shows that it has a pH of 7.20. The situation is discussed with the parents and it is recommended that they proceed with cesarean delivery. A

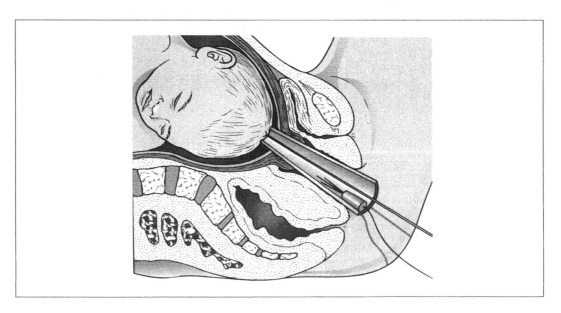

Figure 26.3   Obtaining a fetal scalp blood sample for pH analysis

Source: Callahan TL, Caughey AB, Heffner LJ. Blueprints in obstetrics and gynecology. Malden, MA: Blackwell Science, 1998:24.

final check of the cervix reveals it to still be 5 cm dilated.

T. S. is taken to the operating room and a cesarean delivery is performed. The infant is delivered and found to have three loops of umbilical cord around his neck. These loops are reduced, clamped, and cut. Some meconium staining of the remaining amniotic fluid occurs. The infant is given to the neonatologists, who document that no meconium passed below the vocal cords. When supplemental oxygen is given, the infant quickly becomes responsive. The one-minute and five-minute Apgars are 5 and 9, respectively. The cord blood pH is 7.22. Later that day, the infant is on room air and is oxygenating well with no difficulties.

ARREST OF LABOR/ INDUCTION OF LABOR

Induction of labor may be desired in situations where delivery is recommended due to prolonged gestation; prolonged rupture of membranes; maternal complications such as pregnancy-induced hypertension, diabetes, or renal disease; or fetal demise. Similarly, for women who have an arrest of labor, augmentation of labor may be in order. Labor augmentation is briefly described in Chapter 25. Contraindications to labor induction include situations that also contraindicate vaginal delivery (Table 26.3).

A scoring system was developed in the 1960s as an indicator of success for elective inductions. The Bishop's score (Table 26.4) examines the cervix for evidence of dilation, ef-

Table 26.3 Contraindications to Labor Induction

ABSOLUTE

Placenta or vasa previa

Transverse fetal lie

Prolapsed umbilical cord

Prior classical uterine incision

Active genital herpes infection

RELATIVE

Multifetal gestation

Polyhydramnios

Maternal cardiac disease

Severe hypertension

Breech presentation

Presenting part above the pelvic inlet

Source: Induction of labor. ACOG Technical Bulletin #217. Int J Gyn Ob 1996;53:65–72.

facement, consistency, station, and position and puts a numerical value to these characteristics. Women with a score greater than 8 were found to have a likelihood of vaginal delivery similar to that of those women who underwent spontaneous labor. More recently, cervical ripening has been advanced with preinduction placement of either laminaria that osmotically expand in the cervical canal or prostaglandin preparations. Most commonly used is prostaglandin E_2 gel. When placed into the cervix, it causes local dissolution of collagen and increases the submucosal water. Such cervical ripening agents will often alter the cervix over 24 hours from an unfavorable to a favorable

Table 26.4 Bishop's Scoring System

SCORE	DILATION (CM)	EFFACEMENT (%)	STATION	CONSISTENCY	POSITION OF CERVIX
0	Closed	0–30	−3	Firm	Posterior
1	1–2	40–50	−2	Medium	Midposition
2	3–4	60–70	−1, 0	Soft	Anterior
3	≥5	≥80	+1, +2		

Bishop's score. Use of prostaglandin gel may also increase the rate of entry into labor within the 24 hours following its placement. The major side effect of prostaglandin use is uterine hyperstimulation (six or more contractions in 10 minutes for a total of 20 minutes), which occurs after 1% to 5% of all placements. Maternal effects are generally negligible, but caution is recommended with women with glaucoma, severe hepatic or renal impairment, or adult asthma.

Another common method of initiating labor is the practice of stripping amniotic membranes. This goal is accomplished by placing a finger into the cervical canal to the level of the internal os and vigorously rotating it around the base of the membranes. It is unclear whether the induction of labor follows from the destruction of the amniotic men.branes or from local prostaglandin release. In a woman with a favorable cervix as measured by her Bishop's score, artificial rupture of the amniotic membranes is a method of inducing labor. This technique should be attempted only if the presenting part is applied to the cervix and, therefore, there is minimal risk of umbilical cord prolapse. Its effectiveness is attributable to better application of the presenting part on the cervix (which is felt to increase dilation) and local prostaglandin release.

Oxytocin is a synthetic compound given by intravenous route in the United States to stimulate myometrial contractions. Labor induced by oxytocin is identical to natural, spontaneous labor. Patient's sensitivities to oxytocin vary, however, so careful titration for each individual must be performed. The half-life of oxytocin is 3 to 4 minutes, with a new steady concentration achieved 20 minutes after a change in the infusion rate. The infusion is started slowly (0.5 to 1.0 mU/min) and increased gradually to achieve optimum uterine contractions for labor. Optimal contractions are those that cause progressive dilation of the cervix with passage of the fetus. When a pressure catheter is used, the optimal contraction pattern consists of contractions every 2 to 3 minutes, lasting 60 to 90 seconds, and achieving a maximum intrauterine pressure of 50 to 60 mm Hg and a resting pressure of 10 to 15 mm Hg. The oxytocin doses should be increased at a minimum of 20 minutes, though some protocols prefer 60 minutes between alterations in dosage.

Oxytocin's potential side effects include uterine hyperstimulation, which is treated by reducing the dose until the fetal heart rate and uterine tone become normal. Rapid infusion of oxytocin can result in hypotension. This agent does not cross the placenta and has no direct effect on the fetus. It is structurally related to antidiuretic hormone, and occasionally water intoxication may occur if large amounts of hypotonic solutions are infused with the oxytocin.

ABNORMAL PRESENTATIONS

The presenting fetal part may be an absolute or a relative contraindication to vaginal delivery. Approximately 5% of deliveries are characterized by malpresentation in terms of the presenting part, lie, or flexion attitude. Risk factors for malpresentation include factors that alter the normal polarity of the uterus such as placental location on the cervix, prematurity, polyhydramnios, or multiparity. In addition, fetal conditions such as autosomal trisomies and myotonic dystrophies that leave the fetus with poor muscle tone are associated with a greater incidence of malpresentation.

In an abnormal lie, the alignment of the fetal spine is not longitudinal. A transverse lie occurs when the fetal spine is perpendicular to the maternal spine. An oblique lie occurs when the spine is oriented between longitudinal and transverse, so that the presenting fetal part may be a shoulder or arm. When spontaneous rupture of membranes occurs and no fetal part is filling the pelvis, there is a high risk of cord prolapse. One way to try to correct an abnormal lie prior to labor is to perform external version, whereby the fetus is manipulated by manual pressure on the maternal abdomen into a favorable lie and presentation such as longitudinal and vertex. If external version is impractical or unsuccessful, or if spontaneous rupture of membranes or labor has occurred with a transverse or oblique lie, cesarean delivery is the delivery of choice.

Abnormal deflection attitudes include face presentation. The majority of face presentations will permit vaginal delivery if cephalopelvic disproportion is not present concur-

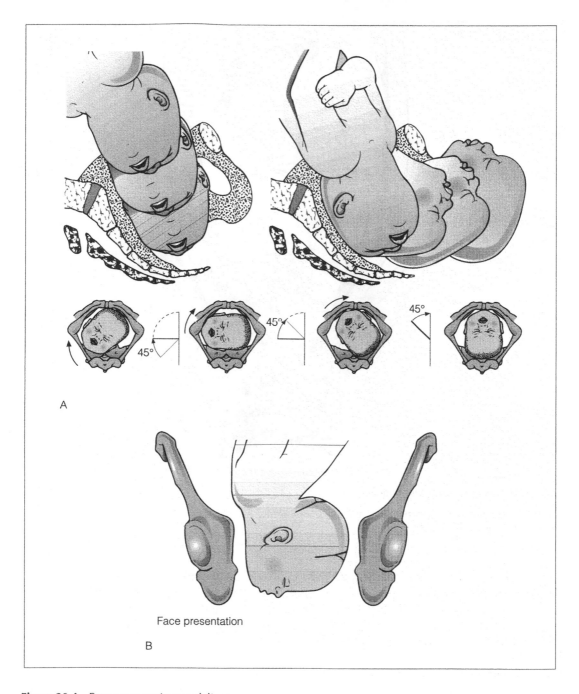

A

B

Face presentation

Figure 26.4   Face presentations at delivery

Source: Callahan TL, Caughey AB, Heffner LJ. Blueprints in obstetrics and gynecology. Malden, MA: Blackwell Science, 1998:47.

rently. Most such cases involve mentum anterior (Figure 26.4). Of those that persist as mentum posterior, cesarean delivery is probably the best option. Compound presentations are those in which a portion of an extremity

prolapses beside the presenting part—most often a hand or arm next to the fetal head (Figure 26.5). Approximately 75% of compound arm/vertex presentations will deliver vaginally, generally with minimal intervention. When in-

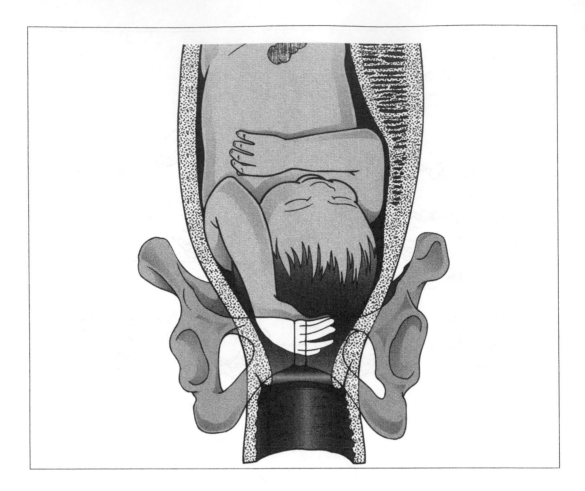

Figure 26.5   Compound presentation at delivery

Source: Callahan TL, Caughey AB, Heffner LJ. Blueprints in obstetrics and gynecology. Malden, MA: Blackwell Science, 1998:48.

tervention is required, cesarean delivery may be the most appropriate choice.

Breech presentation occurs with 3% to 4% of all labors, and is more common with preterm labor than at term. The most common presentation is the frank breech, where the breech presents first with the legs extended and ankles about the face. Less common is the footling breech, where the foot presents before the breech (Figure 26.6). It is associated with the highest incidence of cord prolapse and is a contraindication to vaginal delivery. The least common presentation is the complete breech, where both knees are flexed. Vaginal delivery of a breech presentation is possible provided that the operator is experienced, the presentation is not footling, the infant is term with a flexed head, the estimated fetal weight is be-

tween 2500 and 3800 g, good progress of labor has occurred, and no evidence of fetal distress is apparent. Because of the high rate of morbidity and mortality associated with breech vaginal deliveries (Table 26.5), many clinicians today opt for cesarean delivery of all breech presentations.

Occurring with increased frequency with malpresentation and particularly with premature rupture of membranes is the prolapse of the umbilical cord. This situation represents an emergency, as the presenting part will compress against the cord and restrict blood flow and oxygen to the fetus. If this problem occurs when someone else is present, the current management technique is to place a hand in the vagina and elevate the presenting part to relieve any compression on the umbilical cord

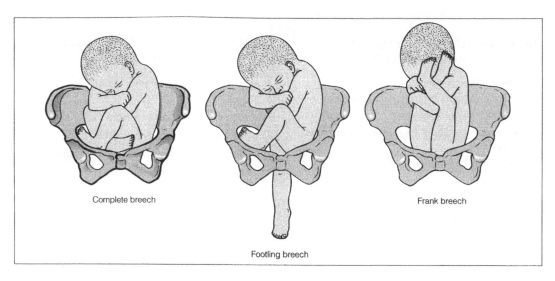

Complete breech

Frank breech

Footling breech

Figure 26.6 Breech presentations

Source: Callahan TL, Caughey AB, Heffner LJ. Blueprints in obstetrics and gynecology. Malden, MA: Blackwell Science, 1998:46.

and then maintain that position until the fetus is delivered via emergency cesarean delivery. When cord prolapse occurs away from a controlled hospital environment, it is almost universally fatal to the fetus.

Table 26.5 Complications Seen with Breech Presentation

COMPLICATION	INCIDENCE
Intrapartum fetal death	Increased 16-fold
Intrapartum asphyxia	Increased 3.8-fold
Cord prolapse	Increased 5- to 20-fold
Birth trauma	Increased 13-fold
Arrest of after-coming head	8.8%
Spinal cord injuries with deflexion	21%
Major anomalies	6%–18%
Prematurity	16%–33%
Hyperextension of the head	5%

Source: Gabbe SG, Niebyl JR, Simpson JL, ed. Obstetrics: normal and problem pregnancies, 2nd ed. New York: Churchill Livingstone, 199:559.

VAGINAL DELIVERY AFTER CESAREAN DELIVERY

CLINICAL CORRELATION

Two years later, T. S. returns to the obstetrician's office and is again pregnant at eight weeks gestational age. She progresses through pregnancy without any complications. As she approaches term, she wants to know about her options for a vaginal delivery. You review her prior delivery and note that she had a low transverse incision in the uterus to deliver her baby.

The high rate of cesarean delivery in the United States is a major health concern. Approximately 20% to 25% of all deliveries in that country take place via the cesarean route. Approximately 40% of these procedures are for repeat cesarean delivery, the most common indication.

Women with a lower segment scar on the uterus, whether transverse or vertical, are potential candidates for a trial of labor (Table 26.6). Multiple prospective studies have revealed a successful vaginal delivery rate after a previous cesarean delivery of 75% to 82%, with a uterine rupture rate of much less than 1%. Clinicians must be familiar with the signs

Table 26.6 Eligibility for Vaginal Birth After Cesarean Delivery

- **Favorable indicators**
  - One previous low-segment transverse cesarean delivery
  - An informed and appropriately counseled patient
- **Expanded indicators**
  - Two or more previous cesarean deliveries
  - Low vertical uterine scar
  - Twin gestation
- **Absolute contraindications**
  - Classical uterine incision
  - T-shaped uterine incision
  - Prior uterine rupture
  - Operative complications at time of first abdominal delivery (i.e., extensive cervical lacerations)
  - Previous uterine surgery with entrance into the uterine cavity
  - "Obvious" cephalopelvic disproportion

Source: Martins ME. Vaginal birth after cesarean delivery. Clinics in Perinatology 1996;23:141–153.

Table 26.7 Signs and Symptoms of Uterine Rupture

- Fetal heart rate abnormalities
  - Fetal bradycardia
  - Rising fetal baseline heart rate
  - Severe variable decelerations
- Disappearance of uterine contractions
- Change in uterine contour
- Ascent of the presenting part
- Abdominal or shoulder pain
- Vaginal bleeding
- Gross hematuria
- Maternal hypotension

and symptoms of uterine rupture so as to detect this complication during labor (Table 26.7). Oxytocin has been shown to be safe in appropriate candidates for vaginal delivery as has cervical ripening with prostaglandin gel.

CLINICAL CORRELATION

After appropriate counseling, T. S. elects to try for a vaginal delivery with her current pregnancy. At 40 weeks gestational age, the cervix is long and closed. Ripening of the cervix with prostaglandin gel is performed. Twenty-four hours later, labor is induced with oxytocin. The cervix at the start of the induction is soft, 50% effaced, and closed. T. S. begins to have regular contractions after 2 hours of oxytocin. At 4

hours, with the presenting vertex at 0 station, an artificial rupture of membranes is performed. T. S. continues to labor with progressive cervical dilation. After 16 hours of labor, she delivers a male infant from a right occiput anterior position with Apgars of 8 and 9 at one and five minutes, respectively. After delivery of the placenta, manual palpation of the lower uterine segment reveals an intact transverse uterine scar.

SUMMARY

Monitoring of the mother and fetus during labor can significantly reduce perinatal mortality. The ability to detect signs of fetal distress early in labor can lead to management of labor with a more favorable outcome. The obstetrician must be familiar with fetal presentations as well, and the risks of malpresentation should be known along with the most effective management strategies for these situations. Being aware of indicators for vaginal birth after cesarean delivery and active management of patients contemplating this route will reduce the repeat cesarean delivery rate.

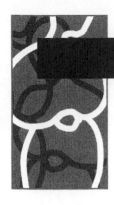

CHAPTER 27

Operative Vaginal Delivery

Alexander M. Burnett

The use of forceps to assist in the delivery of the laboring mother is a skilled technique that is learned through an apprenticeship of observation, participation under skilled guidance, and eventually soloing after adequate observation with knowledgeable assistance. The proper use of forceps can help terminate labor and relieve a mother's fatigue from prolonged pushing in the second stage, can shorten the second stage when medically indicated (such as with maternal cardiac disease), and, when appropriate, may deliver most expeditiously an infant showing signs of distress.

The operator should be thoroughly familiar with the forceps he or she has selected. The fetal head must be engaged, the cervix must be fully effaced and completely dilated, the position of the fetal head must be accurately determined, the fetal membranes must be ruptured, and the operator should have assessed clinically the type of pelvic architecture possessed by the patient. An adequate level of anesthesia should be present for the operative procedure that is contemplated. In most cases, the urinary bladder is emptied.

In August 1994, the *Technical Bulletin* of the American College of Obstetrics and Gynecology enumerated the criteria that the group deemed necessary to justify the use of forceps for delivery. Table 27.1 details these criteria.

In addition to the obstetrical forceps, vacuum cups are also available to assist in the delivery of the infant. These devices vary in terms of their material from rigid metal to soft silicone

and plastic (Figure 27.1). Criteria necessary to justify use of a vacuum cup are similar to those required in a forceps delivery. Vacuum cups offer the advantage of taking up less room and thus reducing maternal trauma, especially in the nulliparous patient who, through prolonged pushing, may have quite edematous vaginal tissue. Their disadvantages include trauma to the scalp of the fetus and the tendency of the cup to pull off with traction.

CLINICAL CORRELATION

M. G. is a 32-year-old, gravida 1 female who is initially seen for prenatal care and noted then to have a height of 5 ft, 4 in, and a weight of 110 lb. During her prenatal course, she gains approximately 20 lb. Clinical evaluation of her pelvis is carried out at approximately 34 weeks gestation. At that time, there is maximal relaxation of her bony pelvis and more adequate clinical evaluation is possible. After the evaluation is carried out, M. G. is noted to have a gynecoid-type pelvis for the following reasons: (1) she has an adequate diagonal conjugate 12 cm or greater; (2) there is no prominence of the ischial spines; (3) she has a moderately wide sacrosciatic notch that is felt to be greater than 2½ fingerbreadths; (4) there is light pubic rami with no narrowing of the public arch; and (5) the intertuberous diameter is relatively wide.

After a prolonged second stage of labor influenced perhaps by an epidural anesthe-

Table 27.1   Classification of Forceps Delivery According to Station and Rotation

TYPE OF PROCEDURE	CLASSIFICATION
Outlet forceps	1. Scalp is visible at the introitus without separating the labia
	2. Fetal skull has reached pelvic floor
	3. Sagittal suture is in anteroposterior diameter or right or left occiput anterior or posterior position
	4. Fetal head is at or on perineum
	5. Rotation does not exceed 45°
Low forceps	Leading point of fetal skull is at station ≥ ±2 cm, and not on the pelvic floor
	a. Rotation ≤45° (left or right occiput anterior to occiput anterior, or left or right occiput posterior to occiput posterior)
	b. Rotation >45°
Midforceps	Station above +2 cm but head engaged
High	Not included in classification

Source: From Cunningham FG, et al. Williams obstetrics, 19th ed. Norwalk, CT: Appleton & Lange, 1993:557.

sia, M. G. is taken to the delivery room for a forceps delivery. She is sterilely prepped and draped. A pelvic examination shows the vertex to be at a +4 station, the cervix is completely effaced and dilated, and the membranes are ruptured. It is possible to palpate the posterior fontanel and fetal ear, and the fetal head is determined to be in a LOA (left occiput anterior) position.

Because of moderate molding of the

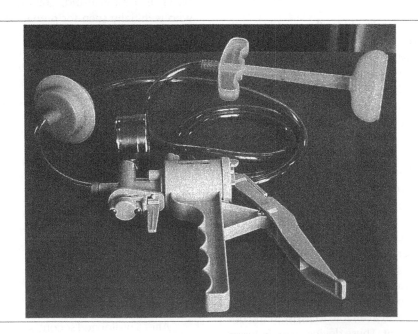

Figure 27.1   Fetal vacuum extractor with hand-held pressure gauge

fetal head, it is felt that Simpson-type forceps would permit a more accurate application to the fetal head. The left or posterior blade is applied initially, followed by the right blade. The blades lock easily. The sagittal suture of the fetus is in line with the handles, and the posterior fontanel of the fetus is one fingerbreadth above the locked blades. Traction is commenced to coincide with the uterine contractions and expulsive efforts of the mother. After three contractions over 10 minutes time, the vertex is crowning and a small midline episiotomy is made. The handles of the forceps are elevated to approximately 45° to aid the extension of the fetal head beneath the pubic arch. After delivery of the fetal head, the remainder of the fetus is delivered with one additional contraction of the uterus. Spontaneous delivery of the placenta occurs, then the cervix and vagina are carefully inspected for any evidence of laceration. None is found, and the episiotomy is closed in layers.

There are four major classifications of the female pelvis, as illustrated in Figure 27.2. The type of pelvis will often determine the type of arrest disorder of labor experienced; it may also determine the type of forceps selected (Figure 27.3).

CLINICAL CORRELATION

A. G. is a 30-year-old, primipara patient who has been followed during her pregnancy for 30 weeks. At 34 weeks gestation, the clinical evaluation determines that it is consistent with a anthropoid-type pelvis for the following reasons: (1) the diagonal conjugate cannot be reached; (2) the ischial spines are prominent and the pelvis seems long and narrow; (3) the sacrosciatic notch is wide—greater than three fingerbreadths; and (4) the pubic arch is narrow.

A. G. comes to the hospital in active labor and progresses rapidly to full effacement and dilation. An epidural anesthetic is administered. After two hours of active pushing, the fetal head has descended to a +4 station. Some late decelerations of the fetal heart are observed, and it is decided that delivery is now appropriate. A. G. is taken to the delivery room, where evaluation of the fetal position shows that the head is at a +4 station but palpation of the posterior fontanel and ear shows that it is in a direct occiput posterior position. Because A. G. is known to have an anthro-

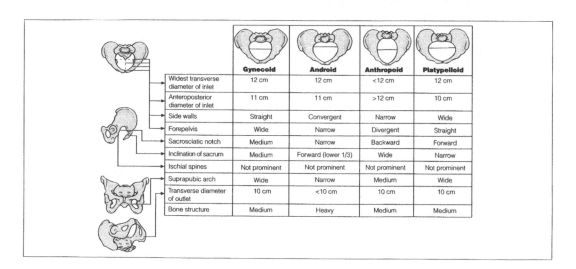

	Gynecoid	Android	Anthropoid	Platypelloid
Widest transverse diameter of inlet	12 cm	12 cm	<12 cm	12 cm
Anteroposterior diameter of inlet	11 cm	11 cm	>12 cm	10 cm
Side walls	Straight	Convergent	Narrow	Wide
Forepelvis	Wide	Narrow	Divergent	Straight
Sacrosciatic notch	Medium	Narrow	Backward	Forward
Inclination of sacrum	Medium	Forward (lower 1/3)	Wide	Narrow
Ischial spines	Not prominent	Not prominent	Not prominent	Not prominent
Suprapubic arch	Wide	Narrow	Medium	Wide
Transverse diameter of outlet	10 cm	<10 cm	10 cm	10 cm
Bone structure	Medium	Heavy	Medium	Medium

Figure 27.2 Categories of the female pelvis

Source: Callahan TL, Caughey AB, Heffner LJ. Blueprints in obstetrics and gynecology. Malden, MA: Blackwell Science, 1998:45.

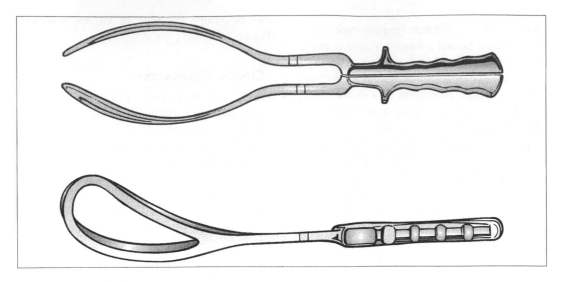

Figure 27.3   Forceps for assisted delivery

Source: Callahan TL, Caughey AB, Heffner LJ. Blueprints in obstetrics and gynecology. Malden, MA: Blackwell Science, 1998:28.

poid-type pelvis, it seems appropriate to deliver this infant as a direct posterior.

The delivery as a direct posterior is more difficult because more soft tissue space is required and extension of the episiotomy is more likely. If directly occiput posterior, the left blade is applied initially; otherwise, the posterior blade is applied first. After the blades are applied but before they are locked, they are depressed against the perineum to bring the handles closer to the posterior fontanel. After the anterior fontanel appears beneath the symphysis, the head is delivered by flexion rather than extension. After delivery of the infant and placenta, careful inspection of the soft parts is carried out—a wise course because of the increased incidence of soft tissue trauma with this delivery technique.

A platypelloid pelvis is one in which the diagonal conjugate is short but the ischial spines are widely spaced. This shape makes it easier for an infant's head to come through the birth canal in a transverse position rather than occiput anterior or posterior. If the degree of width is sufficient, it may be most practical to deliver the infant as an occiput transverse. Op-erative vaginal delivery would utilize Barton's forceps in this situation, with the forceps being applied to the anterior and posterior position with a gentle downward traction. No attempt at rotation is made until the vertex appears at the introitus.

An android pelvis has a short diagonal conjugate with prominent ischial spines and a narrow pubic arch. This structure provides a very tight passageway for the fetal head, and frequently labor is prolonged with extensive molding of the head before delivery. If forceps are applied and no descent is detected with gentle traction, operative vaginal delivery should be abandoned in favor of cesarean delivery.

SHOULDER DYSTOCIA

Shoulder dystocia occurs in approximately 0.5% to 2% of all vaginal deliveries. Its incidence has been reported to increase with macrosomia, obesity, mid-forceps delivery, prolonged second stage of labor, past-datism, excessive weight gain by the mother, and—especially—maternal diabetes mellitus.

Diabetes mellitus, if not well managed, can lead to macrosomic infants who often seem to have larger shoulder girths than their weights alone would dictate. James O'Leary, as reported in the *Journal of Obstetrics and Gynecology*, is presently developing a registry of Zavanelli procedures in the United States. To emphasize the issues that account for the major increase in the incidence of shoulder dystocia, he has coined the mnemonic "DOPE": **d**iabetes mellitus, **o**besity, **p**rolonged pregnancy, and **e**xcess weight gain by the mother.

The major complication of shoulder dystocia is neurologic damage to the brachial plexus, caused by excessive traction on the head when the anterior shoulder becomes trapped behind the symphysis. All traction must be gentle and must be coordinated with contractions and expulsive efforts by the mother (Figure 27.4).

CLINICAL CORRELATION

C. G. is a 35-yearold, gravida 2, para 1, female admitted at 41 weeks gestation with a history of moderate contractions throughout the day. Her one previous pregnancy resulted in a vaginal delivery of an 8 lb, 1 oz, female infant after a four-hour labor. The only complication of that previous labor was a vulvar hematoma.

On her current admission to the hospital, C. G.'s cervix is found to be completely effaced and 6 cm dilated with the presenting vertex at a −1 station. Two hours later, she is found to be completely effaced and dilated. She begins pushing. After 45 minutes of ineffectual pushing, a soft vacuum cup is applied to the fetal head and the head is brought down to the perineum. The head is then allowed to deliver spontaneously. After delivery, it is noted that the head is flush against the perineum. Attempts to deliver the anterior shoulder are unsuccessful. The patient's hips are elevated on a bedpan, her legs are flexed over her abdomen, and suprapubic pressure is exerted—all in an attempt to dislodge the entrapped anterior shoulder. A generous episiotomy had previously been performed. A Woods maneuver is then carried out—that is, pressure on the buttocks with the left hand above and two fingers of the right hand placed on the anterior aspect of the posterior shoulder, with clockwise rotation beyond the 180° arc. The now posterior shoulder cannot be delivered. At this time, restitution of the fetal head, together with flexion and pressure with the palm of the hand, is carried out to return the fetal head to the pelvic cavity. A cesarean section is carried out immedi-

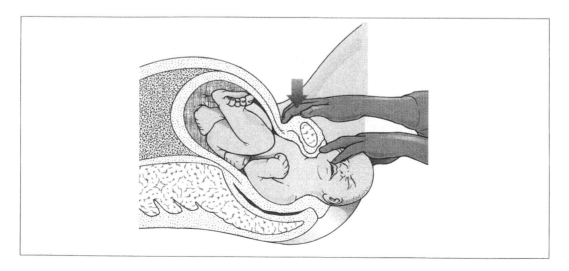

Figure 27.4   Pressure on the maternal symphysis to aid in delivery of the shoulder

Source: Callahan TL, Caughey AB, Heffner LJ. Blueprints in obstetrics and gynecology. Malden, MA: Blackwell Science, 1998:49.

ately, with the delivery of a female infant weighing 4140 g (approximately 9 lb, 1 oz). The Apgars are 5 and 7 at one and five minutes, respectively, with a cord pH of 7.31.

In this case, the initial maneuver carried out was the McRoberts maneuver (Figure 27.5). Exaggerated flexion of the patient's legs resulted in straightening of the sacrum relative to the lumbar spine and consequent rotation of the symphysis pubis cephalad. When the symphysis rotates, it often frees the impacted anterior shoulder without requiring any manipulation of the fetus.

The second procedure, the Woods maneuver, was originally described by C. E. Woods at Nassau Hospital in New York. He compared the trapped shoulder to a screw, suggesting that direct traction merely served to tighten the screw. Woods decided that the best way to correct the cross-thread attitude was the reverse mechanism—bringing the trapped anterior shoulder down to the perineum by exerting pressure on the prior posterior shoulder through a clockwise arc.

When these principal maneuvers proved unsuccessful, a procedure termed the Zavanelli procedure was performed. The maneuver was originally described as the manual replacement of the fetal head after failure to deliver the

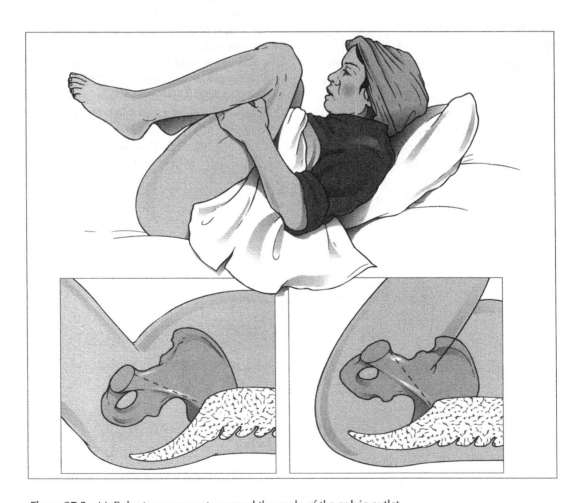

Figure 27.5 McRoberts maneuver to expand the angle of the pelvic outlet

Source: Callahan TL, Caughey AB, Heffner LJ. Blueprints in obstetrics and gynecology. Malden, MA: Blackwell Science, 1998:49.

shoulders and subsequent abdominal delivery. More than 40 cases of successful use of this technique have been described in the U.S. literature.

SUMMARY

Operative vaginal delivery is performed to assist or expedite delivery of the infant. A clear understanding of the physics of delivery are necessary when manipulating the fetal head with either forceps or vacuum cups. Due in part to the potential for complications and consequent litigation, the art of forceps delivery is dying out in the United States. Perhaps with the trend toward reducing the cesarean delivery rate, the future may bring a resurgence of these valuable and—when properly performed—safe techniques to assist in vaginal delivery.

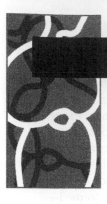

CHAPTER 28

Neonatal Assessment

Alexander F. Burnett

The first month of an infant's life is associated with the highest mortality rate of childhood. The transition from intrauterine to extrauterine life is characterized by profound physiologic changes and requirements for the newborn. Infections, prematurity, and congenital abnormalities are leading contributors to newborn morbidity and mortality. Consequently, it is necessary to evaluate the newborn in such a manner as to recognize potential difficulties as early as possible.

PHYSIOLOGIC CHANGES AT BIRTH

The transition from essentially a parasitic existence to independent existence occurs rapidly at birth. The cardiopulmonary changes are most dramatic, with the blood flow and functioning of the lungs undergoing a complete transformation.

During fetal life, blood flows from the mother through the umbilical vein to the hepatic circulation and directly to the inferior vena cave via the ductus venosus. Once the blood reaches the fetal heart, the majority of blood from the inferior vena cava passes through the foramen ovale to the left atrium, then to the left ventricle and into the main circulation. The venous return via the superior vena cava predominantly goes to the right atrium, then to the right ventricle, then to the systemic circulation by passage through the ductus arteriosus to the aorta (Figure 28.1). Only some 7% of the blood flow goes to the

fetus's fluid-filled lungs. From the aorta, the blood flows to the upper body and brain and to the abdomen and pelvis, eventually reaching the umbilical arteries and returning to the maternal circulation. Because the mother provides oxygen and handles elimination of fetal waste, the blood flow to the lungs, liver, and kidneys of the fetus is minimal during gestation.

At birth, the expansion of the lungs causes the pulmonary vascular resistance to suddenly falls, which in turn increases pulmonary blood flow and return to the left atrium. The increased volume in the left atrium brings about the closure of the foramen ovale because of pressure against the flap valve. This physiologic closure becomes anatomically closed about four weeks after birth in most circumstances. The occlusion of the umbilical arterial flow at birth raises the arterial pressure in the newborn; similar to the closure of the foramen ovale, this event encourages closure of the ductus arteriosus. This process functionally establishes adult-type circulation. Oxygen and prostaglandins are also critical for ductus arteriosus closure. Occasionally, particularly in the premature infant, the ductus arteriosus fails to close in the newborn. Medical therapy with indomethicin will successfully close the ductus in 60% to 75% of these cases, with the remaining infants requiring surgical closure.

NEWBORN ASSESSMENT

Newborn assessment critically evaluates the infant for the normal transition to the mature

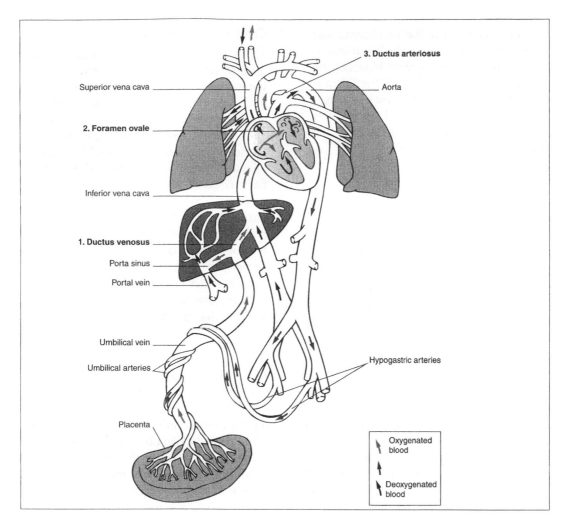

Figure 28.1 The fetal circulation

Source: Gant NF, Cunningham FG, eds. Basic gynecology and obstetrics. Norwalk, CT: Appleton & Lange, 1993:268.

cardiopulmonary circulation. The infant's remnants of the fetal shunts are as follows: the foramen ovale becomes the fossa ovalis; the ductus arteriosus becomes the ligamentum arteriosum; the ductus venosus becomes the ligamentum venosum; the umbilical vein becomes the round ligament of the liver; and the umbilical arteries become the obliterated umbilical arteries.

CLINICAL CORRELATION

P. T. is a 33-year-old, primigravida female at term who has just delivered a living male infant from the right occiput transverse position through a midline episiot-

omy. The obstetrician has clamped and cut the umbilical cord, taken a sample of cord blood and the blood gas, and passed the newborn off to the nurse who begins the assessment. The obstetrician's attention returns to the mother for delivery of the placenta and repair of the episiotomy. Meanwhile, the delivery nurse begins by calculating Apgar scores on the infant at one minute. The newborn is cyanotic in the distal extremities and has a weak cry. His heart rate is 110 beats per minute and strong, however, and the muscle tone appears good. The nurse dries the infant and places him under a radiant heat source.

Gentle suctioning of the oropharynx and nose are accomplished. By five minutes, the distal extremities remain blue, but the baby's cry has strengthened. The infant is brought to the mother's breast as her episiotomy repair is completed. The Apgars are recorded as 8 at one minute and 9 at five minutes.

In 1952, Virginia Apgar developed a method for rapid assessment of the newborn. Unfortunately, this scoring method has since been used as an assessment of potential asphyxia, with which it correlates poorly. Instead, the scoring is a valuable way of assessing resuscitation efforts on the newborn, and evaluating those parts of the physical examination that may signal impending difficulties. Five areas are assessed (as shown in Table 28.1), with each receiving a score of 0, 1, or 2.

RESPIRATORY COMPROMISE

The heart rate is probably the most critical measurement in determining the potential for respiratory compromise. If the heart rate is less than 100 beats per minute and the infant shows either apnea or irregular respiratory efforts, vigorous stimulation of the infant (by rubbing a towel over its back and blowing oxygen on its face) will often lead to a response that improves the condition of the newborn. If the infant fails to respond, bagging with a soft mask over the nose and mouth may be necessary. Adequate bagging will lead to chest expansion, followed by improved color and heart rate. If bagging fails to improve the infant, intubation becomes necessary.

CLINICAL CORRELATION

T. L. is a 22-year-old female who goes into preterm labor at 31 weeks gestation. By spontaneous vaginal delivery, she gives birth to a female infant from the occiput anterior position over an intact perineum. The infant has poor respiratory effort and the heart rate at one minute is 80 beats per minute. Oxygen is administered and the baby is gently stimulated. Despite these measures, respiratory effort is not improved by five minutes and cyanosis is prominent in the extremities. The infant has some nasal flaring and breathing is labored. She is intubated, taken to the neonatal intensive care unit, and a chest X ray is taken. The Apgars are 4 at one minute and 5 at five minutes.

Once intubation occurs, other considerations should include whether the mother has received narcotics close to birth, which might be the etiology of infant's respiratory depression. This condition is treated with naloxone and continued close observation. Prematurity is a very common cause of respiratory difficulties. In such circumstances, inadequate surfactant production may lead to increased alveolar surface tension, which requires increased pressure to maintain the patency of the alveoli. This condition is known as hyaline membrane disease. Typically, the infant with this problem will present with increased respiratory difficulty, tachypnea, nasal flaring, cyanosis, and expiratory grunting. Unless one intervenes, the child may die of exhaustion and asphyxia. Table 28.2 lists the common pulmonary and

Table 28.1 Apgar Scoring System

SIGN	0	1	2
Heart rate	Absent	<100/min	>100/min
Respiratory effort	Apneic	Weak, irregular, gasping	Regular
Reflex irritability	No response	Some response	Facial grimace, sneeze, cough
Muscle tone	Flaccid	Some reflexion	Good flexion arms and legs
Color	Blue, pale	Body pink, hands and feet blue	Pink

Table 28.2 Etiologies of Respiratory Distress

I. Pulmonary
  1. Congenital anomalies
    a. Upper airway obstruction: choanal atresia, laryngeal and tracheal atresia
    b. Tracheoesophageal fistula
    c. Lobar emphysema (congenital)
  2. Developmental
    a. Pulmonary hypoplasia
    b. Hyaline membrane disease
    c. Transient tachypnea
  3. Acquired
    a. Pneumonia
    b. Meconium aspiration
    c. Pneumothorax

II. Cardiovascular
  1. Left-sided outflow tract obstruction
    a. Hypoplastic left heart
    b. Aortic stenosis
    c. Coarctation of the aorta
  2. Cyanotic lesions
    a. Transposition of the great vessels
    b. Total anomalous pulmonary venous return
    c. Tricuspid atresia
    d. Right-sided outflow obstruction

III. Noncardiopulmonary
  1. Hypo- or hyperthermia
  2. Hypoglycemia
  3. Polycythemia
  4. Metabolic acidosis
  5. Drug intoxications, withdrawal
  6. CNS insult: asphyxia, hemorrhage
  7. Neuromuscular disease
  8. Phrenic nerve injury

Source: Adapted from Merenstein GB, Kaplan DW, Rosenberg AA, ed. Handbook of pediatrics, 18th ed. Stamford, CT: Appleton & Lange, 1997:148.

nonpulmonary etiologies of respiratory distress. When the infant has premature lungs, exogenous therapy with surfactant can potentially reduce the pulmonary morbidity and mortality.

PREMATURITY-RELATED PROBLEMS

Prematurity brings other potential problems for the newborn. The smaller size of the premature infant makes thermoregulation more difficult, as the infant has only minimal fat stores. In the intensive care unit, staff must guard against hypothermia. In addition, premature infants have a higher incidence of necrotizing enterocolitis, which is multifactoral in origin. This disease, which involves the immature immune system and infection, is best recognized by its hallmark of intestinal ischemia. A wide range of clinical scenarios are possible with this disease—ranging from mild gastrointestinal upset to fulminant disease with bowel perforation, sepsis, and shock. Radiographic findings may show bowel wall edema or free air in the peritoneum.

Intraventricular hemorrhage is also increased in premature infants, with its most likely cause being ischemia with reperfusion injury in the germinal matrix. Intraventricular hemorrhage is graded from I to IV on the basis of ultrasound findings of the cerebral ultrasound (Table 28.3). The extent of injury will determine the likelihood of long-term neurological sequelae.

CLINICAL CORRELATION

T. L.'s daughter is diagnosed with hyaline membrane disease on the basis of the chest

Table 28.3 Intraventricular Hemorrhage Classification

GRADE	DEFINITION
I	Subependymal hemorrhage
II	Intraventricular hemorrhage without ventricular dilatation
III	Intraventricular hemorrhage with ventricular dilatation
IV	Intraventricular hemorrhage with associated parenchymal hemorrhage

X ray and the physical findings. A surfactant is administered and she is maintained on a ventilator with moderate oxygen demands. In the fourteenth hour of life, the infant experiences a seizure. An ultrasound is performed and reveals a grade IV intraventricular hemorrhage. Supportive measures include continued oxygen therapy and phenobarbital to prevent further seizures. These efforts prove unsuccessful, as the baby again seizes at 22 hours of life. Her pupils are now nonreactive. An electroencephalogram is performed and shows brain damage incompatible with survival. The parents are informed of the findings and prognosis. With the assistance of their religious counselors, the parents elect to discontinue support at 30 hours of life.

NEONATAL JAUNDICE

Neonatal jaundice is a common finding associated with term infants. It is also known as "physiologic jaundice," because most cases occur when the liver is unable to conjugate the excess bilirubin from destruction of red blood cells. The peak serum bilirubin usually occurs at about days 3 to 4 in a term infant and about days 5 to 7 in a premature infant. Peak values should be less than 12.9 mg/dL for term infants and less than 15 mg/dL for premature infants. Pathological causes of jaundice include hemolytic disease (such as Rh and ABO incompatibilities), genetic disorders of hemolysis (such as hereditary spherocytosis), and overproduction from extravasation (bruising) or polycythemia.

Infants who are exclusively breastfed may develop a peak in bilirubin between days 6 and 14 that rises to 12 to 20 mg/dL (called breast milk jaundice). This condition is due to increased intake over the first several days of life when compared with formula-fed infants. Treatment for breast milk jaundice is to increase the frequency of feedings or to supplement breast feedings with formula.

Direct hyperbilirubinemia is rare. Its potential toxicity comes from kernicterus, which is staining of the basal ganglia and hippocampus with resulting severe neurologic sequelae,

including death. Treatment consists of phototherapy, in which the unconjugated bilirubin in the skin is converted into a water-soluble photoisomer and excreted in the bile and urine. If phototherapy does not give a satisfactory response, exchange transfusion may be required to bring the bilirubin down into a safe range. In addition, all infants should receive a dose of vitamin K to prevent hemorrhagic disease of the newborn.

INFECTIOUS COMPLICATIONS

Infectious complications of the newborn are usually due to vertical transmission of maternal infections, including group B streptococcus, gonorrhea, Chlamydia, syphilis, herpes, toxoplasmosis, hepatitis, and human immunodeficiency virus. These infections are covered more fully in Chapters 10 and 23. All infants will receive prophylactic antibiotic ointment in their eyes at the time of birth to prevent neonatal conjunctivitis from *Gonorrhea neisseria*.

CORRELATION OF PHYSICAL/NEUROLOGIC MATURITY WITH GESTATIONAL AGE

For the premature infant, assessment of physical and neurologic maturity is important to correlate with the gestational age. Differences between gestational and physical age or small-for-gestational-age findings may be indicative of a prenatal exposure that has damaged the infant. Such exposures may include maternal hypertension, maternal drug abuse, intrauterine infection, or chromosomal abnormalities. Infants who are deemed large-for-gestational-age suggest that maternal diabetes may be present; they should be observed for neonatal hypoglycemia, hypocalcemia, hyperbilirubinemia, and increased risk of respiratory distress syndrome. Charts are available for determining physical and neurologic maturity, as shown in Figure 28.2.

ROUTINE CARE OF THE TERM INFANT

For the healthy term infant, routine care involves a complete history and physical examination with the following recommendations:

- *Observation:* Should be made and recorded every 8 hours. The neonate gener-

Neuromuscular maturity

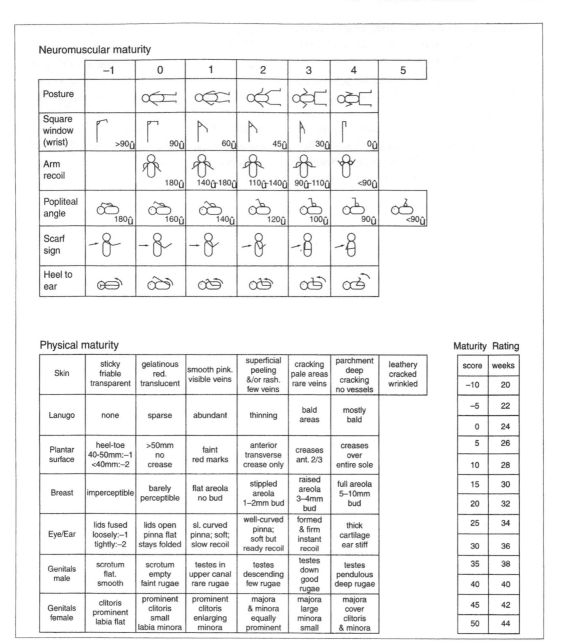

Physical maturity

	-1	0	1	2	3	4	5
Skin	sticky friable transparent	gelatinous red. translucent	smooth pink. visible veins	superficial peeling &/or rash. few veins	cracking pale areas rare veins	parchment deep cracking no vessels	leathery cracked wrinkled
Lanugo	none	sparse	abundant	thinning	bald areas	mostly bald	
Plantar surface	heel-toe 40-50mm:-1 <40mm:-2	>50mm no crease	faint red marks	anterior transverse crease only	creases ant. 2/3	creases over entire sole	
Breast	imperceptible	barely perceptible	flat areola no bud	stippled areola 1-2mm bud	raised areola 3-4mm bud	full areola 5-10mm bud	
Eye/Ear	lids fused loosely:-1 tightly:-2	lids open pinna flat stays folded	sl. curved pinna; soft; slow recoil	well-curved pinna; soft but ready recoil	formed & firm instant recoil	thick cartilage ear stiff	
Genitals male	scrotum flat. smooth	scrotum empty faint rugae	testes in upper canal rare rugae	testes descending few rugae	testes down good rugae	testes pendulous deep rugae	
Genitals female	clitoris prominent labia flat	prominent clitoris small labia minora	prominent clitoris enlarging minora	majora & minora equally prominent	majora large minora small	majora cover clitoris & minora	

Maturity Rating

score	weeks
-10	20
-5	22
0	24
5	26
10	28
15	30
20	32
25	34
30	36
35	38
40	40
45	42
50	44

Figure 28.2   The Ballard score for determining maturity of the infant at birth

Source: Ballard JL, et al. New Ballard Score, expanded to include extremely premature infants. J Pediatrics 1991;119:417.

ally passes meconium in the first 24 hours after delivery. Often the normal infant is permitted to leave the hospital with his or her mother in less than 24 hours.

- *Feedings:* Should be begun immediately. The normal term infant feeds every 2 to 3 hours, with time on the breast increasing from 4 to 10 minutes over the first three days.

- *Laboratory screening:* Should include tests for blood typing, Rh status, and Coombs antibody testing. Most states also mandate testing for phenylketonuria, maple syrup urine disease, homocystinuria, and congenital hypothyroidism.

- *Follow-up:* Should routinely be scheduled within 48 to 72 hours after discharge from the hospital for infants sent home in less than 24 hours. An exception may occur with infants born with cystic fibrosis. Approximately 15% of these infants develop meconium ileus, with delayed passage of meconium or bowel obstruction. Surgical correction may be required.

SUMMARY

The assessment of the neonate is critical to determine whether life-threatening conditions are present. The examination should look for the presence of birth defects or metabolic disorders. Maternal history is important in determining whether additional studies are warranted.

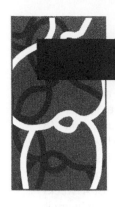

CHAPTER 29

Post-partum Care

The puerperium—the period after delivery—is a time of rapid physiologic changes as the mother's body returns to the pre-pregnancy state. Emotional changes are also frequently observed during this time. Physicians can be of assistance in helping mothers adjust to their new roles, facilitate pair-bonding, and understand the physiologic alterations of this time. In addition, the post-partum period is a good time to educate the patient on contraception, if she desires. In the event of fetal demise, the post-partum period requires sensitivity to the woman's grieving process.

T. P. is a 32-year-old female who delivered a term male infant 12 hours ago via a normal spontaneous vaginal delivery with a second-degree midline episiotomy. She has breastfed twice without difficulty. She is concerned about care for her episiotomy site and has questions about resumption of sexual relations and birth control. In the past, she has used oral contraceptive pills without difficulty; now, however, she is concerned about taking the pills while she is breast feeding. She also has questions about whether she should have her son circumcised.

The puerperium is a time of rapid involution of the uterus and return of the nonpregnant physi-

ology. The uterus will usually involute to normal size by six weeks post-partum. Post-partum discharge, termed lochia, will typically be serosanguinous initially, then become mucopurulent by three to five days post-partum. This discharge may persist for three to six weeks after delivery.

Excessive bleeding during this time may be an indication of retained placental products. This condition is diagnosed by ultrasound, and treatment consists of gentle curettage of the uterus to remove the products, preferably under ultrasound guidance. Bleeding immediately following delivery of the placenta is controlled by contraction of the uterus, causing compression of the vessels. Oxytocin or methylergonovine may be given to stimulate uterine contraction to diminish bleeding.

ENDOCRINOLOGIC DISORDERS IN THE POST-PARTUM PERIOD

If a woman suffers excessive bleeding and shock at the time of delivery, she may later develop ischemic necrosis of the anterior pituitary (Sheehan's syndrome). This syndrome may present immediately as failure to lactate, or it may take several years to be fully expressed. Late-onset evidence of pituitary insufficiency may include loss of axillary and pubic hair, amenorrhea or oligomenorrhea, vaginal atrophy, and hypothyroidism. Treatment involves replacement of hormones lost due to this syndrome.

Autoimmune causes of endocrine dysfunction may also appear or be exacerbated in the post-partum period. During pregnancy, humoral and cellular immunity are suppressed; this suppression may worsen or flare up post-partum. Included in this category of abnormalities are thyrotoxicosis and hypothyroidism.

CONTRACEPTION IN THE POST-PARTUM PERIOD

The return of ovulation is dependent upon whether the woman breast feeds. In those who do not breast feed, ovulation will likely resume by about 10 weeks post-partum. If a woman exclusively breast feeds her child, her likelihood of ovulating in the first six months post-partum is only 1% to 5%.

Myriad contraceptive choices are available in the post-partum period. For the non-breast-feeding woman, the choice should be based solely on her preference. Nevertheless, many clinicians recommend delaying resumption of oral contraceptives for at least two weeks post-partum to avoid a possible increased risk for thromboembolism.

The breast-feeding woman has many options for contraception as well. Oral contraceptives that contain estrogen are not recommended, however, as they may negatively affect milk production. Lactational amenorrhea as a consequence of breast feeding may also prove valuable as a contraceptive measure. During breast feeding, suckling alters the normal pattern of GnRH release, thereby changing the pattern of LH release from the pituitary. For most women, menstruation resumes prior to the return of ovulation; therefore, it is unusual—although not impossible—for breast-feeding women to become pregnant prior to their first menstrual period after delivery.

For women who have completed their childbearing, post-partum tubal sterilization is an option that is quite easy to do at the time of cesarean delivery. It requires a fairly small surgical procedure after vaginal delivery.

Intrauterine devices (IUDs) may also be placed in the post-partum period. Indeed, the highest success rate in terms of IUD retention occurs when these devices are placed within 10 minutes of placental removal. No increase in perforation of the uterus has been noted when an IUD is inserted directly after placental removal. Expulsion rates are higher for IUDs placed between 10 minutes and 48 hours after delivery as compared with insertion during the first 10 minutes. If insertion has not been performed within 48 hours, most physicians would wait until at least 4 weeks post-partum, as the first month after delivery is associated with higher expulsion rates. Copper and progesterone IUDs have no effect on lactation, and breast feeding does not increase the risk of expulsion.

Barrier methods are safe in the post-partum or lactating periods. Progestin-only contraceptives have no effect on lactation. These agents can be administered via pills, injectables, or implants.

Sexual relations may resume as soon as the perineum is no longer uncomfortable. Many women will experience some vaginal dryness in the post-partum period, particularly if they are breast feeding, as this practice contributes to a relative lack of estrogen. Libido is variable in the post-partum, with the majority of women reporting some decrease in sexual desire.

Care of the perineum should include keeping the area clean with either sitz baths or showers, as well as use of appropriate analgesics. In women who have undergone a third- or fourth-degree extension of the episiotomy, stool softeners are also recommended until the area heals. Excessive pain at the episiotomy site may indicate the presence of a hematoma, cellulitis, or necrotizing fasciitis. Therefore, this symptom requires immediate examination of the patient.

The post-partum period can also be a time of emotional stress. Severe fetal malformations or fetal death lead to grieving, which is both appropriate and necessary. Most obstetrical wards now have protocols designed to assist in grieving in a healthy manner (see Chapter 33). The significant changes brought about with a new child can also lead one into emotional turmoil, particularly if the woman has a history of anxiety or depression. Chapter 7 deals more extensively with post-partum anxiety and depression.

CIRCUMCISION

Removal of a newborn male's foreskin is a controversial subject. Historically, this procedure has been done mostly for religious and social reasons. A backlash against the practice has occurred more recently, with opponents claiming that the procedure has no medical benefit and that it is cruel because most newborns were not given any anesthetic prior to the removal of the foreskin. In addition, many argue that circumcision represents mutilation of the male genitalia.

There are, however, some medical arguments that can be made in favor of circumcision. Circumcised men have a lower incidence of cancer of the penis; although this disease is a very rare cancer in the United States, it is a significant health problem in other parts of the world. Since the 1930s, approximately 50,000 cases of cancer of the penis have occurred in the United States, with only about 10 reported in circumcised men. In addition, it has been postulated that the tendency to acquire HIV infection from sexual contact is higher in males who are not circumcised. There is a 10-fold increase in urinary tract infections and complications among uncircumcised men compared with circumcised men. In addition, if a man requires circumcision at an older age, the procedure is associated with more complications and more discomfort than when done in the newborn period. Today, many choose to use anesthesia, most commonly dorsal penile nerve block, in carrying out this procedure, which greatly reduces the discomfort to the newborn male.

The final decision to perform a circumcision is usually made on the basis of either religious or social desires. Typically, parents will elect to have the procedure performed if the father has previously had it done, or if it is the norm in the particular area where the child is likely to grow up. If the parents desire that a circumcision be performed, the procedure may be done by an obstetrician, pediatrician, family practitioner, or urologist, or by a non-physician, particularly for religious purposes. The newborn male should be determined to be healthy by general examination and not have any significant distortion of his genital anatomy prior to undergoing a circumcision.

SUMMARY

The post-partum period is characterized by significant physiologic changes as the body returns to the pre-pregnancy state. It is a time in which physicians should monitor their patients with chronic diseases closely so as to detect alterations or exacerbations to their illnesses, including endocrinologic, cardiac, pulmonary, and psychiatric disorders. The puerperium is also a time to discuss contraceptive options, if the patient desires.

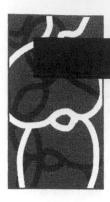

CHAPTER 30

Lactation

Alexander F. Burnett

Breast-feeding makes several very important contributions to the health of a newborn child. To facilitate the breast-feeding process, the physician should be familiar with the physiology of lactation and the mechanics of breast-feeding so as to assist the nursing mother and answer her questions. Breast-feeding should be encouraged because it provides the ideal nutrition to the newborn, along with factors that diminish the child's likelihood of contracting various illnesses. The benefits to the mother include better infant bonding, lactational amenorrhea that may provide contraceptive benefits, and a decreased likelihood of developing ovarian or endometrial cancers. This chapter will review the physiology of lactation, discuss the composition of breast milk and the ways in which that composition changes over time, and describe some of the more frequent difficulties with breast-feeding and their solution. In addition, it is important to remember that virtually all maternally ingested drugs pass to some extent through the breast milk to her offspring. The physician must be aware of which drugs have a high likelihood of harming the newborn.

BREAST PHYSIOLOGY DURING PREGNANCY

The breast undergoes a remarkable transformation over the course of pregnancy. Lobule size increases because of cellular hyperplasia and hypertrophy. A complex interplay of multiple hormones results in mammary growth. In particular, ductal growth is influenced by estrogen, growth hormone, and glucocorticoids. Lobuloalveolar growth is influenced by estrogen, growth hormone, glucocorticoids, prolactin, and progesterone. Lactogenesis—the onset of milk secretion—requires a fully developed mammary gland, prolactin, glucocorticoids, insulin, thyroid hormones, and the withdrawal of estrogen and progesterone. Once lactogenesis has occurred, the level of progesterone receptors in the breast decreases such that this hormone will no longer inhibit lactation if it is reintroduced. Consequently, progesterone contraceptives may be prescribed to the lactating mother without interfering with breast-feeding.

Milk is ejected from the breast by the contraction of myoepithelial cells that surround the alveoli, forcing the fluid out the milk ducts. Oxytocin is the most potent stimulator of these myoepithelial cells. Infant sucking of the breast is necessary to stimulate oxytocin release from the neurohypophysis. Continuing milk production is most dependent on prolactin; if this hormone is inhibited, lactation will cease.

retraction of her nipples. P. T. wonders if she will be able to provide enough milk for her baby or if she will require supplementation. Also, she is concerned that her nipples are abnormal and will not allow the infant to suck properly. She has heard there are some benefits to breast-feeding but wonders if formula might be better for her baby.

COMPOSITION OF BREAST MILK

Breast milk is ideally designed for the developing human. Over time, its composition changes, reflecting the change in nutritional requirements for the infant over time. The initial milk is known as colostrum. It is secreted at a rate of about 40 mL/day for three to four days. It has high levels of protein and salt as well as high numbers of cells such as macrophages, neutrophils, and lymphocytes. When mature milk comes in by the fifth day, it is higher in lactose and fat, but lower in protein and cells. Colostrum offers approximately 54 kcal/dL whereas mature milk provides about 70 kcal/dL.

Infectious diseases in the newborn—including diarrhea, otitis media, upper respiratory tract infections, pneumonia, and urinary tract infections—are all decreased in infants who are exclusively breastfed. That protection is available because human milk is high in antimicrobial factors—most importantly, secretory IgA antibodies that are specific for pathogens in the infant's local environment; anti-inflammatory agents that are probably responsible for decreased necrotizing enterocolitis and diarrhea in breastfed babies; and immunomodulating factors such as cytokines that may contribute to disease prevention after infancy. Breastfed babies have decreased incidence of infections, allergies, and some later-life diseases, such as insulin-dependent diabetes, Crohn's disease, and lymphoma. Table 30.1 presents composition comparison of human milk with typical commercial formula and cow's milk. Table 30.2 lists the secretory IgA antibodies identified in human milk against common microbial pathogens.

MATERNAL CONCERNS

Many women are concerned about their ability to properly and adequately breast-feed their children, particularly with the approach of their first delivery. Prior breast surgery may affect the ability to breast-feed. Breast reduction typically results in a cutting of ducts that could impair lactation. In contrast, breast augmentation surgery should have no effect on lactation, except for the situation where augmentation is performed for some anomaly of the breast that itself may portend decreased lactation potential. Women with inverted or retracted nipples should be successful in breast-feeding if the infant is brought to the breast immediately after birth and not given any bottle supplements. The infant will learn to suck in such a manner as to extract milk from inverted nipples; however, the mother must be prepared to use more diligence in exposing the inverted nipple to the infant (Figure 30.1). Occasionally, use of a breast pump just prior to feeding may help to pull the nipple and aureola out more and to initiate milk let-down.

Breast size has no influence on the ability to breast-feed, and small breasts will supply adequate milk to the infant. If the breast fails to enlarge in a normal manner over pregnancy, however, it may represent an anomaly of the breast that will interfere with lactation. Breastfed infants never need to bottle-feed, and can go directly from breast to cup after about six months of life.

The suckling stimulus is critical to initiate and maintain prolactin release. Consequently, breast-feeding should begin as soon after birth as possible (preferably immediately after birth) and should continue every three to four hours as the infant demands. As the infant ages, the suckling-stimulated release of prolactin becomes less pronounced as a reaction to longer delays between feedings. If a woman is experiencing diminished milk production, she should continue with nighttime feedings or use a breast pump periodically to stimulate prolactin release. The breast pump should be used if the infant is unable to breast-feed due to sickness or hospitalization or as the mother returns to work. Pumping should be performed at three- to four-hour intervals. Freshly expressed breast milk can go unrefrigerated for as

Table 30.1 Comparison of Composition of Mild and Commercial Formula (per 1000 mL)

COMPONENT	UNIT	HUMAN MILK	COMMERCIAL FORMULA	COW'S MILK
Osmolality	mOsm/kg	282	290	275
Energy	kcal	67	67	61
Carbohydrates	g	7.3	7.2	4.7
Fat	g	4.2	3.8	3.4
Minerals				
Calcium	mg	25	51	119
Chloride	meq	1.1	1.5	2.9
Copper	µg	35	41	30
Fluorine	µg	7	20	15
Iodine	µg	7	10	5
Iron	µg	40	150	50
Magnesium	mg	3	4.1	13
Manganese	µg	0.4	3	2–4
Phosphorus	mg	15	39	93
Potassium	meq	1.5	2.0	3.9
Sodium	meq	0.8	1.1	2.1
Zinc	µg	100–300	500	300
Proteins				
Casein	mg	187	1185	2700
Lactalbumin	mg	161	52	400
Total protein	g	0.9	1.5	3.3
Vitamins				
A	IU	155	250	126
B_6	µg	28	40	42
B_{12}	ng	26	150	357
C	mg	4	5.5	0.9
D	IU	1.6	40	42
E	IU	0.32	1.7	0.08
K	µg	0.21	3	6
Folic acid	µg	5.2	5	5
Niacin	µg	200	790	84
Pantothenic acid	µg	225	300	314
Riboflavin	µg	35	100	162
Thiamine	µg	16	65	30

Source: Reproduced with permission. Merenstein GB, Kaplan DW, Rosenberg AA, ed. Handbook in pediatrics, 18th ed. Stamford, CT: Lange Medical Books, 1997:54–55.

long as six hours without significant bacterial growth. Refrigerated expressed breast milk can be stored for as long as 48 hours, and frozen milk can be stored for three to four weeks. Frozen milk should never be microwaved or boiled, but rather should be thawed under warm tap water.

Occasionally, infant malformations may

Table 30.2   Secretory IgA Antibodies in Human Milk Against Common Microbial Pathogens

BACTERIA AND TOXINS	VIRUSES	OTHERS
Escherichia coli	Rotavirus	*Giardia*
Shigella	Respiratory syncytial virus	*Candida albicans*
Salmonella	Poliovirus	
Campylobacter	Other enterovirus	
Vibrio cholerae	Influenza virus	
Haemophilus influenzae	Cytomegalovirus	
Streptococcus pneumoniae	Human immunodeficiency virus	
Clostridium difficile		
Clostridium botulinum		
Klebsiella pneumoniae		

Source: Reproduced with permission. Goldman AS. The immune system of human milk: antimicrobial, antiinflammatory and immunomodulating properties. Pediatr Infect Dis J 1993;12:664–671.

delay breast-feeding. Infants with a cleft palate, for example, may require surgical correction prior to initiating breast- or bottle-feeding. Alternatively, some bottles have been designed to facilitate feeding of infants with a cleft palate that are more squeezable in design. Successful breast-feeding with a cleft lip or palate has been reported.

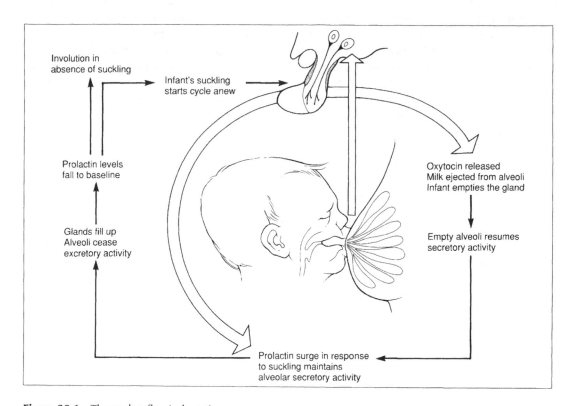

Figure 30.1   The suck reflex in lactation

Source: Gabbe SG, Niebyl JR, Simpson JL, ed. Obstetrics: normal and problem pregnancies, 2nd ed. New York: Churchill Livingstone, 1991:190.

Maternal caloric requirements should not need to increase substantially during breast-feeding, provided that the woman has gained a normal amount of weight over the pregnancy. The majority of fatty acids in milk are derived from maternal stores that are accumulated during pregnancy. If the woman has poor weight gain over gestation, she should maintain an increased caloric intake similar to that during pregnancy. It is reasonable to continue with prenatal vitamins during lactation.

Lactational amenorrhea occurs due to the influence of elevated levels of prolactin, which correlate with diminished estrogen levels. For much of the world, this natural event serves as the only method of family spacing. Ovulation typically returns prior to the first return of menstruation. Although the uterus is usually not in synch with implantation, some 3% to 10% of all women will become pregnant prior to their first menstruation if lactational amenorrhea is the only method of contraception. Women who breast-feed fewer than six times per day are recommended to use alternative forms of contraception during lactation.

Oral contraceptives containing estrogen may have deleterious effects on offspring, although this relationship has not been firmly established and the amount of steroid transferred in breast milk is small. Progestational steroids are recommended as safer contraceptive options during lactation—most commonly, the mini-pill of norgestrel 30 μg/day. Progestational agents are less likely to inhibit lactation than estrogen-containing pills.

In addition to its effects on fertility, inhibition of ovulation during lactation may significantly diminish a woman's lifetime risk of ovarian cancer and endometrial cancer. A decreased incidence of both of these carcinomas is noted with pregnancy and prolonged oral contraceptive use. It appears that lactational amenorrhea and anovulation provide a continued protective effect on the ovaries and endometrium, equal to that imposed by pregnancy.

CLINICAL CORRELATION

P. T. has a history of severe asthma, which has not been a problem thus far during her pregnancy. She is scheduled to deliver in the springtime, which is typically when her asthma flares up along with seasonal allergies. She is concerned about using her medication while breast-feeding and asks your advice.

USE OF DRUGS DURING LACTATION

Any drug ingested by a mother may eventually enter her baby's bloodstream. Absorption by the baby is dependent upon multiple factors, including the concentration of the drug in the maternal serum, its concentration within the breast milk, and the ability of the infant's digestive tract to absorb the substance. Ultimately, a relatively small amount of any maternally ingested drug ever reaches the infant's system. Nevertheless, a number of agents may be harmful and should be avoided (Table 30.3). In P. T.'s case, theophylline appears to be safe during breast-feeding, as are inhalers and bronchodilators.

In certain circumstances, drug passage to the infant is an important therapeutic component in treating the mother's illness. For instance, mastitis is an infection of the breast usually due to bacteria from either the mother's skin or the baby's mouth. Typically, it is treated with dicloxacillin and breast-feeding continues so as to prevent accumulation of infected milk within the milk ducts and treat the infant's mouth. If medical therapy is not successful and an abscess develops, it must be incised and drained.

Some common sense should be used when prescribing drugs during lactation. Any medication that is not absolutely necessary should be avoided. If a topical medication is available for a particular problem, it should be used rather than systemic therapy, as the absorption of the drug into the maternal bloodstream is generally less with the former route of administration. If the mother must take a medication that is contraindicated, she may opt to bottle-feed her child while she is taking the medication and pump her breasts but discard that milk. In most circumstances, the baby will resume breast-feeding once the medication has cleared from the mother's system. Obviously, if multiple drugs are available to treat an

Table 30.3 Use of Drugs During Lactation

Contraindicated

Amantadine	Cocaine	Metamizol
Amiodarone	Dipyrone	Metronidazole
Antineoplastic agents	Gold salts	Radiopharmaceuticals
Bromide	Indandione anticoagulants	Salicylates (large doses)
Chloramphenicol	Iodide	

Potentially Hazardous

Acebutolol	Doxepin	Nicotine/smoking
Alcohol	Ergotamine	Nitrofurantoin
Antihistamine/decongestant	Ethosuximide	Phenobarbital
Atenolol	Fluorescein	Piroxicam
Benzodiazepines	Fluoxetine	Quinolone antibacterials
Chlorthalidone	Lindane	Reserpine
Clindamycin	Lithium	Sotalol
Clonidine	Methimazole	Sulfonamides
Contraceptives	Narcotics	Thiazide diuretics

Probably Safe in Usual Doses

ACE inhibitors	Decongestants, oral	Quinidine
Aminoglycosides	Ergonovine	Salicylates
Anticholinergic agents	Fluconazole	Spironolactone
Anticonvulsants	Histamine H_2-receptor antagonists	Sulfisoxazole
Antihistamines	Metoclopramide	Terfenadine
Antitubercular agents	Nonsteroidal anti-inflammatory agents	Thiazide diuretics (short-acting, low-dose)
Azathiopine	Oxazepam	Tricyclic antidepressants
Barbiturates (*except* phenobarbital)	Phenothiazines	Verapamil
Butyrophenones (haloperidol)	Prophylthiouracil	

Safe in Usual Doses

Acetaminophen	Flurbiprofen	Methylergonovine
Antacids	Heparin	Metoprolol
Caffeine	Inhalers, bronchodilators, corticosteroids	Miconazole
Cephalosporins		Penicillins
Clotrimazole	Insulin	Propranolol
Contraceptives, progestin-only	Labetalol	Theophylline
Corticosteroids	Laxatives	Thyroid replacement
Decongestant nasal sprays	Lidocaine	Vaccines
Digoxin	Magnesium sulfate	Vancomycin
Erythromycin	Methyldopa	Warfarin

Source: Reproduced with permission. Powers NG, Slusser W. Breastfeeding update 2: clinical lactation management. Pediatrics in Review 1997;18:147–159.

illness and one is known to be safe in lactation, then that agent should be selected.

CONTRAINDICATIONS TO BREAST-FEEDING

Few absolute contraindications to breast-feeding exist. Women who are on chemotherapy for cancer should not breast-feed because of the deleterious effects of these agents on newborns. If radiopharmaceuticals are given to the mother, breast-feeding should be terminated until they have been cleared from the maternal system. Illicit drug use should be discussed with the patient and avoided when breast-feeding. Maternal infection with human immunodeficiency virus is a contraindication to breast-feeding, as are active tuberculosis and active herpes simplex virus lesions on the breast. Active infection with hepatitis C has not been shown to be spread through breast milk, and therefore is not a contraindication according to the 1997 Centers for Disease Control guidelines.

If the mother chooses not to breast-feed or has one of the previously mentioned contraindications to breast-feeding, the breasts will involute rapidly, particularly if there has been no suckling to stimulate prolactin secretion. Binding the breasts or application of cold compresses may help with the discomfort of breast engorgement. Bromocriptine, which inhibits prolactin secretion, is no longer recommended to suppress lactation, as many women historically would experience a rebound engorgement after stopping the medication. In addition, bromocriptine is associated with significant side effects in about one-fourth of patients.

SUMMARY

Breast-feeding is nature's way of nourishing the newborn infant. Physicians should encourage this practice due to its proven benefits in terms of improved maternal–infant bonding and decreased infectious and autoimmune diseases in the infant. Many of these benefits will be lifelong.

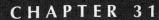

CHAPTER 31

Post-partum Infection

Alexander F. Burnett

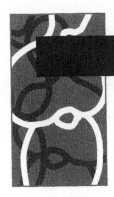

nfections are a significant morbidity occurring in the post-partum period, affecting approximately 5% of all deliveries. The most common infection—endomyometritis—is an infection of the uterus and is usually polymicrobial in origin. This chapter details the signs and symptoms of post-partum infections, describes risk factors for infections, and discusses appropriate therapy for common post-partum infections. The newborn must always be kept in mind with a post-partum infection, as the neonate may be affected during its passage through the birth canal.

DIAGNOSIS OF POST-PARTUM INFECTION

CLINICAL CORRELATION

T. C. is a 24-year-old female, gravida 1, para 1, who delivered 36 hours previously via cesarean section. The indication for cesarean delivery was relative cephalopelvic disproportion with the cervix unchanged at 6 cm dilation despite adequate labor for 14 hours. T. C. delivered a male infant with a weight of 3400 g and Apgar scores of 8 at one minute and 9 at five minutes. Her first temperature elevation occurred 6 hours ago and was 38 °C. Currently, her temperature is 38.6 °C and she feels generalized malaise and feverish.

ENDOMYOMETRITIS

Post-partum fever is defined as two temperatures greater than or equal to 38 °C at least 6 hours apart, occurring between the first and tenth post-partum days. The most common cause is endomyometritis (uterine infection), which occurs after approximately 2% of vaginal deliveries but with a several-fold higher incidence after cesarean deliveries. It is generally a polymicrobial infection, usually involving a combination of aerobic streptococci, anaerobic gram-positive cocci, and aerobic and anaerobic gram-negative bacilli. In most circumstances, endomyometritis is an ascending infection that reflects vaginal flora. When the fever occurs in the first 24 to 48 hours postpartum, group B streptococci must be considered and the neonatalogists made aware of this development so that they can evaluate the newborn.

Risk factors for endomyometritis include cesarean delivery, lengthy duration of ruptured membranes, prolonged labor, low socioeconomic status, and multiple vaginal examinations. Of these considerations, cesarean delivery is the single most important risk factor for infection.

A thorough evaluation of the patient should be performed in an effort to identify the source of infection. A very crude pneumonic is "Wind, Water, Wound, Walking, Wonder drug." Briefly, early temperatures are often related to the lungs (Wind), including atelectasis and pneumonias. In addition, early infections of the urine are common (Water). At three to five days after delivery, fevers may be related to Wound infections. At five to seven days post-partum, temperature elevations may be caused by septic thrombophlebitis (Walking). Finally, after more than one week post-partum, fevers should make one consider drug therapy (Wonder drug) as a possible cause if no other source is evident. This list is very crude, of course, and any type of infection may occur at any time post-partum.

CLINICAL CORRELATION

T. S. is evaluated in her hospital bed. Her current temperature is 38.4 °C, BP = 110/70, P = 105, and R = 16. Her lungs are clear to auscultation and percussion. Her cardiac examination reveals tachycardia without murmurs. There is no costovertebral angle tenderness. A breast examination reveals full, lactating breasts without tenderness or engorgement. An abdominal examination reveals a uterus that is involuting well but tender to moderate palpation. A pfannenstiehl incision has staples in place, and there is no discharge, erythema, or marked tenderness at the wound. The extremities are without edema, cords, or tenderness. Bilateral Homan's sign is negative. A speculum examination reveals a foul-smelling discharge that is purulent from the cervical os; cultures are taken of the discharge. A bimanual examination reveals moderate uterine tenderness without adnexal tenderness. T. S.'s WBC is 14,000/cm³, her hematocrit is 34%, and her platelet count is 154,000/cm³. The differential has a marked left shift with 70% segs and 20% bands. Blood cultures and urine cultures are sent to the lab.

Besides temperature elevation and tenderness, post-partum endomyometritis is often accompanied by a foul vaginal discharge. Cultures are taken as high up into the uterus as possible to avoid vaginal canal contamination. As mentioned previously, most cultures will test positive for multiple organisms, most of which reside normally in the vagina. If group B streptococci infection is suspected, the discharge can be sent for Gram stain, latex agglutination testing, and/or enzyme immunoassay for this organism. A culture of the discharge may prove very helpful in the patient who is not rapidly defervescing, as sensitivities of the found organisms may dictate a change in antibiotic coverage. Occasionally, manual dilation of the cervix is performed to assure adequate passage of the infected contents from the uterus; if the cervix has dilated in labor, this step is generally unnecessary. Blood and urine cultures should be obtained, along with sputum cultures if the patient has a productive cough.

OTHER POST-PARTUM INFECTIONS

Other infections besides endomyometritis that may particularly affect the post-partum woman include breast engorgement and mastitis.

Breast engorgement can be accompanied by high temperature elevations and discomfort of the breasts that are clearly engorged with milk. Milk stasis and engorgement cause an inflammatory response, but typically few white blood cells (WBCs) will be present in the milk expressed from the breasts. Engorgement may lead to infection after about one week post-partum.

Mastitis more frequently occurs in women who are actively breast-feeding. This problem often presents with fevers, pain, and erythema, usually of one breast. The milk should be cultured and the patient begun on antibiotics. It is important for the mother to continue breast-feeding during antibiotic treatment to promote breast emptying and to pass the antibiotic on to treat the mouth of the newborn. Typical offending organisms include *Staphylococcus aureus*, coagulase-negative staphylococci, *Streptococcus* species, and *Escherichia coli*.

TREATMENT OF POST-PARTUM INFECTION

When endomyometritis is established on the basis of clinical signs and symptoms, antibiotic therapy is begun. The typical regimen—which covers the majority of aerobic and anaerobic bacteria responsible for this infection—consists of gentamicin and clindamycin. When the patient defervesces quickly, antibiotics should be continued for 10 to 14 days, switching to oral antibiotics after the patient has gone 48 hours without a fever. If no improvement occurs within 24 to 36 hours, a penicillin may be added to act against enterococcus. If the patient remains febrile at 48 to 72 hours, she should be reevaluated and recultured to look for an alternative source of infection.

Pelvic abscess, which represents a walled-off infection with poor penetration of antibiotics, should be considered. Mastitis and wound infections should also be ruled out.

Wound infections will have erythema and tenderness around the incision. Although opening the wound will often be curative, occasionally antibiotics may be prescribed. The wound should be probed to ensure that the fascial layer is intact. The opened wound can be packed with wet-to-dry dressings and debrided if necessary. Once clean, granulation tissue covers the entire wound, the incision may be reclosed or allowed to close by secondary intent.

A rare, but serious variant of wound infection occurs when an infection of the fascia leads to necrosis—the so-called necrotizing fasciitis. This surgical emergency requires prompt operating room debridement of all affected tissue. In many cases, patients will require grafting to close the large surgical defects created, once they have recovered from the infection. The offending organism is either *Clostridia perfringens* or group A streptococci (although polymicrobial infections may also be present). These pathogens can be differentiated by Gram stain. Gas gangrene with crepitus evident in the area of discoloration is associated with the *Clostridia* species. Both organisms respond to high-dose penicillin with aggressive debridement. Mortality from this condition is high if surgical debridement is not performed quickly.

Infection of an episiotomy site is rare, occurring after only 0.5% of all deliveries. Its signs and symptoms include erythema, edema, and exudate over the episiotomy site and pain in this region disproportionate to that expected. Treatment is generally opening and draining the area, with antibiotics rarely necessary.

CLINICAL CORRELATION

T. S. is begun on gentamicin and clindamycin intravenous antibiotics, with serum testing of gentamicin levels taking place with the fifth dose. She rapidly defervesces over 12 hours and experiences clinical improvement with rapid diminishment of uterine pain. After 48 hours without a fever, she is discharged from the hospital. No additional oral antibiotics are given.

SEPTIC PELVIC THROMBOPHLEBITIS

CLINICAL CORRELATION

P. L. is a 39-year-old female, gravida 3, para 3. It is four days after she underwent a repeat cesarean delivery of a healthy term infant after a 26-hour trial of labor. She has had daily temperature elevations, initially to 38 °C and most recently to 39 °C on post-partum day 4; the elevations occurred despite beginning gentamicin and clindamycin on post-operative day 2 and adding ampicillin on post-operative day 3. Blood cultures from the first two temperature spikes are negative to date. Her WBC is 12,000/cm³. Urine cultures have been negative, and P. L. has not had a productive cough. A chest X ray done on post-partum day 3 was negative for infiltrates or pneumonia. She has no costo-vertebral angle tenderness. Her abdomen is soft and nontender, and there is minimal uterine tenderness. She has negative Homan's signs bilaterally. A pelvic examination fails to suggest a fluid collection. Because of the pattern of the temperature spikes and the failure to respond to antibiotics, a CT scan is performed of the abdomen and pelvis. The examination shows no abscess collection, but there are thromboses of the pelvic veins bilaterally.

An unusual cause of post-partum fevers that are unresponsive to antibiotics is septic pelvic thrombophlebitis. Risk factors for this problem include prolonged labor, malnourishment, anemia, or prolonged rupture of membranes.

Diagnosis is generally made by exclusion after typically infectious etiologies have been ruled out. A CT scan can be helpful in diagnosing thrombi in the pelvic vessels. The patient is begun on heparin (anticoagulation) therapy, and the diagnosis is confirmed when the fevers resolve within 48 to 72 hours. Heparin is usually continued for 7 to 10 days after the patient is afebrile.

CLINICAL CORRELATION

P. L. is administered a bolus of 10,000 units of heparin intravenously and begins receiving a continuous infusion of 1000 units per hour. The APTT is maintained at two times the normal level. P. L.'s fevers resolve completely within 24 hours. She continues taking heparin for seven days and is discharged from the hospital with no further complications.

SUMMARY

Post-partum infection occurs more commonly after cesarean deliveries than vaginal deliveries. Risk factors for endomyometritis include prolonged labor with prolonged rupture of membranes, multiple examinations, and certain characteristics related to the patient's physical well-being at the time of labor and delivery. Prompt attention to fevers with a complete physical examination will often localize the source of infection. Certain infections, including necrotizing fasciitis, are life-threatening and demand immediate surgical debridement. The diagnosis of septic pelvic thrombophlebitis is based on a woman's lack of response to antibiotics without an identifiable source of temperatures. All post-partum infections require notification of the neonatal staff to assess the newborn for possible infection.

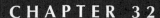

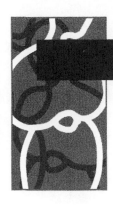

CHAPTER 32

Managing Hemorrhaging Complications in Obstetrics and Gynecology

Luis E. Sanz

I t is important when treating the hemorrhaging patient to consider preservation of life first, and retention of fertility second. The events most frequently associated with bleeding in obstetric patients are uterine atony, ectopic pregnancy, abortions, and lacerations. In the post-partum patient, hemorrhagic shock may be a sequelae infarction of the anterior pituitary (Sheehan syndrome), which may have later endocrinologic manifestations. In gynecologic patients, myomectomies, vaginal surgery, and cancer surgery are the most common causes of bleeding (Table 32.1).

INITIAL MANAGEMENT

It is important to adopt a step-by-step approach in managing the bleeding surgical patient. One should always try the most conservative and least invasive means first so as to avoid major surgical complications. Nonsurgical treatments include fluid and blood replacement, drug therapy, angiography, and selective embolization.

CLINICAL CORRELATION

A 24-year-old G1P1 continues to bleed profusely after removal of the placenta following a vaginal delivery. She had been in a prodromal labor pattern for several days and had experienced regular, strong uterine contractions for 32 hours prior to delivery. The term delivery resulted in the birth of an 8 lb, 6 oz male infant with Apgar scores of 7 at one minute and 9 at five minutes. The third stage of labor lasted eight minutes. Vigorous uterine massage and intravenous Pitocin are effective in stopping the substantial bleeding.

This scenario is consistent with uterine atony, or the inability of the uterus to adequately contract after delivery. This rapid involution of the uterus mechanically constricts the vessels in the endometrium to enable blood flow to cease. Initial attempts to stop post-partum bleeding should include uterine massage to encourage involution. Drug therapy may include oxytocin (Pitocin), methylergonovine maleate (Methergine), or prostaglandins. When necessary, concomitant use of fluid and blood replacement is essential. If these nonsurgical approaches fail to halt the bleeding, angiographic arterial embolization, if available, or surgical intervention should be undertaken quickly before the amount of blood lost results in disseminated intravascular coagulopathy (DIC), which may make it impossible to control the hemorrhage.

SELECTING THE APPROPRIATE SURGICAL PROCEDURE

The choice of the most appropriate surgical procedure depends on the type of injury and the patient's condition and parity. For instance, in an older woman who has given birth

Table 32.1   Conditions That Predispose to or Worsen Obstetrical Hemorrhage

Abnormal placentation
  Placental previa
  Abruption placentae
  Placenta accreta
  Ectopic pregnancy
  Hydatidiform mole
Trauma during labor and delivery
  Episiotomy
  Complicated vaginal delivery
  Low- or midforceps delivery
Small maternal blood volume
  Small woman
  Pregnancy hypervolemia constricted
    Severe pre-eclampsia
    Eclampsia

Uterine atony
  Overdistended uterus
    Large fetus
    Multiple fetuses
    Hydramnios
  Anesthesia or analgesia
  Exhausted myometrium
    Rapid labor
    Prolonged labor
    Oxytocin or prostaglandin stimulation
  Chorioamnionitis
Coagulation defects—intensify other causes
  Placental abruption
  Prolonged retention of dead fetus
  Amnionic fluid embolism
  Severe intravascular hemolysis
  Massive transfusions
  Severe pre-eclampsia and eclampsia
  Congenital coagulopathies
  Anticoagulant treatment

Source: Adapted from Cunningham FG, et al. Williams obstetrics, 19th ed. Norwalk, CT: Appleton & Lange, 1993:820.

to several children and has no desire for future pregnancies, a hysterectomy may stop the bleeding in a more controlled and expeditious manner than hypogastric artery ligation, particularly if one is inexperienced in the latter procedure. On exploration of the abdomen, if an obvious single vessel is identified as the bleeding culprit, isolation and ligation of that vessel would be the appropriate therapy.

A generalized venous bleeding or oozing can often be controlled by applying direct pressure for five to ten minutes. In this situation, it may be helpful to apply a hemostatic agent such as fibrillar collagen before applying pressure to promote local clotting. Another method that is often helpful in the venous oozing patient is the Argon beam coagulator (Figure 32.1), in which the radio frequency current responsible for tissue coagulation is carried through an argon beam rather than oxygen.

This technique has an advantage in that the tissue is not touched directly by the instrument and a more even distribution of the coagulation is possible. This device also produces less thermal injury, which permits its use on the surface of the intestines or major vessels.

ARTERIAL LIGATION

If a specific bleeding vessel is not identified, a reasonable tactic is to diminish blood flow to the uterus by ligating the arteries supplying the majority of blood to this organ (Figure 32.2). A solid appreciation for the anatomical course of the ureter is necessary to identify the hypogastric (internal iliac) or uterine arteries prior to ligating them. In the case of ligation of the uterine artery, the uterus is pushed medially away from the side that will be ligated. The ureter is identified and also retracted medially along with its overlaying peritoneum. With the

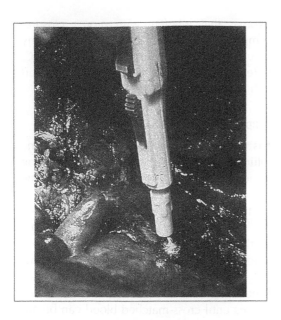

Figure 32.1 Argon beam coagulator

hypogastric artery gently pulled laterally and the ureter pulled medially, it is easy to identify where the uterine artery branches off of the hypogastric artery. The uterine vessel can be skeletonized quickly with a right-angled dissector and then either clipped or sutured. Alternatively, the hypogastric artery may be ligated by identifying the anterior division (again with the ureter in direct visualization) and placing a permanent tie around it.

Both of these techniques decrease the pulse pressure to the uterus and permit normal clotting mechanisms to more readily halt the hemorrhage. Collateral blood flow allows even bilateral hypogastric artery ligation to be performed with preservation of the uterus.

It is important to note that ligation has some potential complications. They include ligation of the external iliac artery, laceration of

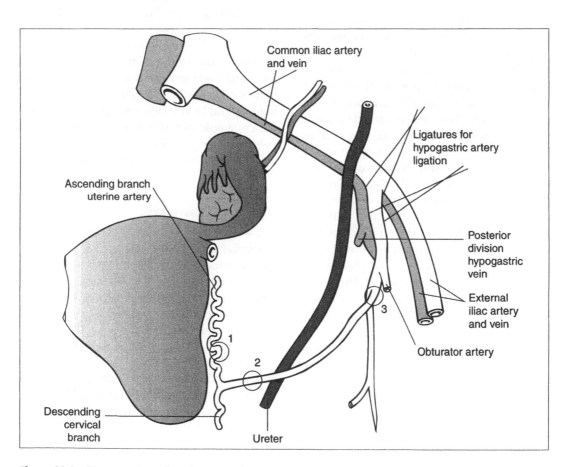

Figure 32.2 Hypogastric and uterine artery ligation

Source: Sanz L, ed. Gynecologic surgery, 2nd ed. Cambridge, MA: Blackwell Science, 1995:6.

the external or internal iliac veins, injury or ligation of the ureters, and retroperitoneal hematoma.

Although preservation of fertility is important, one should not become so committed to saving the uterus as to allow the patient's life to become endangered by massive blood loss or DIC. Continuous communication with the anesthesiologist is critical throughout the surgical procedure. The surgeon should be aware of the amount of estimated blood loss, fluid resuscitation, and blood products given during the procedure to assess the risk of DIC and fluid overload. When massive blood products and fluid are administered, the operative field may display evidence of DIC, such as diminished clotting. This fact should be communicated to the anesthesiologist, and use of other blood products—as fresh frozen plasma and platelets—should be considered. The initial surgical step in a hysterectomy involves identifying and ligating the uterine vessels at the lateral aspect of the uterus. This single step should stop the most significant uterine bleeding. In an emergency situation, a supracervical hysterectomy may be the most expedient way to complete the surgery.

The decision to perform a hysterectomy is more commonly made when the patient has an obstetric condition such as an unresponsive uterine atony, placenta accreta, molar gestation, uterine rupture, extension of uterine incisions with laceration of major vessels, and myomas that interfere with proper closure. Complications of post-partum hysterectomy include infection, a need for transfusion, DIC, ureteral injury, and maternal death associated with massive hemorrhage.

FLUID AND BLOOD REPLACEMENT

It is critical to maintain the patient's plasma volume and oxygen-carrying capacity during an acute bleeding episode. Although volume expansion can be maintained with crystalloid solution, colloids—specifically blood—remain the best solutions for reestablishing the patient's oxygen-carrying capacity. In an emergency situation, whole blood is the product that is most readily available. Rh-negative, O-negative blood is used in life-threatening situations until cross-matched blood can be obtained. In the setting where blood loss is anticipated and evolving over time, packed red blood cells give the highest concentration of red cells per transfusion.

Several different approaches are available for transfusion in the anticipated surgical event, including autologous donation, donor-directed donation, experimental artificial blood, and homologous blood. Depending on the circumstance, autologous blood transfusion may involve preoperative donation or intraoperative or perioperative autotransfusion (Table 32.2).

Preoperative autologous donations can be made as long as five to six weeks prior to elec-

Table 32.2 Blood Component Therapy

PRODUCT	VOLUME	CONTENT	INDICATION	CLINICAL RESPONSE
Red blood cells			To increase oxygen-carrying capacity in anemic women, for hypotension secondary to blood loss	Increase hemoglobin 10 g/L and hematocrit 3%
Whole blood	450 mL	RBCs and plasma		
Packed RBCs	180–200 mL	RBCs with minimal plasma		
Platelets	50–70 mL	$5.5 \times 10^{10}/$ RD unit	To control or prevent bleeding associated with deficiencies in platelet number or function	Increase platelet count 5000–10,000/μL
	200–400 mL	$>3.0 \times 10^{11}/$ SDAP product		Increase platelet count $\geq 10 \times 10^9/$L within 1 hr and $\geq 7.5 \times 10^9/$L 24 hr post-transfusion
Fresh frozen plasma	200–250 mL	Plasma proteins: coagulation factors, proteins C and S, antithrombin	To increase the level of clotting factors in patients with demonstrated deficiency	Increases coagulation factors about 2%
Cryoprecipitate	10–15 mL	Cold-insoluble plasma proteins, fibrinogen, factor VIII, vWF	To increase factors in those with a deficiency of fibrinogen, factor VIII, factor XIII, fibronectin, or von Willebrand factor	

tive surgery. A healthy patient can donate as many as five units of blood during that period but must take iron replacement simultaneously. More units can be donated by the patient over a longer period of time if the blood is frozen.

In intraoperative autotransfusion, blood is aspirated from the noncontaminated field and the red cells are washed in a high-speed ultracentrifuge. The red cells are then combined with normal saline and transfused back into the patient.

Perioperative autotransfusion involves the removal of two units of blood a few hours prior to surgery; those units are stored for transfusion during the elective procedure. This method provides an intravascular hemodilution that diminishes the red cell loss during surgery.

Research continues in the quest to create an artificial red blood cell substitute to eliminate the risks of heterologous transfusions.

ANGIOGRAPHIC EMBOLIZATION

Angiography can be a valuable method of identifying and controlling excessive bleeding in the preoperative or post-operative setting. Bleeding in the pelvis is identified using angiography, with catheters typically being introduced from the contralateral femoral vessels. Under fluoroscopy, dye is injected intravascularly to identify the source of bleeding. Once the particular vessel is located, embolization can be performed with a variety of materials, including steel coils and pellets of gelatin sponge (Figure 32.3). Rapid arterial flow prevents reflux embolization of the proximal vessels. For gynecology, the hypogastric and uterine vessels are the most common targets for embolization.

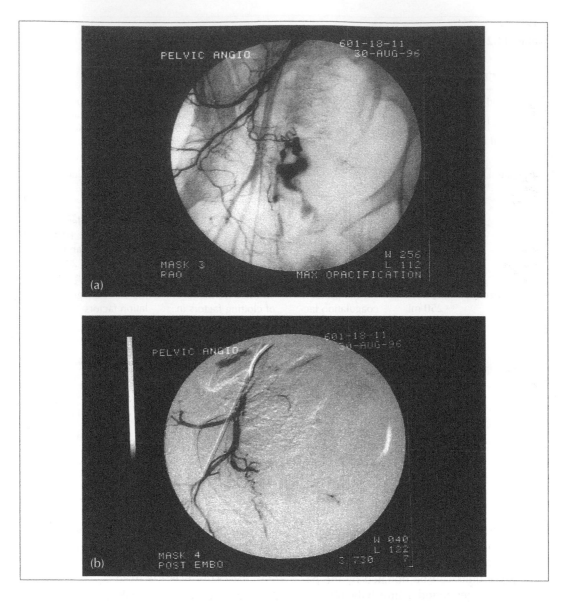

Figure 32.3   (a) Arteriogram demonstrating bleeding from a branch of the hypogastric artery. (b) Arteriogram on the same patient after embolization of a branch of the hypogastric artery.

The morbidity from such procedures is generally minimal. Most complications occur in patients who have significant artherosclerotic vascular disease. The most significant complication from embolization is accidental vessel rupture.

SUMMARY

The most conservative and least invasive procedures to control bleeding should be tried first, depending on the patient's hemodynamic stability. The judicious and rapid use of fluids, oxygen, blood, and blood components while pursuing procedures to control the bleeding are critical to support the patient through the insult.

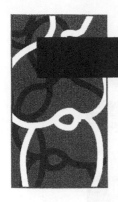

CHAPTER 33

Fetal and Maternal Death

Jean-Gilles Tchabo

FETAL DEATH

The definition of fetal death varies from country to country. Even within the same country, this definition may vary from state to state. These variations are important when one attempts to compare fetal mortality statistics.

The World Health Organization (WHO) defines fetal death as "death prior to the complete expulsion or extraction from its mother, of a product of conception, irrespective of the duration of pregnancy." The death is indicated by the fact that after such separation the fetus does not breathe or show any other evidence of life, such as beating of the heart, pulsation of the umbilical cord, or definite movement of voluntary muscles. Fetal death is further classified as early (less than 20 weeks gestation), intermediate (20 to 27 weeks gestation), and late (28 weeks to term). The fetal death rate is defined as the number of stillborn (born without signs of life) infants per 1000 infants born. The neonatal mortality rate is the number of deaths in the first 28 days of life per 1000 live births. The perinatal mortality combines the number of stillbirths with the number of neonatal deaths per 1000 total births.

The National Center for Health Statistics recognizes fetal death as a death that occurs after 20 weeks pregnancy. Fetal loss before 20 weeks gestation or fetal weight of less than 500 g is defined as abortion. The incidence of fetal death in the United States is 9 per 1000 live births and is decreasing steadily.

It is important to identify the causes of fetal death if at all possible for the following reasons:

- To help the parents understand what led to the demise of their fetus and to alleviate self-imposed guilt.
- To counsel the parents appropriately.
- To manage subsequent pregnancies.

Table 33.1 details the many causes associated with fetal death. The relative frequency of fetal death varies by geographic location. Chromosomal anomalies are present in 70% to 80% of all early gestation fetal losses.

Physical signs of the mother that may be helpful in diagnosing fetal death include decrease or cessation of nausea or breast tenderness in early gestation, or lack or cessation of fetal movement. On physical examination, the lack of uterine growth on serial examinations by the same examiner, and the inability to detect the fetal heart by auscultation at certain weeks in gestation, are suggestive of fetal death. Certain laboratory data, although not very specific, are suggestive and at times confirm fetal death—for example, decreased serial hCG measurements in early pregnancy.

With real-time sonography, a diagnosis can be made with certainty by an experienced sonographer. Fetal heart motion can be seen at seven to eight weeks gestation on abdominal sonogram and even earlier using vaginal probes. Ultrasound not only will confirm the diagnosis but may also determine the etiology by highlighting congenital anomalies, confirming single or multiple gestation, assessing

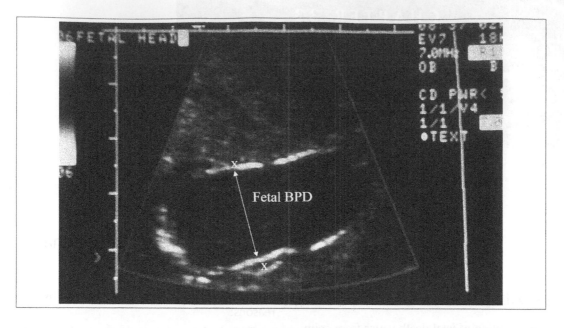

Figure 33.1   Sonogram demonstrating a fetal death in utero. The fetal head has collapsed as demonstrated at the level of the biparietal diameter. A viable biparietal diameter is shown in Figure 6.2.

the fetal age, and examining the intrauterine environment. Common radiographic findings consistent with fetal demise include the Halo sign (scalp edema overlapping the fetal cranial bones), Spalding's sign (abnormal angulation of the fetal spine), and Robert's sign (intravascular gas within the fetus) (Figure 33.1). A thorough maternal history should be taken to eliminate or confirm infectious, immunologic, maternal, or other causes, as outlined in Table 33.1.

At delivery, the fetus, placenta, and membranes should undergo a pathologic evaluation. If any congenital deformity or dysmorphism is present, an X ray of the fetus and a Polaroid picture should be taken for later evaluation by a geneticist. A karyotype should be obtained and infectious causes should be determined.

MANAGEMENT OF FETAL DEATH

As soon as a diagnosis of fetal death has been made by a physician and accepted by the parents, the choice of expectant versus aggressive management must be made. Emotionally, many parents will not tolerate expectant management. In addition, expectant management

may place the mother's health in danger because of fetal death syndrome. The majority of women will go into labor spontaneously within two weeks of fetal death, and fetal death syndrome rarely occurs within four weeks after fetal death. With this syndrome, maternal coagulopathy develops about four weeks after the fetal death. The evolution of the syndrome is gradual, with laboratory tests showing altered levels of hypofibrinogenemia, decreased plasminogen, decreased antithrombin III activity, increased fibrinopeptide A and fibrin split products, and thrombocytopenia. If expectant management is undertaken, assessments of these laboratory results should be done weekly.

The true etiology of the coagulopathy associated with fetal death syndrome has been postulated to be due to tissue thromboplastin release from the decaying fetus, which then leaks into the maternal circulation. The treatment consists of delivery of the dead fetus as soon as possible and supportive therapy of the coagulopathy, such as infusion of fresh frozen plasma, cryoprecipitate, platelets, and blood as needed.

METHODS OF UTERINE EVACUATION

Surgical techniques for aggressive management of fetal death include dilation and evacu-

Table 33.1   Conditions Associated with Fetal Death

Chromosomal

  Autosomal trisomies (e.g., trisomy 13, 18, and 21)

  X-chromosome monosomy

  Triploid and tetrapoid

  Structural abnormalities

    Robertsonian translocation

    Unbalanced reciprocal translocations

Congenital malformations

  CNS abnormalities

    Neural tube defects

    Hydrocephalus

  Cardiac

    Structural defects

    Arrhythmias

  Abdominal wall defects

    Omphalocele

    Gastroschisis

  Genitourinary

    Bilateral renal agenesis

    Obstructive uropathy (posterior urethral valves)

    Infantile polycystic kidney disease

  Skeletal abnormalities

    Dwarfism

    Arthrogryposis

Infectious causes

  Bacterial

    Group B streptococci

    Listeria monocytogenes

    Ascending infection secondary to rupture of membranes

  Mycotic

    Candida albicans

    Coccidiomycosis

  Parasitic infections

    Malaria

    Chaga's disease (*Trypanosoma cruzi*)

    Toxoplasmosis

Viral

  Cytomegalovirus

  Rubella

  Mumps

  Coxsackie B3

  Parvovirus

  Herpes simplex virus

  Syphilis

Immunologic causes

  Isoimmune-mediated

    Anti-D isoimmunization

    Others (anti-kell, anti-Duffy, anti-C, anti-E, and so on)

  Autoimmune

  Systemic lupus erythematosus

  Antiphospholipid antibodies

    Lupus anticoagulant

    Anticardiolipin antibodies

  Anti-SSA antibodies (causing heart block)

Maternal conditions

  Diabetes

  Hypertension

  Trauma (fetomaternal hemorrhage)

  Drug abuse

Placental/umbilical cord

  Placental abruption/infarction

  Placenta previa

  Umbilical cord knots/strictures

  Cord entanglement

  Cord hemangiomas

  Cord prolapse

Other fetal causes

  Intrauterine growth retardation

  Postmaturity

ation of the uterus in early gestation. Experienced and skilled practitioners can use these techniques even in the second trimester. Laminaries can be used to dilate the cervix prior to evacuation. Complications of evacuation of the fetus include cervical laceration and subsequent development of cervical incompetence, uterine perforation, hemorrhage, retained products of conception, infection, and maternal death. The use of ultrasound or contact hysteroscopy when evacuating the uterus in the second or late second trimester will significantly decrease the incidence of uterine perforation or incomplete abortion.

The specimens obtained through these surgical techniques will be in many pieces, making pathologic assessment difficult. In addition, parents may not be able to hold the specimen or take a picture of it, hindering the grieving process.

Hysterotomy, hysterectomy, and laparotomy are rarely indicated. The exceptions involve patients with placenta previa or coexisting gynecological conditions such as cervical carcinoma, cervical myoma obstructing the canal, ovarian malignancy, and abdominal pregnancy.

MEDICAL TECHNIQUES

Labor can be induced by administration of either Pitocin or prostaglandin given by any of several routes, such as intra-amniotic, intrauterine, intracervical, intravenous, intrafetal, oral, or intramuscular. Prostaglandins commonly used include F_2-alpha and E_2. Intra-amniotic injection of urea or saline or prostaglandin, although effective, is discouraged because of the potential for adverse reactions. Potential complications of medical labor induction include uterine rupture, cervical laceration, retained products of conception, hemorrhage, and infection. During induction of labor, the patient should be kept comfortable by repetitive doses of pain medication and treatment of the side effects of the method of induction.

FETAL DEATH IN MULTIPLE GESTATIONS

Fetal death in multiple gestations is rare, having an incidence of 0.5% to 1% of twin gestations. It is more common in monochorionic twins. Management should take into account when in the gestation the fetal death occurs. If it happens close to term, delivery should be accomplished promptly. If it is remote from term, the physician must balance the risk of prematurity of the surviving fetus against the risk of maternal fetal death syndrome. If expectant management is the choice, the patient should receive regular and frequent monitoring by coagulation profile, sonogram, and nonstress testing on the surviving twin.

The surviving fetus may be exposed to the same condition that caused the death of the sibling. If this condition is treatable, it should be corrected promptly. If a monochorionic placentation is present, the risk of intrauterine disseminated intravascular coagulation (DIC) and the surviving twin embolization syndrome is greatly increased. When vascular anastamoses occur within a monochorial placenta, the shared circulation may permit embolization of thromboplastic material from the dead fetus to the living twin. This transfer may promote intrauterine DIC, cortical necrosis, multicystic encephalomalacia, and other structural abnormalities of the surviving twin, even though the mother may suffer no sequelae of DIC.

THE EMOTIONAL IMPACT OF FETAL DEATH

The diagnosis of fetal death puts patients in a state of shock and disbelief. The grief process sometimes starts before the patient comes to the office. A physician should be sensitive, attentive, compassionate, and a good listener and should facilitate—not obstruct—the bereavement process. Although many hospitals have developed protocols for dealing with the grieving process, a physician should be in the forefront and should be able to recognize the signs of pathologic grief and to seek consultation for the patient.

As soon as the patient is stabilized, the delivery should be undertaken. After delivery, the grieving protocol should be followed. The evaluation of the fetus, placenta, and membranes should be discussed openly with the parents. After discharge, regular and frequent contacts should be maintained with the parents and all of their questions should be answered thoroughly. The grieving process may take 6 to 18 months. Patients should be encouraged to complete their grieving prior to the next pregnancy. During the next pregnancy, the patient should be followed closely for signs of anxiety or ambivalence.

MATERNAL DEATH

Maternal death is the death of any woman from a pregnancy-related cause while pregnant or within six weeks of pregnancy termination. A direct maternal death is one due to complications of pregnancy, labor, or puerperium. An indirect maternal death is one due to a nonobstetrical cause that is aggravated by the physiologic effects of pregnancy. A nonmaternal death is death of a pregnant woman from accidental or incidental causes unrelated to the pregnancy itself. The maternal mortality rate is the number of maternal deaths (direct, indirect, or nonmaternal) per 100,000 women of reproductive age. More commonly, it is referred to as the maternal mortality ratio—that is, the number of deaths per 100,000 live births. The deaths may be associated with term pregnancies, abortions, miscarriages, or ectopic pregnancies. Worldwide, only about 1% of maternal deaths occur in developed countries.

The most common cause of maternal mortality in the United States is hemorrhage, which accounts for more than one-fourth of all maternal deaths (Table 33.2). Approximately 35% of hemorrhage-related maternal deaths are due to ruptured ectopic gestations, with most of the remainder attributable to uterine rupture, problems of placentation, DIC, or unspecified uterine bleeding. Thromboembolic phenomena account for approximately 20% of maternal deaths. The majority of these conditions involve pulmonary emboli. Pregnancy is a hypercoagulable state, marked by increases in circulating clotting factors and increased venous stasis due to uterine compression on the inferior vena cava and pelvic vessels. Pregnancy-induced hypertension accounts for some 17% of maternal deaths, followed by infections (13%), cardiomyopathy (5%), and anesthetic complications (2.5%).

Maternal mortality increases with increasing maternal age and with increasing live-birth order. Women who have achieved five or more previous live deliveries have more than double the mortality rates of women on their first gestation. For all age and parity groups, African Americans had roughly three times the maternal mortality rates as Caucasians in the United States from 1987 to 1990. Abortions, including induced (legal and illegal) and spontaneous, preceded approximately 5% of the deaths related to pregnancy, with nearly half of these due to infections.

Table 33.2 Causes of Pregnancy-Related Death by Outcome of Pregnancy, United States, 1987–1990

	LIVE BIRTHS	STILLBIRTH	ECTOPIC	ABORTION	OTHER	TOTAL
Hemorrhage	168	28	148	15	58	417
Embolism	185	11	2	9	79	286
Pregnancy-induced hypertension	190	27	0	1	38	256
Infection	97	20	2	40	32	191
Cardiomyopathy	48	3	0	0	31	82
Anesthetic	22	0	3	7	4	36
Other	87	14	1	9	74	185
Total deaths	797	103	156	81	316	1453

Source: Adapted from Berg CJ, Atrash HK, Koonin LM, Tucker M. Pregnancy-related mortality in the United States, 1987–1990. Obstet Gynecol 1996;88:161–167.

SUMMARY

Maternal mortality is rare in the United States and is generally related to hemorrhage, infection, thromboembolism, or hypertension associated with the gestation. It may occur concomitant with any type of gestation, including abortion or ectopic pregnancy. Fetal mortality is attributable to myriad causes, with chromosomal abnormalities being associated with a high percentage of first trimester losses. Later in pregnancy, infections, hemorrhage, placental accidents, and prematurity are the most common causes of fetal and neonatal demise.

PART IV

Reproductive Endocrinology and Infertility

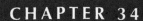

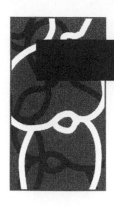

CHAPTER 34

Puberty, Menstrual Cycle, and Reproductive Physiology

Preston C. Sacks

Puberty occurs because of the maturation of the hypothalamic–pituitary–gonadal axis to the adult state of hormonal production. This slow, concerted development is marked by the characteristic advent of secondary sexual characteristics, ultimately making the female reproductively mature. At this point in life, the ovarian follicles, which have been quiescent prior to birth, begin to produce mature ovum on a regular basis so that fertilization may occur. A complicated orchestration of many factors of the axis is responsible for this maturation.

STAGES OF PUBERTY

Puberty involves several stages of development, including adrenarche, gonadarche (including the thelarche and pubarche), and menarche.

ADRENARCHE

Adrenarche, or the maturation of the adrenal gland, initiates puberty. On average, it occurs between ages 6 and 8 in girls in the United States. The adrenal gland regenerates during this time, and production of dihydroepiandrostenedione sulfate (DHEA-S), DHEA, and androstenedione increases until girls reach ages 13 to 15. Adrenarche may play a role in sensitizing the axis to gonadotropin stimulation.

GONADARCHE

Initially, increased gonadotropin-releasing hormone (GnRH) levels occur during sleep.

Levels of luteinizing hormone (LH) and follicle-stimulating hormone (FSH) also begin to rise during sleep; initially, however, they remain at prepubertal levels during waking hours. Increases in gonadotropin begin to appear at about ages 8 to 10, resulting in the beginning rises in serum estradiol.

The development of the breast bud (the start of thelarche) begins at approximately age 11 as a result of estradiol stimulation; it represents the first phenotypic expression of secondary sexual characteristics. Breast development has been studied extensively, and normal stages of development, termed Tanner stages, have been elucidated (Figure 34.1).

Pubarche (the onset of pubic and axillary hair) usually follows thelarche, beginning at about age 12. This hair growth is believed to result from the action of circulating androgens. Pubarche also has a characteristic pattern of development and has been staged by Tanner (Figure 34.2).

MENARCHE

The onset of menses is the culmination of the earlier events involved in puberty. Initially, anovulatory cycles are common and menses may be irregular. The average age of onset of menarche in the United States is approximately 12 to 13 years (Figure 34.3). It generally takes a year for cycles to become consistently ovulatory and regular. Menarche will be delayed until the child reaches a critical mass of roughly 105 lb. Probably the total fat content is the crucial factor, with research suggesting that

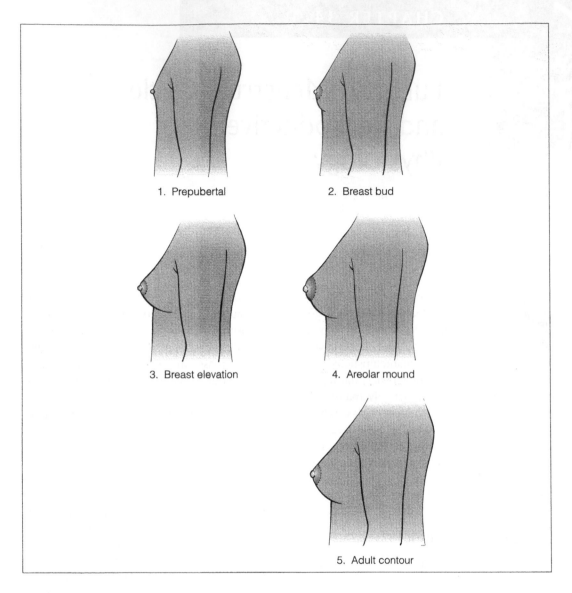

Figure 34.1   Tanner stages of breast development

Source: Callahan TL, Caughey AB, Heffner LJ. Blueprints in obstetrics and gynecology. Malden, MA: Blackwell Science, 1998:128.

a minimum of 22% body fat is required before menses will begin. Abnormalities in the onset of menses may be the first sign that the girl may have a genital abnormality.

REPRODUCTIVE PHYSIOLOGY

Reproduction involves the passage of genetic material to the next generation. The reproductive process involves many steps. Although some of these stages have been well characterized in humans, many steps have been characterized in lower animals and extrapolated to the human model. A significant number of unanswered questions remain, however. Therefore, it is helpful to review the reproductive process by enumerating some facts. Significant unanswered questions and clinical correlates are mentioned in the ensuing discussion.

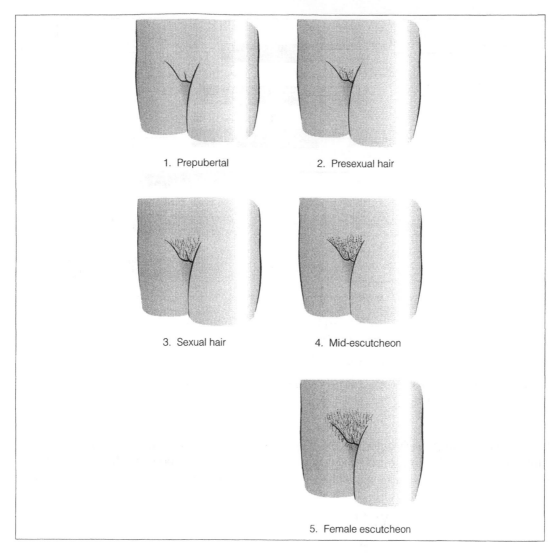

1. Prepubertal

2. Presexual hair

3. Sexual hair

4. Mid-escutcheon

5. Female escutcheon

Figure 34.2   Tanner stages of pubarche

Source: Callahan TL, Caughey AB, Heffner LJ. Blueprints in obstetrics and gynecology. Malden, MA: Blackwell Science, 1998:129.

WOMEN ARE BORN WITH ALL OF THEIR OOCYTES

Whereas men produce sperm on a daily basis, women are born with all of their oocytes. At the ninth week of gestation, the germ cells migrate from the yolk sac to the genital ridge and undergo rapid mitosis. This process continues until the twentieth week of gestation, when the number of oocytes peaks at 4 to 6 million. These oocytes have entered the first meiotic division, and their development remains arrested at this stage. In the ensuing weeks of pregnancy, rapid atresia occurs; by the time of birth, the number of oocytes has been reduced to 1 to 2 million. By puberty, further atresia reduces this number to 500,000 oocytes. During the average reproductive lifespan, 300 oocytes will reach full maturity and be ovulated. The other oocytes undergo atresia. Women therefore reach puberty with less than 10% of their initial oocytes.

When no further oocytes are present in the ovary, estradiol production falls and menopause ensues. The median age of menopause in the United States is 52 years old. Any factor that destroys or removes the oocytes completely will induce menopause, regardless of

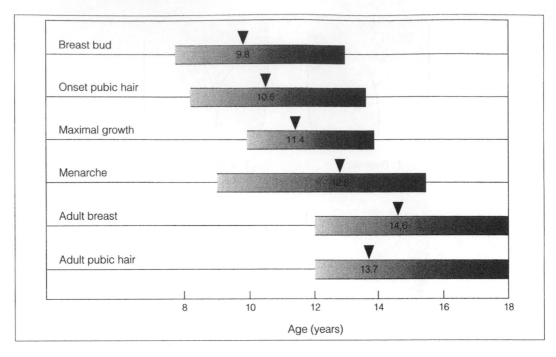

Figure 34.3 Timeline of pubertal events

Source: Callahan TL, Caughey AB, Heffner LJ. Blueprints in obstetrics and gynecology. Malden, MA: Blackwell Science, 1998:127.

the age of the woman. Such factors include the surgical removal of the ovaries and toxic exposures, such as radiation and chemotherapy.

THE MENSTRUAL CYCLE

The menstrual cycle is a coordinated series of events that occur on a regular basis and affect the sex organs of the female, with ovulation being followed by menstruation if fertilization of the ovum does not occur (Figure 34.4). The normal cycle has a duration of 28 ± 4 days, and will occur on a regular basis in a regularly ovulating female. It is divided into the follicular phase and the luteal phase. By convention, the first day of the menstrual cycle is the onset of menstrual bleeding. Ovulation in a 28-day cycle will occur about day 14.

THE FOLLICULAR PHASE

At the completion of the menstrual cycle, progesterone and estrogen withdrawal lead to the sloughing of the endometrium. This drop in estrogen levels permits a gradual rise in FSH, which in turn recruits several follicles for maturation. The developing oocyte is packaged in a

unit referred to as a follicle. The follicle consists of three main components: the oocyte, a fluid-filled space (antrum), and two types of hormone-producing cells (granulosa and theca) (Figure 34.5). The follicle exists to maintain a microenvironment suitable for protection and maturation of the oocyte. This microenvironment changes in response to the hormonal fluctuations of the menstrual cycle. FSH is responsible for increasing estradiol production from the granulosa cells that surround the follicle; it also induces the aromatization of androgens to estrogens. As a consequence of FSH's action, the microenvironment of the developing follicle is transformed from an androgenic milieu to an estrogenic milieu. As a result, serum estrogen levels begin to rise. These hormones serve as a negative feedback to FSH secretion and, at midcycle, induce a surge of LH release from the pituitary. Inhibin, which is released from granulosa cells under the stimulation of FSH and LH, will also negatively affect FSH secretion. With the decline in FSH levels, only the dominant follicle, which has adequate numbers of FSH receptors, continues to develop. The other follicles become atretic.

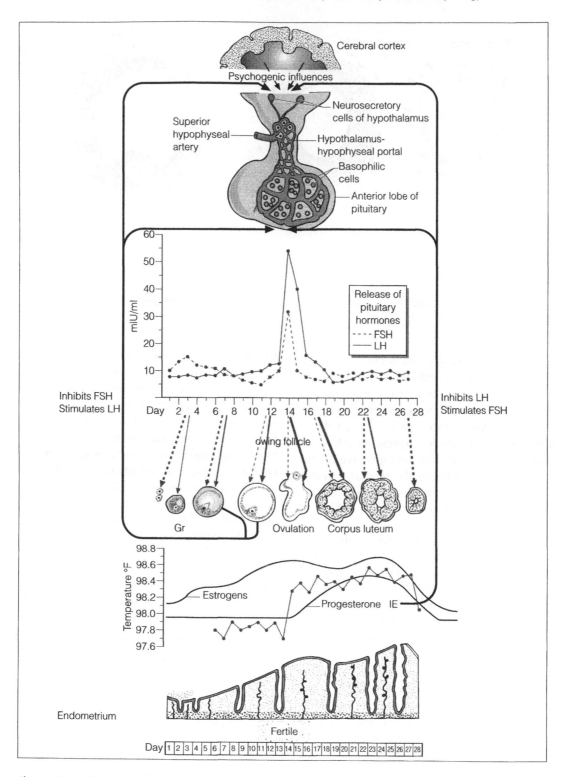

Figure 34.4 The normal menstrual cycle

Source: Callahan TL, Caughey AB, Heffner LJ. Blueprints in obstetrics and gynecology. Malden, MA: Blackwell Science, 1998:130.

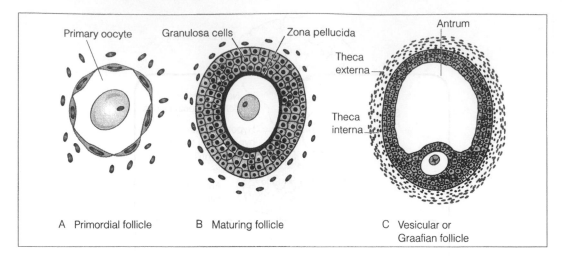

Figure 34.5   The developing ovarian follicle

Source: Callahan TL, Caughey AB, Heffner LJ. Blueprints in obstetrics and gynecology. Malden, MA: Blackwell Science, 1998:131.

The process of follicular recruitment actually begins three months prior to ovulation, with the expression of FSH receptors on the granulosa cells of the recruited follicle. Before recruitment takes place, the granulosa cells of a resting follicle do not express receptors for FSH. They are therefore unresponsive to the hormonal conditions in the woman's body. Once the receptors are present, however, the follicle can respond to serum levels of FSH by producing estradiol.

On the second or third day of the menstrual cycle, the pituitary gland releases a large amount of FSH to stimulate the recruitment of follicles. Measuring the amount of FSH released gives insight into the process of recruitment and the overall health of the ovaries. The typical amount of FSH required to recruit follicles in health ovaries is 6 to 10 mIU/mL (as measured in a radioimmunoassay). If the serum level of FSH on the second or third day of the menstrual cycle exceeds 20 mIU/mL, ovarian dysfunction is present. Women with this type of problem have greatly reduced pregnancy rates.

Estradiol Action

Estradiol stimulates production of cervical mucus, proliferation of the endometrium, and suppresses the release of FSH. The amount of estradiol produced by the developing follicles increases during the follicular phase of the menstrual cycle. Some of this estradiol is released into the systemic circulation.

In the reproductive process, estradiol serves three important functions. First, it stimulates the production of thin, elastic cervical mucus. This watery mucus permits the sperm to pass into the uterine cavity. Second, it increases the mitogenic activity of the basal cells in the endometrium, with proliferation of these cells creating a thickened uterine lining. These endometrial cells form a glandular pattern and begin to express receptors for progesterone. Third, estradiol exerts negative feedback on the release of FSH. Rising estradiol levels inhibit the production, release, and bioactivity of FSH. The result is a perceived decrease in FSH at the level of the granulosa cells.

Selection of a Dominant Follicle

By the sixth or seventh day following the onset of menstruation, one follicle has begun to express more receptors for FSH. This follicle is able to maintain estradiol production, despite the declining levels of FSH in the serum. The oocyte contained in this dominant follicle is the one that will be ovulated that cycle. All other follicles undergo atresia, and their oocytes will never reach maturity.

Ovulation

At midcycle, estrogen levels peak, which in turn stimulates an LH surge 38 to 48 hours before ovulation. This LH surge induces the resumption of meiosis in the ovum, and it stimulates the granulosa cells and theca cells of the follicle to produce progesterone and androgens, respectively.

The mature follicle is about 20 mm in diameter. Proteolytic enzymes and prostaglandins facilitate its rupture with extrusion of the egg (Figure 34.6). The egg is captured by the fimbriae of the fallopian tube and moved along the lumen of the tube by cilia.

THE LUTEAL PHASE

The second half of the menstrual cycle—the luteal phase—is characterized by increased progesterone production by the corpus luteum, which is the remnant of the follicle that has released its ovum. Production of progesterone climbs during the luteal phase. This elevation in the progesterone level in turn leads to an elevation in basal body temperature (see Chapter 37). The corpus luteum has a finite lifespan of approximately 14 days unless stimulation by human chorionic gonadotropin occurs. With the regression of the corpus luteum and the ensuing decline in progesterone levels, the endometrium sloughs and menses begins.

THE ENDOMETRIUM

The menstrual cycle influences the status of the endometrium through the circulating sex steroids. The follicular phase of the ovary corresponds to the proliferative phase of the endometrium. During the first half of the cycle, estrogen stimulates rapid growth and brings about increased mitotic activity of the endometrial glands and stroma. The luteal phase corresponds to the secretory phase of the endometrium, in which progesterone limits the height of the endometrium by antagonizing the effects of estrogen. Progesterone exerts its influence on estrogen by decreasing estrogen receptor replenishment and increasing the conversion of estradiol to estrone (a weaker form of estrogen). Withdrawal of estrogen and progesterone at the end of the cycle result in spiral vessel spasm and local ischemia, leading to breakdown and sloughing of the endometrium.

The average amount of blood lost at the time of menses is approximately 35 mL. This blood should be dark and nonclotting. Cessation of bleeding occurs because of hemostasis and vasoconstriction. The uterus will typically contract to constrict the endometrial vessels, which may be felt by the woman as uterine cramps.

FERTILIZATION

During intercourse, sperm are deposited in the vagina. The physical conditions in the vagina are not favorable for sperm survival, and sperm will normally die within 12 hours. Many are able to swim to the cervical canal and reach the cervical mucus, however. Unlike the harshly acidic vaginal secretions, midcycle cervical

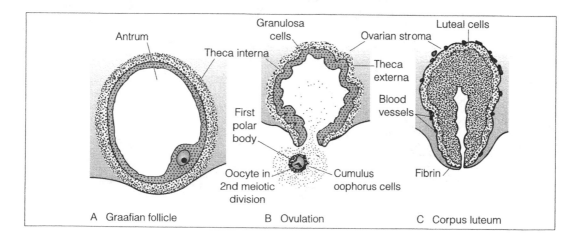

Figure 34.6 Follicular rupture

Source: Callahan TL, Caughey AB, Heffner LJ. Blueprints in obstetrics and gynecology. Malden, MA: Blackwell Science, 1998:131.

mucus is neutral in pH, and sperm may readily survive in the cervical canal for 72 hours. In fact, recent evidence suggests that the sperm may remain viable for six days, providing a very large "window of opportunity" for fertility. The size of this "window of opportunity" is important in the field of natural family planning. Couples who attempt to prevent pregnancy by abstaining from sexual intercourse during the fertile period should not have intercourse for at least six days prior to ovulation.

Once ejaculated, the sperm are not fully capable of fertilization. Instead, they must undergo a series of maturational steps known as capacitation. During capacitation, the sperm alter their swimming pattern and lose the outer coating on the head (acrosomal cap). This loss of the acrosomal cap exposes proteins that will recognize the zona pellucida of the oocyte.

PENETRATION OF THE OOCYTE

Following ovulation, the oocyte remains in the ampullary region of the fallopian tube. Chemotactic factors attract spermatozoa to the mature oocyte. The acrosomal cap actively binds the sperm to the zona pellucida. This binding is receptor-mediated, and the zona pellucida receptor is species-specific. As a consequence, it prevents cross-species fertilization.

After traversing the zona pellucida, the sperm head reaches the membrane surrounding the oocyte (oolemma) (Figure 34.7). The membrane surrounding the sperm head fuses with the oolemma, and the DNA contained

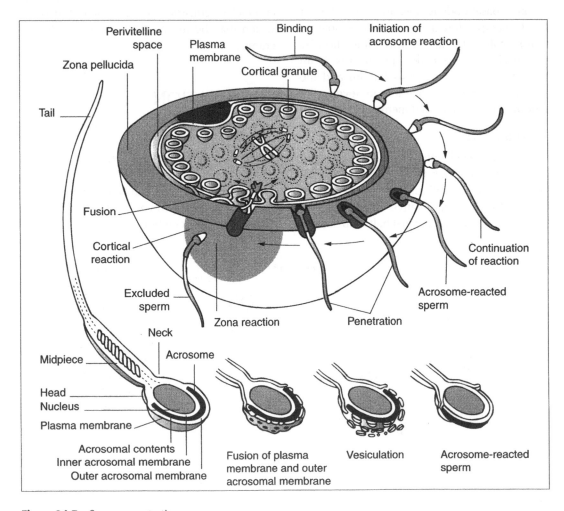

Figure 34.7   Sperm penetration

Source: Wasserman PM. Fertilization in mammals. Sci Am 1988;259:78.

within the sperm head is incorporated into the cytoplasm of the oocyte by pinocytosis. The oocyte then directs the sperm DNA to decondense, and a membrane is created surrounding the decondensed DNA (nuclear membrane). At this stage, the oocytes contains two pronuclei: one containing DNA from the oocyte and one containing DNA from the sperm. Substances released with the acrosomal reaction induce the zona reaction in the zona pellucida, whose inner portion becomes impenetrable to sperm, thereby blocking polyspermy.

Over the next 12 to 24 hours, these nuclear membranes dissolve and the chromosomes align to produce a metaphase plate. Subsequently, cellular division produces a two-cell embryo.

IMPLANTATION OF THE BLASTOCYST

The embryo continues to divide for three to four more days. It begins to form an inner cell mass and a fluid-filled cavity becomes visible. At this stage, the embryo is referred to as a blastocyst. The blastocyst travels through the isthmus of the fallopian tube and reaches the endometrial cavity. It will remain in the uterine cavity for 24 to 48 hours before attaching itself to a particular site in the endometrium. The forces that control the attachment of the embryo to the endometrium (implantation) are poorly described.

ROLE OF HUMAN CHORIONIC GONADOTROPIN

Following implantation, trophoblastic cells of the developing embryo produce a glycoprotein known as human chorionic gonadotropin (hCG). Significant amounts of hCG are released into the systemic circulation. This protein binds to specific receptors in the corpus luteum and stimulates the continued production of progesterone.

The trophoblast produces hCG as early as seven days after ovulation. Levels become detectable in the serum after 9 to 10 days. Normally, hCG levels should double every three days. Lower values are associated with abnormal pregnancies. Ectopic pregnancies frequently have slower doubling rates in hCG level, though not always. Multiple gestations may have faster doubling rates.

SUMMARY

Many steps are involved in the process of reproduction. Although some steps have been well studied in humans, others have been evaluated only in animal models and the information subsequently extrapolated to humans. Further research and advances in assisted reproductive technology should eventually increase our understanding of the reproductive process.

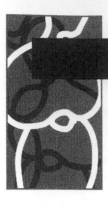

CHAPTER 35

Evaluation of the Infertile Couple

Megan E. Breen

Infertility is defined as 12 months of unprotected intercourse without conception. Primary infertility occurs in couples who have never conceived. Secondary infertility involves couples who have achieved a prior conception. Approximately 20% to 25% of couples will encounter difficulties with fertility at some point in their lives. In a normal population, 80% would conceive within one year of unprotected intercourse. Fecundability is the probability of conception within one menstrual cycle; in normal populations, the fecundability rate is 25%. Fecundity is the percentage of live births per menstrual cycle.

BACKGROUND

Two important considerations for an infertile couple are maternal age and duration of infertility. Many more women today are delaying childbearing. In the United States, one of every five women now bears her first child after the age of 35 years. Increasing maternal age is associated with impaired fecundity as well as an increase in early pregnancy loss. Impaired fecundity is likely in only 4% of 15- to 24-year-old women. This rate increases to 13% in 25- to 34-year-old women, and leaps to 30% in 35- to 44-year-olds. Similarly, the rate of miscarriage increases from 10% for 30-year-old women to 18% for women in their late thirties and 34% for women in their early forties. Current theory suggests that the available ova are less functional in older women. Notably, older women have improved fertility rates when they use donor eggs from younger women. A smaller effect is seen with advanced paternal age.

Lifestyle also affects fertility. Although only cigarette smoking has been clearly implicated in delayed conception and increased infertility, other behaviors may also contribute to fertility problems. For example, marijuana use inhibits GnRH production in both men and women. Alcohol, cocaine, and tight clothing all decrease spermatogenesis in men. Environmental exposures may also have an effect, though their role is not yet understood.

CLINICAL CORRELATION

M. D., a 28-year-old, gravida 0, woman, presents to her gynecologist's office with the complaint of infertility. She and her husband have been trying unsuccessfully to conceive for more than 12 months. Neither she nor her husband has a history of prior pregnancies.

PGynHx: M. D. has had regular menstrual cycles since she was 13 years old, occurring every 27 to 30 days and lasting 5 days, accompanied by menstrual cramps. She is not aware of any midcycle pain. M. D. has had three sexual partners since she first became sexually active at age 20, and she has used oral contraceptives in the past without difficulty. She does not have a history of abnormal Pap smears or sexually transmitted diseases. She is otherwise healthy, with no known drug allergies, and is not currently taking any medications. M. D. does not smoke and does not currently use alcohol or drugs.

M. D.'s husband's history is also unremarkable. He is a healthy, 33-year-old man with no prior surgeries or medical conditions. He denies any history of mumps or sexually transmitted diseases. He does not use tobacco, alcohol, or drugs.

CAUSES OF INFERTILITY

Fertility can be compromised in several different areas (Table 35.1). Appropriate questions in the work-up include the following:

- Are sperm available and normal?
- Is the area of ovum transport (fallopian tubes) normal?
- Is ovulation occurring?
- Is the endometrium receptive for a fertilized zygote?

The evaluation should begin with the least expensive and least invasive tests, including semen analysis, basal body temperature charts, post-coital tests, and hysterosalpingogram.

These tests can identify problems in 80% of all couples.

MALE FACTORS

Many factors in a couple's failure to conceive may be related to male infertility (Table 35.2). The World Health Organization has set standards for a normal semen analysis (Table 35.3).

Oligospermia is a decrease in the sperm count to less than 20 million/cm^3. It may occur because of exposure to excessive heat (for example, from saunas or tight-fitting clothes) or because of consumption of alcohol, marijuana, or toxins. A varicosity of the spermatic vein (varicocele) may be a surgically correctable cause of decreased sperm count and decreased motility. Hyperprolactinemia and hypogonadotropic hypogonadism are rare causes of diminished sperm production that can be managed medically.

Azoospermia is an absence of sperm, which could be a sign of gonadal failure or outflow obstruction. If the sperm volume is too small, the male patient may have an obstructive disorder or retrograde ejaculation. Agenesis of the seminal vesicles may be evaluated ultrasonographically. If the volume is too great, a dilutional effect can be observed. Excess WBCs may indicate the presence of an infection.

Table 35.1   Common Causes of Infertility and Basic Diagnostic Tools

ETIOLOGY	INCIDENCE* (%)	BASIC INVESTIGATIVE TOOLS
Male factor	40	Semen analysis
		Postcoital test
Ovulatory factor	15–20	Basal body temperature
		Serum progesterone
		Endometrial biopsy
Peritoneal factors	40	Laparoscopy
Uterine-tubal factor	30	Hysterosalpingogram
		Laparoscopy ± hysteroscopy
Cervical factors	5–10	Post-coital test

*Multiple factors are identified in 20% of cases.

Source: Adapted from Hacker N, Moore JG. Essentials of obstetrics and gynecology, 3rd ed. Philadelphia: WB Saunders, 1992:611.

Table 35.2 Common Causes of Male Factor Infertility

Endocrine disorders

    Hypothalamic dysfunction (Kallman's)

    Pituitary failure (tumor, radiation, surgery)

    Hyperprolactinemia (drug, tumor)

    Exogenous androgens

    Thyroid disease

    Adrenal hyperplasia

Abnormal spermatogenesis

    Mumps orchitis

    Chemical/radiation/heat exposure

    Varicocele

    Cryptorchidism

Abnormal motility

    Varicocele

    Antisperm antibodies

    Kartagener's syndrome

    Idiopathic

Sexual dysfunction

    Retrograde ejaculation

    Impotence

    Decreased libido

Source: Adapted from DeCherney A, Pernoll M. Current obstetric and gynecologic diagnosis and treatment. Norwalk, CT: Appleton and Lange, 1994:998.

Table 35.3 Values for Semen Analysis

PARAMETER	NORMAL VALUE
Volume	1.5–5 cm³
WBCs	< 1 million/cm³
pH	7.2–7.8
Sperm concentration	> 20 million/cm³
Forward motility	> 50%
Normal morphology	> 50%

Her husband's examination by a urologist is completely normal. His semen analysis is also within normal limits

Cervical Factor

A post-coital test is performed around the time of ovulation. It examines both the cervix's function and the sperm's ability to reach the cervix. The function of the cervix is to line up live sperm, reserve those sperm in its crypts, and filter out debris. When estrogen levels peak immediately prior to ovulation, this surge causes the cervix to produce copious, clear, watery mucus. A sample of cervical mucus is taken two to eight hours post-intercourse. The stretch quality—known as spinbarkeit—is evaluated by lifting the cover slip from the slide where the mucus is placed. A stretch of 8 to 9 cm is normal under estrogen influence. If the mucus is allowed to dry, ferning patterns may be observed. Both the number and forward motility of the sperm are examined. Six to ten sperm/hpf and 60% forward motility are considered adequate. If the infertility appears to have a cervical factor, then the cervical mucus may be bypassed by intrauterine insemination (IUI).

Mycoplasma and ureaplasma have been cultured from the cervix as well as the male tract, and infection with these organisms has been associated with infertility. Nevertheless, these organisms' role as causative agents in infertility has not been clearly established. Likewise, treatment of these infections has not clearly been shown to increase conception.

FEMALE FACTORS

The female factor in infertility is evaluated through several different methods. The first step involves physical examination.

CLINICAL CORRELATION

M. D. is examined but shows no obvious abnormalities. She is 5 ft, 6 in, and weighs 135 lb. She has a normal hair growth and hair pattern. There is no thyromegaly. M. D. does not have galactorrhea. Her pelvic examination reveals normal external genitalia, a normal-appearing cervix, and a uterus and ovaries that are palpably normal, mobile, and nontender. The remainder of the examination is unremarkable.

CLINICAL CORRELATION

M. D. schedules a post-coital examination after the urologic examination is completed. The speculum examination reveals copious amounts of clear mucus, with a spinbarkeit of 9 to 10 cm. On microscopic examination, more than 10 sperm/hpf are observed. Approximately 75% of the sperm are moving in a forward direction. There are no WBCs present. The couple is informed that the examination shows no abnormalities.

Disorders of Ovulation

Abnormal ovulation accounts for 40% of all female infertility. As with other aspects in the evaluation of infertility, simple tests to determine ovulation should be performed first. Most women with regular cycles and premenstrual symptoms (cramping, bloating, irritability) will have monthly ovulation, but as many as 5% of women with these symptoms will be anovulatory.

The basal body temperature (BBT) chart graphs daily temperature. The woman takes her temperature each morning before arising from bed, using a thermometer graduated to 0.1 °F calibrations. The resultant curve over the course of the cycle should show a nadir at the LH surge, followed by a subsequent rise in temperature two to three days later, reflecting increased progesterone levels. Some women, however, do not detect a distinct nadir; others may show a slow, gradual increase in temperature during the luteal phase.

BBT charts can predict ovulation within two to three days. Intercourse is recommended every 36 to 48 hours from three to four days prior to expected ovulation to two days after ovulation. Only two months of recordings should be necessary, and episodes of bleeding and intercourse may also be charted (Figure 35.1).

Another technique that has been used involves the measurement of urine LH. This method detects an elevation after the LH surge.

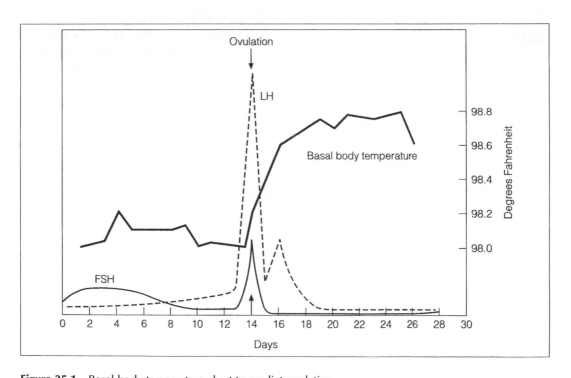

Figure 35.1   Basal body temperature chart to predict ovulation

Source: Callahan TL, Caughey AB, Heffner LJ. Blueprints in obstetrics and gynecology. Malden, MA: Blackwell Science, 1998:151.

Unreceptive Endometrium

Luteal-phase defects are abnormalities of the corpus luteum function that lead to insufficient progesterone production. In this case, the endometrium matures inappropriately so that it is not suitable for implantation. The easiest way to measure the adequacy of the corpus luteum is to measure serum progesterone during the luteal phase. A normal value would be greater than 10 ng/mL one week after ovulation. Endometrial biopsy to determine endometrial response to progesterone is a less reliable approach. Treatment for low progesterone during the luteal phase includes intravaginal progesterone suppositories and/or clomiphene citrate.

Tubal Factor

Abnormalities of the fallopian tubes account for 35% of all cases of infertility. These tubes may be damaged by prior pelvic infections, ectopic pregnancies, peritoneal infections, or endometriosis. In a hysterosalpingogram (HSG), radio-opaque dye is injected through the cervix to fill the uterine cavity; this dye spills out of the tubes and into the peritoneal cavity under fluoroscopy. Either a water-based or oil-based contrast medium may be used. The HSG may reveal intrauterine defects such as acquired intrauterine adhesions (Asherman's syndrome) or submucous myomas that may affect fertility. Although tubal obstructions are revealed by this technique, it may yield false-positive results because of tubal spasm. An HSB is performed after menstruation, during the midfollicular phase but before ovulation, when the endometrial lining is thin. Many defects detected by HSG can be corrected via hysteroscopy, such as submucous myomas or uterine adhesions. The HSG itself may improve fertility by washing out any mucus plugs within the fallopian tubes.

If the patient's history suggests pelvic inflammatory disease, some clinicians will check the sedimentation rate. If this rate is elevated, the problem may be treated with antibiotics prophylactically.

After all other preliminary tests have been performed, a laparoscopy may be carried out as the next level of testing. If a mass is present or the physical examination detects tenderness, a laparoscopy may be preferable to HSG initially. Although it is invasive and involves general anesthesia, this technique results in positive findings in 50% to 70% of all infertility cases. The most frequent abnormalities are pelvic adhesions, which can be lysed under laparoscopy, and endometriosis, which can be fulgarated. Following resection of fine adhesions, the pregnancy rate is reported to be 50%. Dye can be injected through the cervix and watched under laparoscopy to detect it traversing the tubes and spilling into the peritoneum. The tubes can be examined, and any patient with severe tubal disease may be offered in vitro fertilization.

Approximately 10% to 15% of couples have unexplained infertility. That is, all of the tests appear normal, yet the couple is still unable to conceive. In unexplained infertility the fecundity rate drops to 1.5% to 3%. Options for these couples include superovulation with intrauterine insemination or in vitro fertilization, both of which have a 40% pregnancy rate within six months. If unexplained infertility has existed for more than three years, the overall prognosis of conception is poor.

SUMMARY

Couples find the problem of infertility to be emotionally and financially draining. It is often unexpected and can impose significant strains on a relationship. The physician must offer emotional support during the work-up for these couples. The work-up should occur in a well-organized, step-by-step fashion to discover the cause of infertility with the smallest number of tests and costs possible. The physician must be able to present all of the options available to the couple as determined by the cause of infertility. The various treatments for infertility are described in Chapter 36.

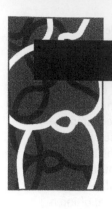

CHAPTER 36

Assisted Reproductive Techniques

Melvin H. Thornton

In vitro fertilization (IVF) and related assisted reproductive technologies (ART) have attained a preeminent role in the management of infertility. Since the first successful human pregnancy following IVF in 1978, ART has become widely available and is used extensively around the world. In the United States alone, more than 5600 live deliveries annually result from ART procedures. Indications for ART include infertility related to tubal disease, endometriosis, sperm defects, unexplained infertility, and ovarian failure. To fully understand the principles behind ART (particularly IVF), it is necessary to be familiar with the process of fertilization and embryogenesis (Table 36.1).

Oocytes are derived from oogonia as a result of two meiotic divisions. In the male, four spermatid are formed from a single germ cell. In the ovary, a single oocyte is formed from each oogonium; the excess genetic material is contained in two polar bodies, each of which is extruded as a result of one meiotic division. Meiosis resumes only in the oocyte contained in a dominant follicle and only after adequate stimulation of the follicle by luteinizing hormone (LH) or human chorionic gonadotropin (hCG). The first polar body is then extruded before ovulation. Although the oocyte passes into the second metaphase, meiosis is again arrested and does not resume until a spermatozoon successfully penetrates the oocyte. The second polar body is thus extruded only after fertilization (Figure 36.1).

Before fertilization can occur, the sperm must undergo the acrosome reaction. This reaction releases proteolytic enzymes contained within the acrosome that surrounds the sperm head (Figure 36.2). These enzymes digest the glycoprotein matrix (zona pellucida) that envelopes the oocyte. Capacitation—a biochemical prerequisite to the acrosome reaction—is achieved in vivo by sperm contact with the female reproductive tract. In vitro capacitation may be achieved by exposing the sperm to protein-containing buffers or culture media. The hyperreactive motility of sperm that results from capacitation, combined with the zonal digestion performed by the acrosomal proteins, facilitates the transport of sperm through the zona pellucida.

After successful penetration by a spermatozoon, the oocyte undergoes a cortical reaction. During this process, the contents of ooplasmic cortical granules are extruded into the perivitelline space (the space between the oocyte plasma membrane and the zona pellucida). The zona undergoes a zona reaction, which causes the zona to harden and prevents further penetration by sperm, thus limiting polyspermy.

Embryo cleavage follows successful fertilization, with subsequent mitotic cell divisions occurring at approximately 12- to 14-hour intervals (Figure 36.3). The blastocyst stage is achieved approximately five days after fertilization—approximately the same amount of time required for the embryo to reach the uter-

Table 36.1   Drugs Used in the Treatment of Infertility and in Assisted Reproductive Technologies

COMMERCIAL NAME	GENERIC NAME	MECHANISM
Clomid/Serophene	Clomiphene citrate	Antiestrogen, stimulates follicular development for ovulation induction
Pergonal	Human gonadotropins	Purified FSH/LH, stimulates follicular development during ovulation induction
Danocrine	Danazol	Androgen derivative, decreases FSH and LH used to treat endometriosis
hCG	Human chorionic gonadotropin	Triggers ovulation
Lutrepulse	Pulsatile GnRH	Stimulates release of FSH/LH from pituitary
Lupron	Leuprolide acetate	GnRH agonist, decreases estrogen levels, shrinks fibroids, causes regression of endometriosis

ine cavity. Implantation takes place seven to nine days after ovulation. At that time, hCG may first be detected in the circulation.

CLINICAL CORRELATION

E. L. is a 28-year-old nulligravida who presents with a complaint of 2½ years of unprotected intercourse without conception. She also has a history of chlamydia salpingitis requiring hospitalization at age 22. Her infertility work-up included documentation of normal ovulatory menstrual cycles, and her husband was found to have a normal semen analysis. A hysterosalpingogram revealed bilateral hydrosalpinges, with dilation and obstruction at the fimbriated ends.

Today, the technique of IVF with embryo transfer is widely used to treat infertile couples. Although the method was originally restricted to women who had no functioning oviducts as a result of severe tubal disease, it is now employed to help women with endometriosis, and couples with male factor or unexplained infertility. Because the rate of pregnancy following IVF is directly related to the number of embryos placed in the uterine cavity, most IVF centers utilize some form of ovarian hyperstimulation to increase the number of oocytes obtained at the time of follicle aspiration. Stimulation protocols typically use intramuscular injections of human menopausal gonadotropins (hMG), which consist of FSH and LH. Follicular growth is monitored on a frequent basis with transvaginal ultrasound and serum estradiol levels until follicle maturity is documented. Maturation occurs when the follicle reaches a size of 17 to 18 mm with total serum estradiol levels approaching 200 pg/mL per mature follicle.

Follicle aspiration is performed via transvaginal ultrasound needle guidance through the vagina into the cul-de-sac. Following their retrieval, the oocytes are cultured in a rigidly controlled, sterile laboratory environment. After 6 to 12 hours of incubation, sperm prepared by a washing procedure are added to the culture medium. Eighteen hours later, the oocytes are observed to determine whether fertilization has occurred. Fertilized oocytes are then cultured for another 24 to 48 hours. One to four normally cleaving embryos are then placed into the uterus of the patient in a sterile environment.

Embryo placement takes place via a small catheter placed through the cervical canal. The number of embryos transferred depends upon the age of the patient. Because women older than age 40 have decreased implantation rates relative to younger women, most IVF centers transfer four or more embryos to those

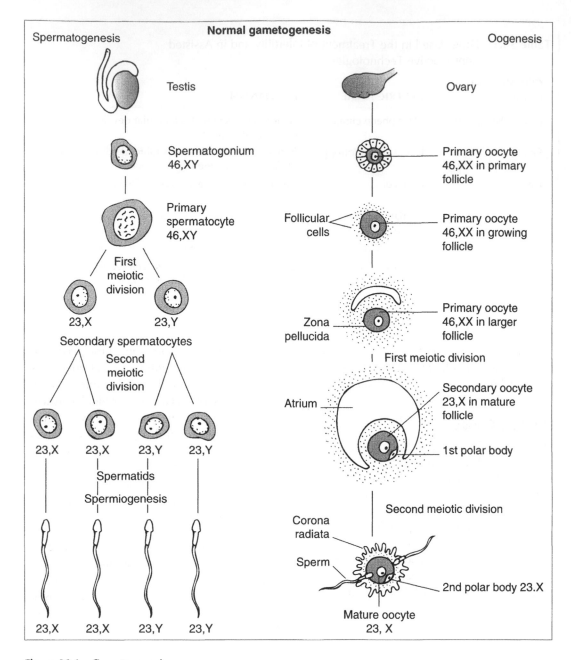

Figure 36.1   Gametogenesis

Source: Cunningham FG, MacDonald PC, Leveno KJ, Gant NF, Gilstrap LC, ed. Williams obstetrics, 19th ed. Norwalk, CT: Appleton and Lange, 1993:41.

women unless donor oocytes are used. The embryos that are not transferred during the initial cycle are cryopreserved and may be transferred in a subsequent spontaneous ovulatory cycle.

Recently, advances in male infertility have made possible the harvesting of spermatozoa from the testes and subsequent microinjec-

tion of the sperm into the cytoplasm of the oocyte (called intracytoplasmic sperm injection [ICSI]). This technique can be used for males with very low sperm counts, retrograde ejaculation, or even azospermia when spermatids can be harvested from the testes. It also bypasses the acrosomal reaction. ICSI will most likely play a larger role in ART in the future. For

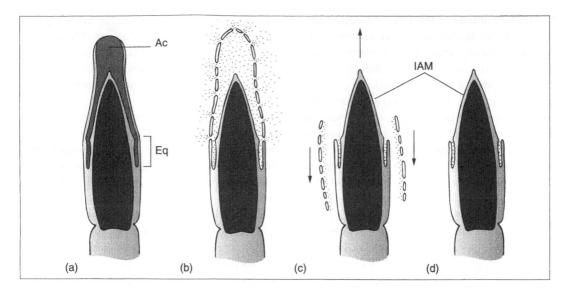

Figure 36.2 Diagrams showing the progression of a typical acrosome reaction. Ac, acrosomal cap; Eq, equatorial segment of the acrosome; IAM, inner acrosomal membrane.

Source: Knobil E, Neill JD, ed. The physiology of reproduction, vol. I. New York: Raven Press, 1988:148.

men with low sperm counts, the sperm may be washed of the seminal plasma and then injected into the uterine cavity (intrauterine insemination) to present a higher percentage of the sperm to the oocyte. Intrauterine insemination is also used to bypass the cervix if a cervical factor is associated with the infertility, such as unfavorable cervical mucus, cervical stenosis, or surgical absence of the cervix.

A modification of in vitro fertilization, called gamete intrafallopian transfer (GIFT), can be used if the infertile woman has functioning oviducts. With this technique, both oocytes and sperm are placed into the oviduct

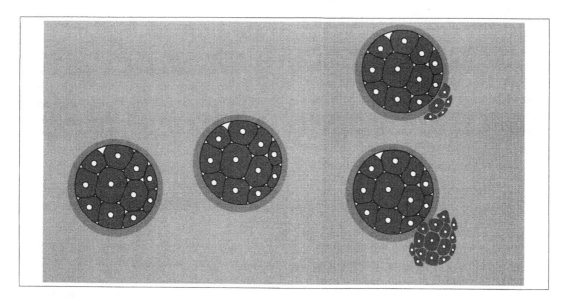

Figure 36.3 Cleaving human embryos at 48 hours after follicle aspiration

Source: Mishell DR, ed. Infertility, contraception, and reproductive endocrinology, 3rd ed. Cambridge, MA: Blackwell Science, 1991:148.

through a catheter at the time of laparoscopy. Although this technique avoids in vitro fertilization, embryo culturing, and embryo transfer into the uterus, ovarian hyperstimulation and oocyte retrieval are still required.

The Society for Assisted Reproductive Technology (SART) conducts annual surveys to assess the effectiveness of the various assisted reproduction techniques. The 1996 SART survey reported that the live delivery rate per ovum retrieved was 26% for IVF and 29% for GIFT. Data from this survey also indicated that the likelihood of delivering a term infant is lessened with both techniques if the woman is 40 years of age or older or if the semen samples contain a decreased number of sperm or percentage of motile sperm. The pregnancy rate per treatment cycle will remain constant for approximately six cycles. After six cycles, the cumulative pregnancy rate is approximately 60%. Women should be counseled that the chance of pregnancy occurring with IVF after six previous failed cycles is very low.

CLINICAL CORRELATION

A 30-year-old woman with primary infertility has been told that she will require IVF to become pregnant. She and her husband have questions regarding pregnancy outcome and the risk of multiple gestation after IVF.

It is important to counsel couples regarding pregnancy outcome when they are considering any of the ART options to help them conceive. With any form of ART resulting in a singleton gestation advancing to the second trimester, the perinatal outcome, mean birth weight, congenital malformations, and complications of pregnancy or labor are no different than those observed in the normal fertile population. Therefore viable singleton pregnancies occurring after ART should not be considered high-risk pregnancies. On the other hand, there is an increased risk of spontaneous abortion and preterm delivery among women with multiple gestations conceived by ART. All types of ART with ovarian stimulation are followed by a relatively high incidence of multiple gestation. The majority of these pregnancies consist of twins (25%), with triplets (4%) and higher-order gestations (1%) occurring less frequently. Furthermore, some 4% of all IVF-assisted pregnancies are tubal pregnancies, with 1% being combined ectopic and intrauterine pregnancies.

Higher-order pregnancies (such as quadruplets) are associated with poor maternal and fetal outcomes, including preterm delivery, prolonged hospitalization, pre-eclampsia, polyhydramnios, and post-partum hemorrhage. The relative risk of perinatal morbidity and mortality from prematurity among quadruplets is high. Fetal reduction or the termination of one or more of the fetuses is an alternative for the patient that may increase the chance of a successful pregnancy outcome. Currently, the most widely used technique for fetal reduction consists of injection of potassium chloride into the fetal thorax by ultrasound guidance, inducing cardiac asystole. This procedure is most often performed at 10 to 13 weeks to balance the risk of spontaneous abortion against the risks of termination of fetuses in the second trimester. The total rate of pregnancy loss has been reported to be 5% to 10% when an experienced practitioner carries out the procedure. The small placental mass that is present at 10 to 13 weeks of gestation reabsorbs after fetal death.

CLINICAL CORRELATION

An infertile couple is preparing to undergo an ART procedure to achieve pregnancy. They are trying to choose between two ART programs. The principal difference between the two options is that one offers embryo cryopreservation and the other does not. They consult with their referring gynecologist, seeking answers to some general questions about cryopreservation of embryos and oocytes.

Cryopreservation of human embryos was introduced for several reasons: to meet specific needs associated with IVF, such as avoiding the transfer of an excessive number of fresh embryos and reducing the risk of multiple gestations; to decrease the number of ART treatment cycles needed for pregnancy; and to decrease the overall cost of ART. To date, these goals for human embryo freezing have largely been met. Approximately 70% of all human embryos retain their viability after thawing. In 20% to 40% of IVF cycles, extra embryos are available for freezing. The total pregnancy rate from a single stimulated IVF cycle in which extra embryos were cryopreserved is 32% (19% fresh embryos and 13% thawed embryos).

It is uncertain how long human embryos can remain viable in terms of their capability to produce normal offspring. To date, normal human pregnancies have resulted from embryos that have been stored in liquid nitrogen for as long as 10 years. If pregnancy occurs after transfer of a cryopreserved embryo, the fetus does not appear to suffer any deleterious effects. A birth defect rate of 0.8% per neonate delivered after the transfer of thawed embryos has been reported.

DONOR OOCYTES

CLINICAL CORRELATION

A 30-year-old woman who has previously undergone chemotherapy for non-Hodgkin's lymphoma has now developed premature ovarian failure. Her FSH levels have exceeded 100 mIU/mL on several occasions, and she has been amenorrheic for one year. She visits her gynecology to discuss whether she might possibly become pregnant.

Women with ovarian failure are most likely to achieve pregnancy through IVF with donor oocytes. The success rate with surrogate oocytes from young (less than 34 years old) female donors is excellent, ranging from 25% to 40% live births per treatment cycle. In general, women younger than age 35 are sought as oocyte donors to maximize success rates and to minimize the risk of chromosomal anomalies in resulting pregnancies. All potential donors must have a normal medical history, uneventful physical examination, and a genetic history that is free of risk factors for significant inherited diseases. Laboratory studies to screen

oocyte donors include a complete blood count and blood type, HIV testing, and blood studies to minimize the risk of syphilis and hepatitis B and C. In addition, a psychological evaluation to uncover risk factors that may make the oocyte donor unsuitable is recommended.

The oocyte donor undergoes controlled ovarian hyperstimulation. Next, the donor oocytes obtained through standard transvaginal aspiration are inseminated with the recipient's male partner's sperm. The resulting embryos are then transferred to the hormonally synchronized recipient or cryopreserved for future use.

The recipient requires exogenous hormone therapy to simulate the natural ovarian cycle and thereby produce the endometrial proliferation, secretory changes, and subsequent endometrial receptivity necessary for embryo nidation. Estrogen may be administered either orally or transdermally. Progesterone is administered beginning on cycle day 15 by intramuscular injection or vaginal suppositories. Effective replacement protocols result in estradiol levels during the late follicular and mid-luteal phases of more than 200 pg/mL and 100 pg/mL, respectively. Progesterone levels of 20 ng/mL or greater in the mid-luteal phase are considered adequate. Before the actual cycle of embryo transfer, the recipient usually undergoes a preparatory cycle to document the adequacy of her response through an endometrial biopsy.

With IVF, embryos are generally transferred at the two- to eight-cell stage. Higher pregnancy rates are achieved when embryo transfer occurs on day 17, 18, or 19 of the recipient's simulated cycle. After the embryo transfer, the recipient undergoes luteal supplementation of exogenous hormones as previously described. A serum pregnancy test is checked 10 to 12 days after embryo transfer. If pregnancy has not occurred, the exogenous hormone therapy is discontinued and menses occurs.

If the recipient conceives in an oocyte donation cycle, the exogenous estrogen and progesterone regimen is continued at doses similar to those used in the replacement cycle. In a pregnancy achieved through oocyte donation, the serum estradiol level is maintained at more than 300 pg/mL and the progesterone level at more than 20 ng/mL in the first 8 to 10 weeks. At approximately 10 to 12 weeks, the placental output of steroid hormones should be sufficient to maintain an ongoing pregnancy, and the exogenous hormones are discontinued.

The success rate of IVF with donor oocytes is clearly higher than that achieved with routine IVF because in the former procedure the embryos are derived from relatively young, normal females and transferred to an endometrium that has been exposed to physiologic levels of estrogen and progesterone. Most ART programs that perform IVF with donor oocytes have observed a pregnancy rate that is about double that seen with standard IVF procedures. In the United States as a whole, the rate of pregnancies achieved with standard IVF ranges from 10% to 20%.

OVARIAN HYPERSTIMULATION SYNDROME

CLINICAL CORRELATION

A 35-year-old woman with distal tubal disease undergoes an IVF cycle. Controlled ovarian hyperstimulation is achieved with daily injections of human menopausal gonadotropins. The embryo transfer occurred three weeks ago, and the patient now presents with bloating, lower abdominal discomfort, and nausea, but no vomiting. A pregnancy test is positive. Ultrasonography reveals two small intrauterine gestational sacs, enlarged ovaries, and increased free peritoneal fluid (ascites). The hematocrit is 41%, and serum potassium concentration is 4.1 meq/L.

Ovarian hyperstimulation syndrome (OHSS), in its mild form, is a relatively common complication of controlled ovarian hyperstimulation. Although severe OHSS is uncommon, its symptoms can be disabling and even life-threatening. Controlled ovarian hyperstimulation, such as that utilized during clinical IVF and other ART procedures, is associated with mild to moderate OHSS in many patients and with severe OHSS in approximately 1% of patients. Severe cases usually require hospitalization.

The magnitude of the ovarian response, as determined by the number of preovulatory follicles and serum estradiol levels, roughly correlates with the likelihood that OHSS will develop. Predisposing factors include young age and polycystic ovaries on ultrasonography, as both of these factors increase the chance that a patient will develop more follicles and higher estrogen levels. The likelihood that clinical OHSS will develop, however, varies widely. In most cases, symptoms begin five to six days after ovulation or follicle aspiration; they may appear earlier among patients with more severe degrees of the syndrome. Pregnancy, with its attendant stimulation of the corpus luteum by hCG, typically exacerbates the syndrome. When pregnancy occurs, symptoms may not abate until 8 to 10 weeks of gestation.

OHSS begins with lower abdominal discomfort, which is commonly described as a swelling or bloating and is thought to be related to ovarian enlargement. Increased capillary permeability results in exudation of fluid from the vascular space into extracellular areas. Clinically, the fluid first appears in the peritoneal cavity, but it may also be noted as a pleural or rarely pericardial effusion and generalized edema. This third spacing may result in intravascular fluid depletion, which is clinically detected as oliguria and may be measured indirectly as hemoconcentration. Patients commonly complain of nausea and vomiting. In extreme cases, the patient may require hospitalization for fluid replacement. Although the pathophysiology of OHSS is not well understood, it appears that the primary disturbance involves increased capillary permeability. Several biochemical mediators have been proposed as being responsible for the clinical picture associated with this syndrome.

Most cases of OHSS can be managed on an outpatient basis. Criteria for hospitalization are not absolute but include respiratory compromise, intractable vomiting, ketonemia, and hyperkalemia. Oliguria and hemoconcentration are also indications for hospitalization. In extreme cases, intravascular dehydration may lead to renal failure or thrombotic events. Treatment of OHSS, even during hospitalization, is supportive and focuses on alleviating symptoms and correcting the intravascular depletion.

SUMMARY

Assisted reproductive techniques continue to improve and become more refined. The myriad options available to infertile couples include ovarian stimulation, in vitro fertilization, use of donor sperm, use of donor oocytes, ICSI, surrogacy, embryo freezing, and newly emerging techniques. The process of trying to conceive can be both emotionally and financially draining, however, and it is not always free of complications (such as those linked to ovarian hyperstimulation). Physicians should be familiar with the techniques and options available to their infertile patients.

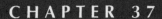

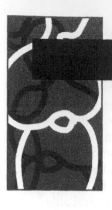

CHAPTER 37

Contraception, Sterilization, and Abortion

John K. Jain

Contraception includes a variety of reversible methods by which a couple can prevent an unwanted pregnancy. Sterilization is intended to be a permanent, irreversible method of contraception. Elective abortion represents a less-desirable alternative to proper contraception, but nevertheless may be used as a last resort when a method of contraception fails.

CLINICAL CORRELATION

W. C. is an 18-year-old, gravida 0, college freshman who presents to the student health center requesting a method of contraception. She has had one lifetime sexual partner but has not been sexually active since moving to college.

In discussing contraceptive choices, it is important to explain that a variety of methods exist, each having specific advantages and disadvantages. Contraceptive effectiveness is usually judged by measuring the number of unintended pregnancies that occur during a specific period of exposure to a contraceptive method. Both the Pearl Index, which is defined as the number of failures (pregnancies) per 100 woman-years of exposure, and the Life Table Analysis, which calculates a failure rate (pregnancy rate) for each month of contraceptive use, are used to calculate contraceptive efficacy.

Other important aspects of contraceptive efficacy relate to method failure and use failure. Method failure refers to the expected failure rate of a contraceptive method when used correctly; such rates are established in clinical trials. Use failure rates are often higher than method failure rates because they depend on actual experience and are prone to human error (Table 37.1).

Available contraceptive methods include barrier methods, injectable and implantable methods, the intrauterine device (IUD), and the oral contraceptive pill (OCP). The following areas should be covered when counseling a patient about selection of a contraceptive method:

- The mechanism of action and effectiveness of each method.

- The ability of the method to protect the user against sexually transmitted diseases (STDs).

- The side effects and contraindications for specific contraceptive methods.

- The time needed to return to fertility after use of the method ends.

BARRIER METHODS

Barrier methods include the male and female condoms, spermicides, the diaphragm, the cervical cap, and the sponge. Spermicides may be used either alone or in combination with a physical barrier. Barrier methods work by inhibiting passage of sperm to the upper genital tract of the female or by inactivating sperm. Because these methods are highly

Table 37.1 Overview of Contraceptives

CONTRACEPTIVE	MECHANISM OF ACTION	FAILURE RATE (% OF WOMEN WITH PREGNANCY)	PROTECTION AGAINST STDs	SIDE EFFECTS AND CONTRAINDICATIONS
None		85.0	None	
Oral contraceptive pill	Inhibition of GnRH release (inhibit follicular growth and ovulation); less favorable cervical mucus; less favorable endometrium for implantation	3.0	Slightly decreased PID by increasing cervical mucus	Breakthrough bleeding, amenorrhea, weight gain, thrombo-embolism (rare) Contraindications: thrombophlebitis, thromboembolic disorders, cerebral vascular disease, coronary occlusion, impaired liver function, breast cancer, pregnancy, undiagnosed vaginal bleeding, smokers older than age 35
Intrauterine device (IUD)	Create inflammatory response in endometrium that impairs implantation and is toxic to sperm	<1.0	Increased risk of PID during first 20 days after insertion; thereafter, same as no contraceptive	Copper IUDs have lower rates of ectopic pregnancy than no contraceptive Progestin IUDs have higher rates of ectopic pregnancy than no contraceptive Increased uterine bleeding, actinomycosis, uterine perforation with IUD Contraindications: pregnancy, acute PID, post-partum endometritis, cervical or uterine cancer, undiagnosed vaginal bleeding, previously inserted IUD that has not been removed
Norplant	Inhibits LH surge, thickened cervical mucus, atrophy of endometrium	0.2	Same as no contraceptive	Menstrual irregularities Contraindications: thromboembolic disease, active liver disease, undiagnosed vaginal bleeding, breast cancer

Table 37.1 *(Continued)*

CONTRACEPTIVE	MECHANISM OF ACTION	FAILURE RATE (% OF WOMEN WITH PREGNANCY)	PROTECTION AGAINST STDs	SIDE EFFECTS AND CONTRAINDICATIONS
Depo-Provera	Same as Norplant	0.3	Same as no contraceptive	Contraindications: pregnancy, undiagnosed vaginal bleeding May have prolonged (>9 months) delay in fertility after last injection
Barrier methods	Barrier for sperm to contact oocyte			
Diaphragm		18.0	About 50% reduction in transmission of STDs	Only side effects are associated with latex allergy
Condom		12.0		
Cervical cap		18.0		No contraindications
Withdrawal		18.0	Same as no method	
Periodic abstinence		Lowest expected:		
Calendar method		9.0		
Ovulation method		3.0		
Symptothermal		2.0		
Post-ovulation		1.0		

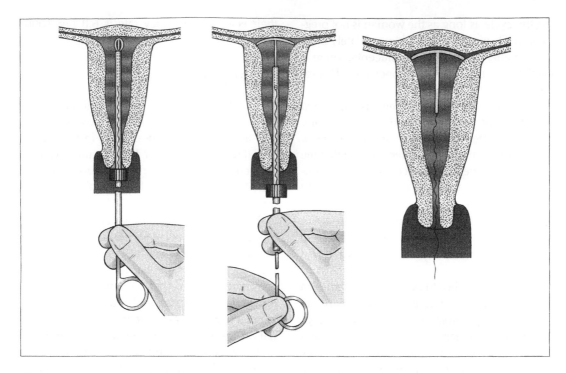

Figure 37.1 Placement of an IUD

Source: Callahan TL, Caughey AB, Heffner LJ. Blueprints in obstetrics and gynecology. Malden, MA: Blackwell Science, 1998:156.

user-dependent, the typical failure rates in the first year of use range from 12% to 28%.

Condoms, diaphragms, and spermicides provide protection (approximately a 50% reduction) against STDs and upper genital tract infection (pelvic inflammatory disease [PID]). The condom has also been proven to prevent HIV infection. There are no specific side effects to these products except allergy to latex or the spermicide. Return to fertility is obviously immediate once the method is stopped.

INTRAUTERINE DEVICES

Two IUDs are used in the United States: the TCu-380A, a copper-containing IUD approved for 10 years of use, and the Progestasert, a progestin-releasing IUD approved for 12 months of use. IUDs work principally by acting as a foreign body in the endometrium and creating a sterile inflammatory response (Figure 37.1). This inflammatory response is toxic to sperm. The progestin-releasing IUD also acts locally on the endometrium to make it unsuitable for embryo implantation. The typical fail-

ure rate during the first year of use with an IUD is 3%, comparable to the failure rate observed with oral contraceptive pills.

The use of IUDs greatly decreased in the 1980s after one type of IUD, the Dalkon Shield, was found to be associated with a high incidence of pelvic infections. The problem with this device related to its multifilamented tail, which served as a pathway for bacteria to colonize and ascend into the upper genital tract. Unlike the Dalkon Shield, modern IUDs are associated with a risk of pelvic infection only during the first 20 days following insertion. In studies by the World Health Organization, the risk of PID was increased 6-fold during the 20 days after insertion; beyond this time, PID was extremely rare. The results of this study underscore the importance of carefully screening patients for evidence of STDs prior to inserting an IUD. IUDs do not provide protection against STDs and should not be used by women with current or history of PID.

IUDs are typically placed during the menses. Nevertheless, studies have shown that they are effective when placed at any time during the cycle as long as the woman is not pregnant. IUDs may be inserted immediately postpartum after removal of the placenta. There is no delay in return to fertility once an IUD is removed.

The most common side effects associated with IUDs are increased uterine bleeding and increased menstrual pain (dysmenorrhea). These symptoms usually decrease with time and can often be treated successfully with nonsteroidal anti-inflammatory drugs (NSAIDs) and reassurance. As many as 5% of patients will expel the IUD in the first year of use. For this reason, it is important for the patient to confirm the presence of IUD strings on a monthly basis.

If a woman should become pregnant with an IUD in place, it is more likely to be an extrauterine pregnancy (ectopic pregnancy). Nevertheless, when compared to noncontraceptive users, who have an ectopic pregnancy rate of 3 to 4.5 per 1000 woman-years, users of the TCu-380A have an ectopic rate of only 0.2 per 1000 woman-years. In other words, the overall incidence of an ectopic pregnancy is decreased because the IUD provides excellent contraception. In contrast to the TCu-380A, users of progestin-releasing IUDs have a twofold increase in risk for an ectopic pregnancy—

their ectopic pregnancy rate is 6.8 per 1000 woman-years.

NORPLANT

Norplant is a system of six silastic capsules, each containing the progestin levonorgestrel, that are implanted subdermally in the upper arm (Figure 37.2). After the capsules are implanted, levonorgestrel freely diffuses through the silastic shell and establishes stable concentrations in the blood within 24 hours. Norplant is thought to prevent pregnancy by inhibiting the LH surge necessary for ovulation and thickening the cervical mucus, thereby forming a more formidable barrier to sperm. It also causes atrophy of the endometrium, thereby preventing implantation. Because this contraceptive system does not rely on patient participation, its first-year use failure rate approximates its true method failure rate of 0.2%. Norplant does not provide protection against STDs.

The most common side effect associated with Norplant is menstrual irregularity, which occurs in 80% of users during the first year of use. Unlike oral contraceptive pills, where the steroid hormones are not taken for seven days at the end of each cycle to allow for a men-

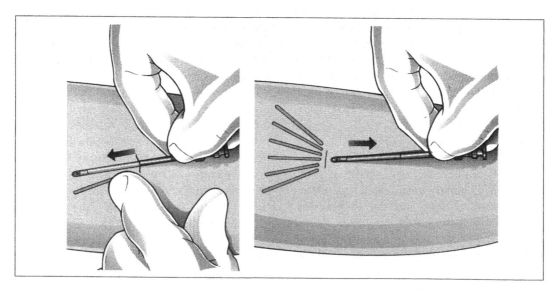

Figure 37.2   Placement of Norplant contraceptive pellets

Source: Callahan TL, Caughey AB, Heffner LJ. Blueprints in obstetrics and gynecology. Malden, MA: Blackwell Science, 1998:159.

strual period, the steroid hormone in Norplant, levonorgestrel, is released continuously. As a result, the endometrium sheds unpredictably, leading to menstrual irregularities. Patients also complain that the implants can be seen under the skin or palpated by their partners. In rare circumstances, one or more of the implants may become displaced. This problem portends a more difficult removal and may require an extensive surgical procedure.

Norplant is contraindicated in women who have active thrombophlebitis or thromboembolic disorders, undiagnosed genital bleeding, active liver disease, liver tumors, or known or suspected breast cancer. Within 48 hours of its removal, levonorgestrel levels in the plasma are undetectable. Consequently, there is no delay in the return to fertility after cessation of this method.

DEPO-PROVERA

Depo-Provera is an injectable form of contraception that consists of the progestin medroxyprogesterone acetate. It is administered as an intramuscular injection every three months. Depo-Provera works by blocking the LH surge necessary for ovulation; in addition, it thickens the cervical mucus and alters the endometrium so as to prevent implantation. Like Norplant, Depo-Provera requires very little patient participation and is therefore associated with a very low first-year failure rate of 0.3%. This contraceptive method does not provide protection against STDs.

The major problems with Depo-Provera are irregular menstrual bleeding (which affects as many as 70% of users in the first year), breast tenderness, weight gain, and depression. The incidence of irregular bleeding drops to 10% after the first year. As many as 80% of users do not have a period (amenorrhea) by five years of use. This method is contraindicated in pregnancy and in unexplained genital bleeding.

One significant problem with Depo-Provera is the delay in return of fertility. Although the pregnancy rate by 18 months after the last injection is 90%, a nine-month delay to conception occurs after the last injection. Return to a normal menstrual pattern is also delayed by 12 months after the last injection in 25% of Depo-Provera users.

ORAL CONTRACEPTIVE PILLS

OCPs consist of either (1) a combination of ethinyl estradiol and one of several progestins or (2) progestin alone. They work by inhibiting the LH surge necessary for ovulation, an effect of the progestin component, and by modulating GnRH release and pituitary FSH production necessary for folliculogenesis, an effect of the estrogen component. Additionally, OCPs alter the cervical mucus, making it less penetrable by sperm and induce atrophic changes in the endometrium that limit embryo implantation.

OCPs have a first-year failure rate of 3%. In addition to providing effective contraception, these pills have other, noncontraceptive benefits. For example, their use is associated with a lower incidence of endometrial and ovarian cancer, fewer ovarian cysts, and regulation of menses with less flow and menstrual pain. Although OCPs are associated with a greater incidence of lower genital tract chlamydial infections, they decrease the incidence of upper genital tract infection (PID), probably an effect of thicker cervical mucus and less menstrual flow.

Side effects linked to OCPs include breakthrough bleeding (which can usually be treated with a seven-day course of supplemental estrogen), amenorrhea, and weight gain (although this relationship has not been confirmed in clinical studies). Absolute contraindications to OCPs are a result of the estrogen component; they include thrombophlebitis, thromboembolic disorders, cerebral vascular disease, coronary occlusion, impaired liver function, known or suspected breast cancer, undiagnosed vaginal bleeding, known or suspected pregnancy, and being a smoker older than age 35. There is no delay in the return to fertility in women who discontinue the pill so as to become pregnant.

No evidence supports the claim that OCPs are a cause of secondary amenorrhea. The incidence of post-pill amenorrhea is approximately 0.8%—the same as the incidence of spontaneous secondary amenorrhea.

OCPs are effective in the first cycle of use so long as the pills are started no later than the fifth day of the cycle and no pills are missed. If the pills are started on the first day of menses (day 1 start), protection is immediate. In the United States, most women prefer to start on the first Sunday after their menses so that their menstrual period does not fall on a weekend day. Women who do not want to have a menstrual period for an extended time, such as during a vacation, can prevent a period from occurring by skipping the seven inactive pills and starting a new pill pack after the last active pill is taken.

If a woman misses one pill, she should take it as soon as she remembers and take the next pill as scheduled. If a woman misses two pills during the first or second week of her cycle, she should take two pills for two days and then finish the pack. A back-up contraceptive method, such as a condom, should be used for the duration of the cycle. If the two pills were missed during the third week and she is a Sunday starter, she should take a pill daily until Sunday and then start a new pack. In addition, she should use a back-up method immediately and for the next seven days. If she is a day 1 starter, she should start a new pack and use a back-up method immediately and for the next seven days. If three or more pills are missed and the women is a day 1 starter, she should start a new pack and use a back-up method immediately and for the next seven days. If she is a Sunday starter, she should continue to take a daily pill until Sunday, then start a new pack; she should also use a back-up method immediately and for seven days thereafter.

STERILIZATION

Sterilization is meant to be a permanent, irreversible method by which a woman or a man can prevent pregnancy. It is the most popular method of contraception in the United States, being used by approximately 25% of all people who employ some sort of contraceptive technique.

The most commonly used method of sterilization is female sterilization. In this surgical procedure, the patency of the fallopian tube is disrupted by excision, ligation, cauterization, or occlusion by rings or clips (Figure 37.3). The 10-year cumulative failure rates for female tubal sterilization methods range from 0.75% for unipolar cauterization to 3.65% for the Hulka-Clemens clip. As many of 50% of the failures are attributable to suboptimal surgical technique. The surgical risks associated with these procedures are low.

Disruption of the vas deferens in the male —that is, a vasectomy—is safer, easier, and less expensive than female tubal sterilization and has a low first-year failure rate of 0.15% (Figure 37.4). With this type of sterilization, men can continue to ejaculate and not notice a decrease in the volume of semen, since it is produced distal to the testes.

Sterilization methods are best suited for the couple who have completed their family. Some women and men do seek reversal of sterilization, typically if they have remarried. Successful pregnancy is achieved in approximately 50% of women and men after sterilization reversal.

EMERGENCY CONTRACEPTION

The use of large doses of estrogen within 72 hours of unprotected intercourse has been shown to prevent pregnancy. Emergency contraception is thought to work by inhibiting implantation. Although several regimens are available, the most commonly used option consists of two tablets of Ovral, each contain-

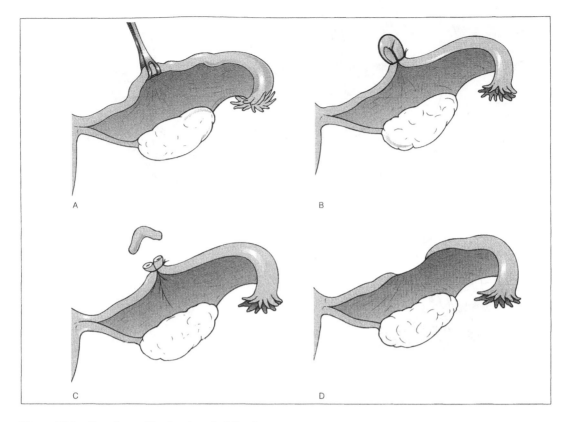

Figure 37.3   Female sterilization by tubal ligation

Source: Callahan TL, Caughey AB, Heffner LJ. Blueprints in obstetrics and gynecology. Malden, MA: Blackwell Science, 1998:161.

ing 50 µg of ethinyl estradiol, followed by two more tablets taken 12 hours later. Nausea, vomiting, and headache are common side effects with this regimen. This method should not be used by women who have contraindications to OCPs.

CLINICAL CORRELATION

When W. C. returns to college, she resumes taking her OCPs. That month, she notes her menstrual period to be delayed and unusually light. She begins another pack of OCPs but fails to have a period at the end of the cycle. Additionally, she notes mild nausea in the morning and breast tenderness. Fearing an unwanted pregnancy, W. C. purchases a home pregnancy kit and tests her urine; the results are positive. W. C. does not desire this pregnancy and is concerned that the fetus might have been harmed by exposure to the steroid hor-

mones of the OCPs. She presents to the student health center for counseling and referral for an abortion.

Urine pregnancy kits detect the beta subunit of human chorionic gonadotropin (hCG). This hormone is secreted by the trophoblastic cells of the developing pregnancy. Home pregnancy tests are sensitive enough to detect β-hCG by the first missed menstrual period—a time corresponding to two weeks following conception and four weeks after the last menstrual period. Pregnancy can be confirmed by visualizing the early gestational structures with the aid of an ultrasound. The earliest gestational structure that can be visualized sonographically is the gestational sac. This structure is usually identifiable by the fifth gestational week. In early pregnancy, trophoblastic tissue grows rapidly. This tissue secretes hCG, which acts on the corpus luteum so as to maintain the

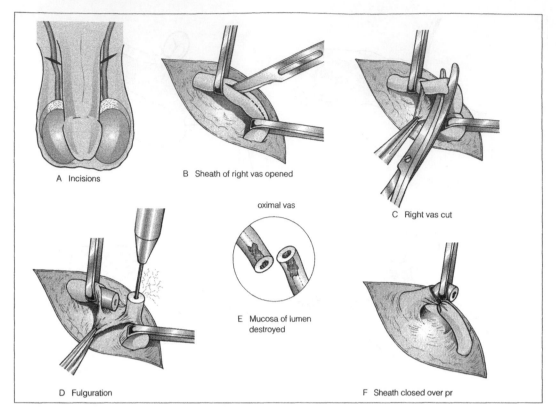

A Incisions

B Sheath of right vas opened

C Right vas cut

oximal vas

E Mucosa of lumen
destroyed

D Fulguration

F Sheath closed over pr

Figure 37.4   Male sterilization by vasectomy

Source: Callahan TL, Caughey AB, Heffner LJ. Blueprints in obstetrics and gynecology. Malden, MA: Blackwell Science, 1998:162.

progesterone production needed to support the growth of the pregnancy.

No conclusive evidence exists proving that exposure of the fetus to contraceptive steroids in early pregnancy is teratogenic. Consequently, first trimester exposure to contraceptive steroids is not a medical indication for an abortion.

Of the approximately 1.5 million abortions performed in the United States annually, 90% are completed in the first trimester of pregnancy. The most frequently used method is dilation and suction curettage (D&C). In this procedure, the physician first dilates the cervix with metal dilators and then introduces a plastic tube (cannula) attached to suction into the uterus to evacuate the uterine contents (Figure 37.5). When performed by an experienced physician, this procedure carries a very low risk of complications.

Medical methods to abort a pregnancy in

the first trimester are not yet available in the United States. The "French abortion pill," RU-486 (mifepristone), is a progesterone-antagonist that is used in combination with a prostaglandin agent to induce abortion up to nine weeks of gestational age. With this method, the woman experiences uterine cramping and bleeding and passes the pregnancy in a manner similar to a miscarriage. This method is successful approximately 95% of the time and avoids the need for a surgical procedure.

The remaining 10% of abortions performed in the United States are performed in the second trimester of pregnancy. The most commonly used method for terminating second trimester pregnancies involves the surgical method of dilation and evacuation. This method is similar to the D&C, except that larger-bore cannulas and other accessory instruments are used to completely remove the pregnancy from the uterus. Because of the

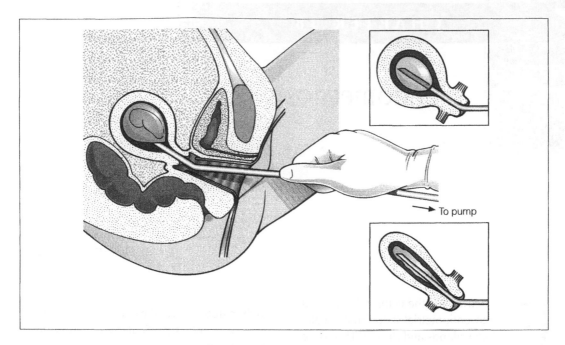

To pump

Figure 37.5   Voluntary abortion with suction curette

Source: Callahan TL, Caughey AB, Heffner LJ. Blueprints in obstetrics and gynecology. Malden, MA: Blackwell Science, 1998:165.

more advanced gestational age and size of the uterus, this procedure carries significant risks if performed by an inexperienced operator. Catastrophic complications such as bowel injury and profound hemorrhage have been associated with dilation and evacuation.

Medical methods to terminate pregnancies in the second trimester are available in the United States. These methods utilize synthetic prostaglandins that are administered either vaginally or intramuscularly. Prostaglandin agents promote uterine contractions that ultimately lead to expulsion of the pregnancy.

SUMMARY

Contraception, sterilization, and abortion have been reviewed in this chapter. In counseling a woman on contraceptive options, it is important to individualize the contraceptive choice, taking into account desire for future fertility and risk of exposure to STDs. Abortion is a less-desirable alternative to contraception. Although first trimester abortion is associated with a very low risk of complications, it should be viewed as a last resort for family planning.

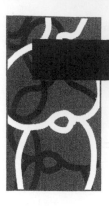

CHAPTER 38

Endometriosis

Alexander F. Burnett

Endometriosis is the ectopic location of benign endometrial tissue that usually includes glands and stroma. This tissue responds to the normal hormones of the female reproductive cycle with cyclic growth and sloughing (hemorrhaging). The sequelae of this process may include pelvic pain, adhesions, infertility, dysmenorrhea, dyspareunia, and the creation of pelvic tumors (endometriomas). Alternatively, this disease may remain silent.

Endometriosis is a disease of reproductive-age women, with the highest incidence occurring in women in their late twenties and early thirties. It is estimated that 1% of all reproductive-age women have endometriosis, and as many as 8% of gynecologic hospital admissions are related to this disease.

in dyspareunia over the entire course of the month, which is particularly painful with deep penetration.

PATHOGENESIS OF ENDOMETRIOSIS

There are three generalized theories as to the genesis of endometriosis. The first, and widely accepted, theory focuses on retrograde menstruation. According to this theory, the endometrial contents pass retrograde through the fallopian tubes at the time of menstruation. The tissue then implants on the peritoneal surfaces and is able to survive there. The most common sites for endometriosis are the ovaries, uterine ligaments, and pelvic peritoneum, all of which are in close proximity to the fallopian tubes (Figure 38.1). Distant sites may also be involved, including anywhere in the abdomen, the lymph nodes, the extremities, the lungs, and other portions of the female genital tract. Supportive evidence for the theory of retrograde menstruation includes the results of animal studies in which the uterine outlet was obstructed, permitting the menstrual contents to pass out the fallopian tubes. In these experiments, endometriosis successfully developed in the pelvic peritoneum.

A second theory of endometriosis points to the spread of the endometrial tissue via lymphatics or hematogenous routes. This theory helps to explain the occurrence of metastatic

CLINICAL CORRELATION

M. R. is a 29-year-old, gravida 0 female who comes to see her gynecologist complaining of progressively painful menses. She reports menarche at age 13, with regular menses every 28 to 30 days and lasting 4 days. During her teenage years, she states that her menses were not particularly uncomfortable. Over the past six years, however, they have become increasingly painful with a tender feeling throughout her pelvis. She occasionally experiences blood in her stool during her menses. In addition, intercourse during this time is extremely painful, and she reports moderate increase

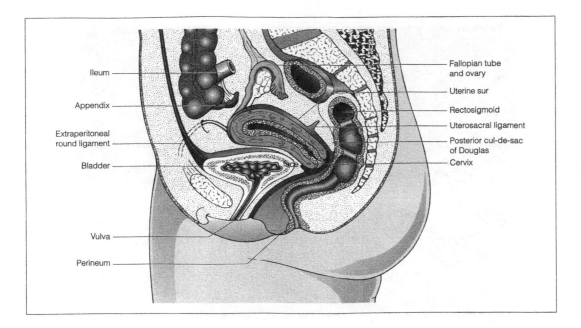

Figure 38.1   Common sites of endometriosis

Source: Callahan TL, Caughey AB, Heffner LJ. Blueprints in obstetrics and gynecology. Malden, MA: Blackwell Science, 1998:94.

endometriosis, such as to the lungs. A third theory involves metaplasia of the coelomic epithelium, which ultimately develops into endometrial tissue. If this theory were valid, one would expect global development of endometriosis throughout the abdominal as well as thoracic cavities. This condition rarely—if ever—occurs, however.

DIAGNOSIS

A presumptive diagnosis of endometriosis may be made on the basis of symptomatology. Nevertheless, a pathologic diagnosis should be confirmed before any therapeutic intervention is undertaken. Most frequently, a diagnosis is made via laparoscopy for evaluation of pelvic pain or infertility. The characteristic lesion will appear as a "powder burn" that is caused by hemorrhage within the endometriotic implant. The appearance of endometriosis may also take a variety of other forms, including clear lesions, clear adhesions, or a collection within the ovary of hemorrhagic material (the so-called endometrioma or "chocolate cyst") (Figure 38.2). When the diagnosis is in doubt, a confirmatory biopsy should be performed. The

extent of endometriosis is characterized using a scoring system developed by the American Fertility Society (Table 38.1).

Because of irritation of the coelomic epithelium by endometriosis, the CA-125 serum marker is frequently elevated. This elevation can occasionally present a diagnostic dilemma, particularly in the older reproductive-age woman who has an adnexal mass. Ultrasound evaluation can often give a reasonable assessment as to whether the mass has the characteristic appearance of an endometrioma (an endometriotic collection on the adnexae) or appears to be more consistent with a carcinoma.

CLINICAL CORRELATION

M. R. has a blood sample drawn. Her CA-125 level is 65 µg/mL. A preoperative ultrasound is negative for any pelvic masses. She undergoes laparoscopy that reveals extensive endometriosis over both ovaries and in the cul-de-sac. Filmy adhesions are found between the right fallopian tube, right ovary, and right pelvic peritoneum. Dense adhesions are present on the

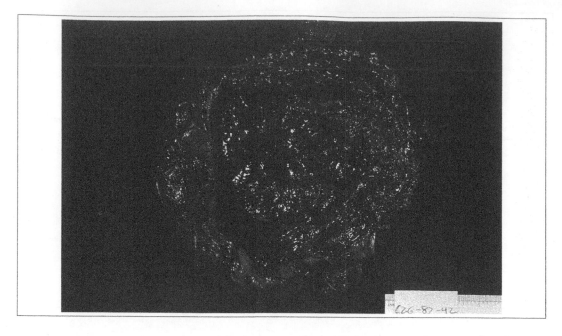

Figure 38.2   An ovarian endometrioma. This cyst was originally filled with dark brown, viscous fluid, representing old blood. The fluid is frequently described as resembling chocolate.

left ovary, enclosing approximately one-half of the ovary. Lysis of adhesions is performed under laparoscopy, as is fulguration of endometriotic implants using electrocautery. At the completion of surgery, dye is injected through the uterus and spills out of both fallopian tubes (chromopertubation).

POST-OPERATIVE THERAPY

The decision about the type of post-operative therapy to pursue will depend on whether the patient has a current complaint of infertility, whether she wishes to retain her fertility potential even though she is not interested in becoming pregnant at this time, or whether she has no further reproductive desires and wishes a definitive surgical procedure be performed.

INFERTILITY TREATMENT

Endometriosis plays a more complex role in infertility than merely creating adhesions that would prevent normal egg and sperm transport. In many cases, minimal adhesive disease is accompanied by an inability to become pregnant. Theories about the cause of this infertility suggest that an immunologic factor or factors may interfere with normal ovulatory function, normal tubal motility, normal implantation, or sperm motility (Table 38.2).

With mild to moderate endometriosis (AFS Stage I and II), five approaches have been advocated in an effort to overcome infertility:

- Observation

- Fulguration

- Laser

- Danazol

- GnRH agonist

Other causes of infertility, which may respond well to therapy, must also be ruled out.

Observation appears to be a reasonable approach to dealing with infertility after making a diagnosis of endometriosis, in that little evidence supports the use of a more active approach to improve a woman's chance of conception. Laparoscopic fulguration of minimal endometriosis may be beneficial if all evidence of endometriosis can be removed; on the other hand, cauterization (burning) of the peritoneum has the potential to result in increased scarring and possible damage to other

Table 38.1 Revised American Fertility Society Classification of Endometriosis

ENDOMETRIOSIS	LESS THAN 1 CM	1–3 CM	MORE THAN 3 CM
Peritoneum			
Superficial	1	2	4
Deep	2	4	6
Ovary*			
Superficial	1	2	4
Deep	4	16	20
		PARTIAL	COMPLETE
Posterior cul-de-sac obliteration		4	40

ADHESIONS	LESS THAN 1/3 ENCLOSURE	1/3–2/3 ENCLOSURE	MORE THAN 2/3 ENCLOSURE
Ovary*			
Filmy	1	2	4
Dense	4	8	16
Uterine tube*			
Filmy	1	2	4
Dense	4[†]	8[†]	16

Scoring: Stage 1 disease (minimal) = 1–5; Stage 2 (mild) = 6–15; Stage 3 (moderate) = 16–40; Stage 4 (severe) = more than 40.

*Each ovary and uterine tube is scored separately.

[†]If the fimbriated end of the tube is completely enclosed, the score is 16.

Source: Reproduced with permission from DeCherney A, Pernoll M. Current obstetric and gynecologic diagnosis and treatment. Norwalk, CT: Appleton and Lange, 1994:806.

organs. Although laser therapy for minimal endometriosis has not been proven to improve fecundity rates, it has been reported to reduce pain associated with endometriosis.

Danazol, a synthetic steroid, reduces pre-ovulatory FSH and LH surges, which in turn reduces the serum levels of estradiol, thereby inhibiting the formation of endometriotic implants. Danazol is also a potent androgen-agonist, producing the side effects commonly related to excess levels of androgen. Conception rates after stopping Danazol appear to be no higher than those found in women who were merely observed after their diagnosis of endometriosis.

GnRH agonists function to create a pseudo-menopause. Theoretically, their use should inhibit any growth of endometriosis after the initial diagnosis is made. Some advocate a short course (three months) of therapy with these agents after diagnosis, although this strategy has not been proven to improve fertility in cases of mild to moderate endometriosis.

In moderate to severe endometriosis, conservative surgical therapy aims to restore the

Table 38.2 Conception Rates After Conservative Treatment of Endometriosis

EXTENT OF DISEASE	CONCEPTION RATES (%)
Mild	75
Moderate	50–60
Severe	30–40

anatomy, eliminate adhesive disease, and remove as much endometriotic tissue as possible. This surgery, combined with hormonal therapy post-operatively to diminish the return of endometriosis, may improve a woman's chances at reproduction.

RETENTION OF FERTILITY

For the woman who wishes to retain her fertility, but does not desire to become pregnant immediately, therapy is aimed at reduction of pain and stabilization or reduction of endometriosis. Continuous treatment with oral contraceptive pills or oral progesterone is the first choice in therapy for these patients.

Danazol and GnRH agonists may be effective as well. Given the higher cost and increased side effects of these agents, however, they should be reserved for those cases that fail to respond to the other therapies. GnRH agonists will induce a menopausal condition that is effective in eliminating the symptoms of endometriosis. This measure is temporary, however, and symptoms generally resume with menses. In addition, GnRH therapy results in accelerated bone demineralization and loss of the cardioprotective effects of estrogen. Because of the potential for significant bone loss, GnRH therapy is used for a maximum of six months. It is therefore a temporizing therapy for endometriosis rather than a definitive treatment.

DEFINITIVE TREATMENT/NO FERTILITY POTENTIAL

In severe disease in women who no longer wish to maintain their fertility potential, total abdominal hysterectomy and bilateral salpingo-oophorectomy may be considered for treatment of pelvic pain. Studies have shown that, with removal of the uterus and ovaries, as many as 90% of women remain symptom-free. If the ovaries remain in place, 60% of women report a return of the symptoms of pelvic pain.

ADENOMYOSIS

Adenomyosis occurs when the myometrium contains endometrial stroma and glands. The exact etiology of this condition remains unknown. It is estimated that this condition is present in some degree in 60% of all uteri. Accompanying the endometrial presence in the myometrium is a compensatory hypertrophy of the myometrium. The classic triad of symptoms is abnormal uterine bleeding, secondary dysmenorrhea, and an enlarged, tender uterus. MRI, and to a lesser extent HSG, may be able to detect adenomyosis. The mainstay of therapy for this condition is hysterectomy. No effective medical therapy is currently available, although antiprogestational agents such as RU-486 hold promise for the future.

CLINICAL CORRELATION

M. R. recovers quickly from her laparoscopic procedure. She is placed on continuous oral contraceptive pills and allowed to have a withdrawal bleed by discontinuing the pills every three months for one week's duration. This regimen continues to maintain her in a pain-free state for two years. Her dysmenorrhea is reduced to minimal discomfort, and her dyspareunia is eliminated.

SUMMARY

Endometriosis is a common problem in reproductive-age women. Symptoms may be either absent or quite severe. Therapy should be directed at improving fertility or treating symptoms, based on the patient's desires in this regard. Surgical therapy must also take into consideration the patient's fertility desires. Often these patients require a combination of surgical and hormonal treatments.

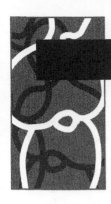

CHAPTER 39

Menopause

Alexander F. Burnett

Menopause is defined as the permanent cessation of menses due to depletion of ovarian follicles with a resultant lack of production of estradiol. Although women are born with approximately 1 to 2 million ovarian primordial follicles, only a few hundred follicles remain at the time of menopause. These few remaining follicles are poorly responsive to gonadotropin stimulation; hence ovulation ceases and ovarian estrogen and androgen production decline. Ovulation first becomes erratic and unpredictable, and then finally ceases altogether.

The mean age of menopause is approximately 51.3 years. In general, a woman is considered to be menopausal if she is 45 years of age or older with 6 to 12 months of amenorrhea. Less than 1% of women younger than 40 years old are menopausal. A number of factors may be associated with an earlier menopause, including smoking, previous hysterectomy, undernourishment, thin stature, and living in high altitudes.

Perimenopause—the period just prior to menopause—is characterized by menstrual irregularities and transient signs and symptoms of menopause. On average, perimenopause begins at 47.5 years and lasts about four years. Ovulation may occur unpredictably during this time, resulting in erratic bleeding. The term "climacteric" refers to the transitional period during which the woman moves from reproductive life to menopause. Two long-term sequelae of estrogen deprivation—osteoporosis and cardiovascular disease—are responsible for a large portion of morbidity and mortality in this group. The physician caring for these women needs to understand the risks and benefits of estrogen replacement therapy and must be able to inform his patients about their hormone replacement options.

HISTORY AND PHYSICAL EXAMINATION

The history taking should help to determine whether the patient has symptoms suggestive of estrogen deprivation. Early symptoms of decreased estrogen production consist of hot flushes, insomnia, and psychological symptoms such as depression or anxiety. Intermediate sequelae include symptoms of urogenital atrophy, such as dyspareunia, vaginal irritation, dysuria, urinary frequency, and urinary urgency. Long-term sequelae of estrogen deprivation consist of osteoporosis and cardiovascular disease.

Past medical history should cover conditions that may contraindicate the use of estrogen therapy, including breast cancer, advanced-stage endometrial cancer, severe hypertriglyceridemia, current liver or gallbladder disease, or a history of estrogen-related thromboembolism (Table 39.1). The presence or history of breast or endometrial cancer, both of which are felt to be estrogen-related, has in certain circumstances become merely a relative contraindication, as some patients receive greater benefits than relative risk from hormonal replacement. Women with a history

Table 39.1   Contraindications to Hormone Replacement (Estrogen) Therapy

Absolute

Current breast cancer

Current endometrial cancer

Acute liver disease

Acute thrombophlebitis or thromboembolic disorders

Undiagnosed vaginal bleeding

Known or suspected pregnancy

Relative

Triglycerides >250 mg/dL (increased risk for pancreatitis)

History of breast or endometrial cancer

Chronic liver disease

Large uterine leiomyomata

Endometriosis

History of thrombophlebitis or thromboembolism

History of cerebral vascular accident

Recent myocardial infarction

Hyperlipidemia

Pancreatic disease

Gallbladder disease

Familial hypertriglyceridemia

Hypertension aggravated by estrogen

Migraine headaches

Hepatic porphyria

of osteoporosis, tobacco use, high blood pressure, and cardiovascular disease may particularly benefit from estrogen replacement.

Lifestyle questions, such as the patient's degree of physical activity and diet, are important factors in the prevention of osteoporosis over which the patient has direct control. Issues of alcohol or excess drug (including prescription drug) use should be addressed as well; these considerations are frequently overlooked in the older patient. Domestic violence is not uncommon among the elderly, often as a result of the actions of a child or caretaker.

Areas on the physical examination that most often reflect the effects of estrogen depri-

vation include the breasts and genitalia. Atrophic changes are commonly observed in the vagina, cervix, and vulva in post-menopausal women who do receive estrogen replacement therapy. Pap smears should continue into the menopause. The bimanual and rectovaginal examinations are particularly important for detecting ovarian masses, uterine enlargement, or occult fecal blood—all signs suggestive of carcinoma. Screening guidelines developed by the American Cancer Society for use with elderly women call for yearly mammograms, sigmoidoscopy every three to five years beginning at age 50, and yearly fecal occult blood testing. Lipid profiles should be performed every three to five years in the postmenopausal patient.

THE PERIMENOPAUSE

CLINICAL CORRELATION

Mrs. H. is a 47-year-old, white female, G2P2, who presents with a complaint of abnormal vaginal bleeding. She has had normal regular menses her entire life until about six months ago, when she began missing periods. She also experienced increased flow when her menses did occur, including the passage of large clots for 10 to 14 days. She is currently sexually active but does not use any contraception. Mrs. H. denies any hot flushes, changes in sleep patterns, alterations in urinary habits, or vaginal dryness. Her past history is unremarkable.

On examination, Mrs. H.'s blood pressure is 120/60. Her breasts have diffuse fibrocystic changes without any dominant masses. On pelvic examination, the external genitalia appear normal, and the vagina is moist, well rugated, and of normal size, shape, and consistency. The ovaries are normal size and nontender. A rectal examination reveals no masses, and the stool guaiac is negative.

MANAGEMENT AND TREATMENT

The menstrual irregularities described by this patient are most consistent with either dysfunctional uterine bleeding secondary to anovulation or endometrial hyperplasia or carcinoma. Sampling of the endometrium can usually be performed in the office with a small curette or pipette biopsy instrument. Prior to the biopsy, a pregnancy test should be performed, as the patient can still potentially conceive. A Pap smear and endocervical curettage should also be done to rule out cervical carcinoma as the etiology of her bleeding. A thyroid-stimulating hormone (TSH) level screens for thyroid disorders that may contribute bleeding irregularities.

CLINICAL CORRELATION

The endometrial biopsy results show a proliferative endometrium without hyperplasia or carcinoma. The Pap smear and endocervical curettage are normal. Mrs. H.'s mammogram and TSH test results are also normal.

Three options can be presented to the patient with dysfunctional perimenopausal bleeding. The first option is to give no therapy and allow menopause to progress over time. The second option is to offer cyclical progesterone withdrawal, which will counteract the action of estrogen on the uterine lining. When given for 10 to 14 days each month, progestins will lead to synchronous shedding of the endometrial lining and reduce the risk of developing hyperplasia/cancer. The third option is to offer low-dose oral contraceptive therapy to minimize the growth of the endometrium and regulate the patient's bleeding. In the perimenopausal period, oral contraceptives also provide the added benefit of birth control in women who may still ovulate occasionally.

CLINICAL CORRELATION

After careful consideration, Mrs. H. decides to commence low-dose oral contraceptive therapy. She returns in three months for a check of her blood pressure, which is normal, and reports that her menses have become regular and are lighter in flow amount and duration. She is concerned about how long she can take oral contraceptive pills and how will she know when she is menopausal.

One way of assessing whether the woman has gone into the menopause is to periodically measure her FSH and LH levels on day 5 of the placebo pill week. The patient can be switched to standard hormone replacement therapy when both values become elevated into the menopausal range.

THE MENOPAUSE

CLINICAL CORRELATION

Mrs. D. is a 60-year-old, thin, white female, G0, with a last menstrual period about 10 years ago who complains of vaginal dryness, irritation, and chronic discharge. She is also troubled by dysuria, urinary frequency, and urinary urgency. Mrs. D admits to hot flushes but states that they have been improving somewhat. She denies being sexually active because she has little desire and because intercourse is extremely painful for her due to her vaginal dryness.

Mrs. D.'s medical history is significant in terms of hypertension, for which she takes multiple medications, and adult-onset diabetes, for which she takes oral hypoglycemics. Her surgical history includes a recent (benign) breast biopsy. She is a heavy smoker and leads a sedentary lifestyle. Her family history includes a sister who died at age 60 from breast cancer and a strong family history of cardiovascular disease. She denies any prior abnormal Pap smears or gynecologic complaints.

On physical examination, Mrs. D. is found to be 5 ft, 3 in tall and weighs 100 lb. Her blood pressure is 150/90. Her breast examination reveals a scar from her recent biopsy, but is otherwise negative. The vulva is thin and flat with almost total eradication of the labia. The vaginal mucosa is thin and pale without visible rugations. The cervix is pale and atrophic and is flush with the vagina. On bimanual examination, the uterus appears small, mobile, and nontender. The ovaries are not palpable. Stool guaiac is negative.

MANAGEMENT AND TREATMENT

Vasomotor instability (hot flushes) are experienced as a sudden sensation of intense warmth of the upper body with a visible flush ascending from the thorax to the neck and face; this sensation is followed by profuse sweating. These flushes may last anywhere from a few seconds to several minutes. They originate in the hypothalamus, when an inappropriate excitation of the heat release mechanisms causes a decline in the core body temperature. Generally these flushes are precipitated by a fall in estrogen levels and an LH surge. Hot flushes commonly occur at night and can result in poor sleep, insomnia, fatigue, irritability, impaired memory, and impaired concentration.

Estrogens are more than 95% effective in relieving hot flushes. Estrogen also appears to play a role in maintaining memory and may be important in the prevention of Alzheimer's disease. Other medications, such as clonidine and aldomet, are used in cases where estrogen replacement therapy is contraindicated. These medications act centrally to effect the release of neurotransmitters and successfully relieve symptoms in 35% to 40% of patients. In addition, Bellergal (a combination of atropine and phenobarbital), Danazol, and progesterone may help in reducing hot flushes. One-half to three-fourths of all menopausal women experience hot flushes.

Clinical Correlation

Mrs. D.'s examination is consistent with the sequelae of hypoestrogenism. She has previously demonstrated the early symptoms of hypoestrogenism (vasomotor instability, insomnia) and now complains of intermediate symptoms of urogenital atrophy.

Urogenital atrophy is another sequelae of estrogen deprivation. The labia, vagina, bladder, and urethra are all estrogen-dependent tissues. Estrogen promotes growth and cornification of the vaginal epithelium. These epithelial cells are rich in glycogen, a substance that is metabolized by the lactobacillus bacteria to create an acidic environment that prevents bacterial overgrowth and infection. During menopause, less vaginal transudate is produced and therefore less natural lubrication is provided. The vaginal tissue may become thin, less elastic, and friable, leading to symptoms of vaginal dryness, pruritus, burning, discharge, bleeding, and dyspareunia. Dyspareunia will often result in decreased libido in the postmenopausal woman. The bladder mucosa may also thin, causing the urine to come into direct contact with the sensory nerves of the bladder, which in turn increases dysuria, urinary frequency, and suprapubic discomfort. Urinary incontinence may occur with thinning of the urethral mucosa. The incontinence may result from genuine stress urinary incontinence, a condition attributable to relaxation and laxity of the pelvic support secondary to lack of estrogen. Alternatively, incontinence may have a detrussor instability component, caused by the previously mentioned direct contact of the sensory nerves of the bladder with the urine due to bladder mucosal thinning. Six to 12 months of estrogen replacement is necessary to achieve full alleviation of atrophic symptoms. Vaginal lubricants during intercourse can be used while the hormones are taking time to work.

With menopause, the breasts decrease in size and the ducts atrophy. The breasts are increasingly replaced with fatty tissue. Elasticity of the skin of the breasts, like the elasticity of the skin elsewhere on the body, is diminished and results in sagging of the breasts.

Decreased libido may result from many of the menopausal symptoms described—especially vaginal dryness, decreased sleep and irritability, and decreased androgen (testosterone) production by the ovaries. Testosterone supplementation plus estrogen replacement may be necessary to restore libido in some women.

Long-term sequelae of estrogen deprivation include osteoporosis and cardiovascular disease. During the menopause, a woman's risk of heart disease rises rapidly to reach the same risk level associated with men. In fact, 500,000 women die each year from cardiovascular disease. Estrogen therapy in the menopause can decrease cardiovascular mortality by as much as 50%. Although estrogen lowers the low-density lipoprotein (LDL) fraction and increases the high-density lipoprotein (HDL) fraction of cholesterol, an improvement in the lipid profile explains only 35% to 50% of this reduction. In addition, estrogen retards the atherosclerotic process and promotes vasodilatation, which may lower blood pressure. It also results in reduced platelet adhesion and aggregation by increasing prostacyclin levels. Left ventricular diastolic filling and stroke volume are increased by a direct ionotropic effect of this hormone.

Estrogen administration is the standard therapy for prevention of osteoporosis. Osteoporosis is a disease of reduced skeletal mass accompanied by microarchitectural deterioration of the skeleton that results in increased bone fragility and greater risk of fracture. The loss of estrogen is accompanied by increased bone resorption and decreased bone formation. Other risk factors for osteoporosis include tobacco use, thin stature, poor calcium intake, alcohol use, sedentary lifestyle, and a family history of osteoporosis. The bone loss during the menopause is primarily trabecular bone, which is metabolically active. Some 25% of women older than age 60 have evidence of vertebral fractures; 50% of women older than age 75 exhibit this condition. The average woman will shrink 2.5 inches during the menopause and will experience cortical bone loss. Ultimately, 25% of women older than age 80 will experience hip fracture, with one in six such fractures proving fatal.

Adequate calcium intake is necessary to stave off osteoporosis. Women in the menopause taking estrogen should consume 1000 to 1500 mg of calcium daily. In addition, weight-bearing exercises for 30 minutes, three times per week, are necessary to maintain bone density. For the patient with limited exposure to sunlight, vitamin D supplementation should be provided.

Bone density measurements can predict a woman's risk of osteoporotic fractures. Dual-photon absorptiometry reports the measurement of bone density as a deviation from the mean for young adults. Each standard deviation reduction in bone mass doubles the patient's risk of fractures. Most commonly, measurements are taken at the hip and spine. By definition, osteoporosis involves bone mass density 2.5 or more standard deviations below the mean. Mrs. D. has many risk factors for osteoporosis, including smoking, sedentary lifestyle, thin, and not taking calcium supplements. Most compelling is the statement that she has "shrunk"—objective evidence of significant bone loss.

One of the most common reasons for refusing estrogen replacement is a fear of breast cancer. From an overall health point of view, 23% of women will die from cardiovascular disease and only 4% will die from breast cancer. Large, controlled trials have failed to show a causative relationship between estrogen use and the development of breast cancer. That is, estrogen does not appear to cause breast cancer, but it will promote the growth of such cancer after it has developed. This lack of a causative relationship appears to hold even for those women with a strong family history of breast cancer.

CLINICAL CORRELATION

Mrs. D. has a normal mammogram, a normal Pap smear, and a normal screening flexible sigmoidoscopy. Her cholesterol is 250, with an HDL component of 30 and an LDL component of 120. Her triglyceride level is 150. Bone densitometry studies document significant bone loss to date. She agrees to begin estrogen replacement therapy.

Estrogen therapy can be administered in different forms and via a variety of routes (transdermally, orally, vaginally). Standard therapy involves oral daily administration of 0.625 mg of conjugated estrogen. A progestin should be administered to those women who have an intact uterus to prevent unopposed estrogen from causing hyperplasia or carcinoma of the endometrium. These hormones can be given sequentially or continuously. Many women like the convenience of taking both estrogen and 2.5 mg of medroxyprogesterone acetate on a daily basis. With this regimen they will quickly become amenorrheic and should have no further bleeding abnormalities.

CLINICAL CORRELATION

Because Mrs. D. does not wish to have any vaginal bleeding, she opts for continuous estrogen/progesterone therapy. She is instructed to return in three months for follow-up with a blood pressure check.

Her follow-up blood pressure is 140/80. Mrs. D. admits to some irregular spotting during the first two months of therapy, which has since ceased. She has experienced improvement in her vaginal and bladder symptoms, and is aware that more time is necessary for complete resolution of these symptoms. Her hot flushes have completely resolved. She is instructed to call if she experiences any further bleeding. She will follow up with yearly examinations, and bone density measurements will be repeated in one to two years to document the lack of progression of her osteoporosis.

Additional therapies may be viable alternatives in patients with contraindications to estrogen replacement therapy. Bisphosphonates are analogues of pyrophosphate that affect the osteoclasts decreasing bone resorption. The net result is increased bone mineral density and a decreased fracture rate. Alendronate (Fosamax) is the most widely used of the bisphosphonates. Studies have documented a significant decreased risk of fracture for osteoporotic women taking this drug as compared with placebo. Calcitonin inhibits the action of osteoclasts and may play a role in the future in fracture prevention. Hormones that have mixed estrogen-agonist/estrogen-antagonist activity, such as tamoxifen and raloxifene, may also prove beneficial in preventing post-menopausal osteoporosis. The benefit of sodium fluoride remains controversial.

SUMMARY

The menopause is a time of significant change for a woman. The withdrawal of estrogen has effects on the genitourinary system, the cardiovascular system, the bones, and the psychological system. Estrogen replacement is advised in women without contraindications to the medication and should remain a life-long supplement.

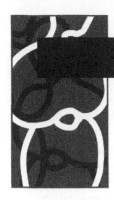

CHAPTER 40

Hirsutism and Virilization

Megan E. Breen

Hirsutism is the abnormal presence of excess hair. Virilization is a more extreme condition where secondary female sexual characteristics may be lost. Many women will come to their physicians complaining of unwanted hair growth only after cosmetic measures have failed. While this condition is often distressing to the patient, it may also be a marker for more serious conditions.

PHYSIOLOGY

The number of hair follicles is established from 8 to 22 weeks gestational age in the fetus. Although no differences in the number of hair follicles are found between men and women; racial differences are noted. For example, Asian people have relatively fewer hair follicles per unit measured, whereas Mediterraneans have relatively more hair follicles per unit measured.

The sebaceous unit of the hair shaft contains androgen receptors. Testosterone is converted to dihydrotestosterone (DHT) by the enzyme 5-alpha-reductase. DHT, which is twice as potent as testosterone, functions primarily locally. Two types of hair exist: (1) vellus hair, which has fine, unpigmented shafts, and (2) terminal hair, which has thick, coarse, pigmented shafts. Vellus hair is transformed into terminal hair by the action of testosterone. Once hair has the terminal phenotype, it will remain terminal even if testosterone is withdrawn. Hair growth will continue indefinitely unless the dermal papilla of the hair follicle is destroyed.

Nonendocrine factors that influence hair growth include destructive measures such as radiation and decreased circulation. In addition, some medications (for example, phenytoin and minoxidil) may increase hair growth. Likewise, systemic endocrinopathies such as acromegaly can increase hair growth. Hypothyroidism may result in thick, coarse, scalp hair with decreased axillary and pubic hair and loss of hair from the lateral third of the eyebrow.

Normally, androgens will stimulate growth of thicker, darker, coarser hair, with an increased rate of growth being observed everywhere except the scalp. Estrogens have the opposite effect, creating lighter, finer hair with a slower growth rate. Progestins have no effect on hair growth. Increased hair production and alteration to an adult distribution follows an orderly pattern during puberty. Familiarity with the Tanner staging of pubertal hair growth (see Chapter 34) may provide clues about abnormal hormone production in the young woman.

CLINICAL CORRELATION

P. C. is a 28-year-old, African American woman who presents to her gynecologist complaining of increased hair growth that is noticeable on her chest. This growth has been gradually increasing over the past two years. P. C. bleaches and plucks her facial hair but became disconcerted by the appearance of chest hair. She has not noticed any change in body habitus, muscle distribution, or breast size. She denies any balding or deepening of her voice. Acne, however, has been present for years.

Her menses began at age 15 and have never been regular. The flow may be heavy or light but is not associated with cramping. She is sexually active and currently uses condoms for contraception. Coitarche was at age 19, and she has had two lifetime partners. She is otherwise healthy and does not see any doctor other than her gynecologist.

ANDROGEN SOURCES IN WOMEN

In normal women, the total testosterone level is 0.2 to 0.3 mg/dL. The adrenal glands and the ovaries contribute equal amounts of testosterone, except during midcycle when ovarian production increases. Approximately half of the testosterone is derived from peripheral conversion of androstenedione. Dihydroepiandrostenedione-sulfate (DHEA-S) is almost exclusively produced by the adrenal gland, but mild to moderate increases may be noted in patients with polycystic ovaries (Figure 40.1).

Normal women may have the same total testosterone level as hirsute women, with the difference being noted in the amount of free testosterone. Unbound or free testosterone accounts for 1% of total testosterone in normal women but rises to 2% of total testosterone in affected women. The unbound form is the active form of the hormone. In the hirsute woman, peripheral conversion of androstenedione accounts for only 25% of the total testosterone with the remainder coming from the ovary. Sex-hormone binding globulin (SHBG) is the transport protein produced by the liver that binds testosterone and estradiol. Estrogens will increase SHBG amounts and androgens will decrease SHBG amounts. Shifts in sex steroid levels, such as an increase in testosterone, may decrease SHBG-binding sites for the androgens and therefore result in increased levels of free testosterone, which may further decrease SHBG levels.

EFFECTS OF ANDROGEN EXCESS

One of the earliest signs of excess androgen levels is acne. Later, hirsutism with an increase in male hair patterns (including scalp alopecia) may be seen. Menstrual irregularities may occur. Lipid profiles are adversely affected, with increased triglycerides and LDL cholesterol and decreased HDL cholesterol being noted. In extreme cases of androgen excess, as seen with a testosterone-producing ovarian tumor such as an arrhenoblastoma, virilism may occur. Virilization may be accompanied by clitoromegaly, breast atrophy, increased muscular mass, and masculinization of the body habitus (Figure 40.2).

Polycystic ovarian syndrome (PCO) is a situation where the ovaries fail to ovulate in the normal fashion. Women affected by PCO classically have hyperandrogenism and some degree of hirsutism with menstrual disturbances (oligomenorrhea or amenorrhea). Commonly, the patients are obese. The irregular menses reflect anovulation, and symptoms often begin shortly after menarche. Typically, the serum LH is elevated relative to the FSH concentration, often at a 3:1 ratio. Elevated levels of serum testosterone are common—particularly the unbound or free testosterone—but rarely to levels exceeding 150 ng/dL. Adrenal androgens may also be mildly elevated. In addition, women with PCO may develop insulin resistance through an unknown mechanism.

Because women with PCO do not have effective levels of FSH or experience an appropriate LH surge at midcycle, they generally do not ovulate. On ultrasound, the ovaries will often show small cysts of multiple follicles just below the cortex (hence the name "polycystic"). On gross examination, the cortex is smooth and thickened, without evidence of breaks in the surface due to ovulation.

The etiology of PCO is unknown but certainly multifactorial. Improvement in the endocrinologic abnormalities associated with PCO is seen in patients who lose weight. Wedge resection of affected ovaries or electrocautery drilling of the affected ovaries has also been shown to improve symptoms and stimulate ovulation. Oral contraceptive pills are effective in regulating menstrual cycles. This

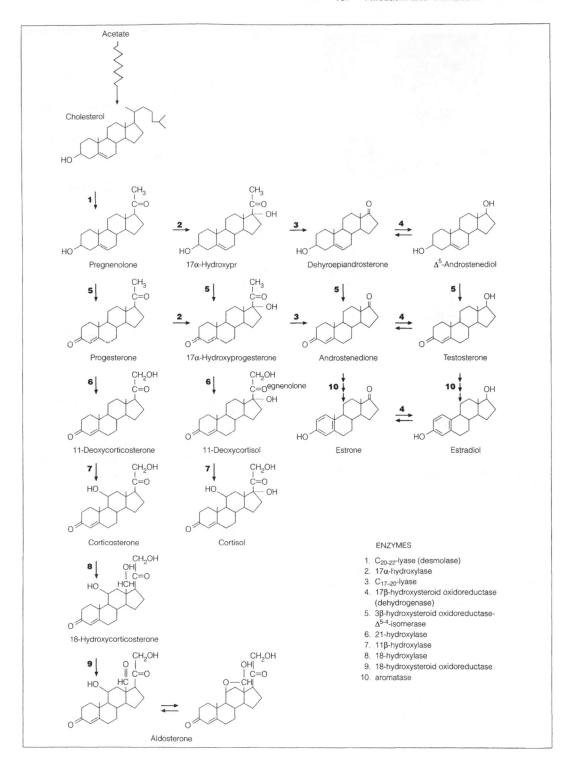

Figure 40.1 Biosynthetic pathways for production of estrogens, progestins, and androgens

Source: Callahan TL, Caughey AB, Heffner LJ. Blueprints in obstetrics and gynecology. Malden, MA: Blackwell Science, 1998:146.

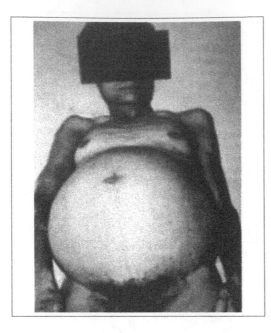

Figure 40.2 A woman with an androgen-producing ovarian tumor. She is clearly masculinized by the male hormones of the tumor.

Source: Morrow CP, Curtin JP, ed. Synopsis of gynecologic oncology, 5th ed. Philadelphia: Churchill Livingstone, 1998:286.

consideration is important because women with PCO face an increased risk of endometrial hyperplasia and carcinoma with chronic elevations of circulating estrogens and amenorrhea. Clomophine citrate is prescribed to stimulate ovulation in those patients who wish to conceive. This agent binds to estrogen receptors in the hypothalamus, inhibiting the negative feedback of estrogen. As a result, gonadotropins are released, leading to ovulation.

Congenital adrenal hyperplasia (CAH) is a deficiency in cortisol biosynthesis. It most commonly involves a 21-hydroxylase deficiency. A lack of this enzyme results in inhibition of cortisol production, which in turn leads to overproduction of adrenocorticotropin hormone (ACTH) because of the lack of negative feedback from cortisol. This condition may be present at birth with masculinization of the female infant and ambiguous genitalia. One form of CAH is associated with salt-wasting at birth that may prove fatal if it goes undetected. Milder, adult-onset forms of CAH will typically present with symptoms of androgen excess. Treatment consists of replacing the deficiency

of glucocorticoids and/or mineralocorticoids as needed.

CLINICAL CORRELATION

Physical examination: BP, 128/80; height, 5 ft, 3 in; weight, 170 lb.
HEENT: bleached hair noted on cheeks, chin, and upper lip.
Neck: no thyromegaly.
Chest: scant amount of hair distribution on the chest.
Breasts: no galactorrhea.
Abdomen: male escheon pattern of hair distribution on the lower abdomen.
External genitalia: no clitoromegaly or other evidence of virilism.
Bimanual examination: normal-sized uterus and ovaries.
    The remainder of the examination is unremarkable.

ETIOLOGY OF ANDROGEN EXCESS

The various sources of androgen excess are listed in Table 40.1. The rapidity with which androgen excess develops may also aid in the

---

Table 40.1 Sources of Androgen Excess

1. Testosterone	50% from peripheral conversion of androstenedione
	25% directly produced by the adrenal gland
	25% produced by the ovary
2. DHAS	100% produced by the adrenal gland
3. DHA	90% produced by the adrenal gland
	10% produced by the ovary

Therefore, the sources are:

• Adrenal gland	Tumors, hyperplasia
• Ovary	Tumors, hyperstimulation
• CNS	Overproduction of ACTH (Cushing's disease)
• Ectopic ACTH	Tumors

differential diagnosis. Rapid hirsutism or virilization is most commonly seen with tumors. Chronic conditions such as PCO tend to produce a more gradual development of androgen excess. Table 40.2 lists the differential diagnoses employed with androgen excess.

SCREENING

The screening laboratory studies for hyperandrogenism will help to determine the source of androgen excess (Table 40.3). Testosterone, prolactin, LH, FSH, DHEA-S, and 17-OH progesterone are all adequate laboratory tests for the initial work-up. High levels of testosterone suggest the presence of an androgen-secreting tumor (either adrenal or ovarian). High levels of prolactin suggest prolactinoma. Elevated LH with normal FSH is suggestive of PCO. Elevated DHEA-S indicate a problem of adrenal origin. High levels of 17-OH progesterone are consistent with 21-hydroxylase deficiency, which is the most common cause of congenital adrenal hyperplasia.

CLINICAL CORRELATION

The patient's initial laboratory evaluation returns with the following results: LH, 15.6 mIU/mL (0.6–12.5); FSH, 5.9 mIU/mL (<0.6–9.13); testosterone, 85 ng/dL (25–95); androstenedione, 135 ng/dL (65–270); TSH, 1.9 mIU/mL (0.4–5.5); DHEA-S, 4.1 µg/mL (0.7–4.5); prolactin, 17 ng/dL (<25); 8 A.M. 17-OH-progesterone, 0.8 ng/dL (<2).

THERAPY

All therapy should be targeted toward any specific cause identified. If an ovarian or adrenal tumor is identified, surgical management is indicated. If Cushing syndrome is found, the source of cortisol production should be determined. If CAH is recognized, dexamethasone 0.125 mg qhs is given, with the dose being slowly advanced until levels are suppressed to mid-normal values. Oral contraceptives and GnRH agonists may be used as well. Idiopathic hirsutism may be successfully treated in the same manner as PCO.

In hirsutism, the source of androgens must be suppressed to prevent additional production. Oral contraceptives are the mainstay of therapy. These agents lower LH levels, and most androgen production is LH-dependent. The level of free testosterone is decreased by increasing the SHBG levels with oral contraceptives. The adrenal source of androgens is also decreased when DHEA-S are reduced by 50%. At the level of the hair follicle, 5-alpha reductase is inhibited and progestin within the oral contraceptive pill will directly compete for the androgen-binding site.

Table 40.2   Differential Diagnosis in Androgen Excess and Hirsutism

Ovarian

Severe insulin resistance

Virilizing ovarian tumors

   Sertoli-Leydig tumors

   Thecomas

   Hyperthecosis

Adrenal

Congenital adrenal hyperplasia

   21-hydroxylase deficiency

   3 β-hydroxysteroid dehydrogenase deficiency

   11-hydroxylase deficiency

Cushing's disease

Ectopic adrenocorticotropin-secreting tumors

Virilizing adrenal tumors

Combined Ovarian and Adrenal

Polycystic ovary syndrome

Functional hyperandrogenism

Table 40.3   Laboratory Screening for Androgen Excess

Hirsutism	Testosterone, DHEA-S, 17-OH progesterone
Irregular menses	Thyroid function tests, prolactin
R/O adrenal causes	Dexamethasone suppression test
Metabolic abnormalities	Three-hour glucose challenge, fasting lipids

If the patient is unable to tolerate oral contraceptives, Depo-Provera may be used. This agent provides less of a decrease in LH, albeit a still significant decline. Although SHBG levels are diminished, testosterone clearance is increased, leading to lower amounts of free testosterone.

Both oral contraceptives and Depo-Provera take six months before any benefits become visible. Acne is the first sign to show improvement; hirsutism often takes 6 to 12 months to begin to improve.

Specific antiandrogen medications have been used to decrease hair growth:

- Spironolactone is an aldosterone antagonist diuretic that competitively inhibits the androgen receptor on the hair follicle.

- Cyproterone acetate is a progesterone with antiandrogen effects. It blocks androgen receptors and inhibits gonadotropin secretion.

- GnRH agonists should be used only in resistant cases. A higher level is required in these patients than in patients who require only estrogen suppression; for this reason, testosterone levels should be monitored. Patients who receive GnRH agonists will require estrogen add-back therapy, and this therapy is quite expensive.

- Finasteride has been used for benign prostatic hypertrophy. It directly inhibits 5-alpha reductase and may hold some promise for the treatment of hirsutism in women.

Once the patient has been treated for six months, further hirsutism should not occur if the androgen levels remain suppressed. A hair follicle that has been changed from vellus to terminal hair can be removed only if the dermal papilla is destroyed, however. Electrolysis can accomplish this goal as a permanent hair removal therapy.

CLINICAL CORRELATION

P. C. begins oral contraceptive pills and spironolactone. One year later, after electrolysis, the patient is quite pleased with the cosmetic results. She is counseled about her increased risk of cardiovascular disease and begins a program of regular exercise and diet restriction. Her lipid screen and glucose challenge are both normal.

SUMMARY

The evaluation of the patient with androgen excess as demonstrated by hirsutism should follow a systematic approach with a history and physical examination and appropriate laboratory studies. It is critical to determine that the source of the androgen production is not a tumor; this cause can usually be ruled out by the serum hormone levels. Therapy is directed at correction of the source of the androgen excess and then at cosmetic issues related to the hirsutism.

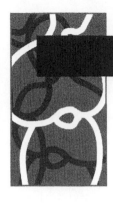

CHAPTER 41

Amenorrhea and Abnormal Uterine Bleeding

Alexander F. Burnett

AMENORRHEA

Amenorrhea is defined as a lack of menstrual flow. It has an incidence of 5% in reproductive-age women. The only times at which amenorrhea is physiologic and therefore "normal" are during the prepubescent period, pregnancy, lactation, and menopause. Amenorrhea is not a diagnosis or a disease, but rather a symptom of a pathologic process occurring at some level in the reproductive tract.

Amenorrhea is classified as primary or secondary, depending upon whether the patient has been menstruating in the past. Primary amenorrhea is the absence of menarche by age 16 in a woman with normal secondary sexual characteristics, or no menses by age 14 in a woman lacking secondary sexual characteristics. Secondary amenorrhea is the absence of menses for six months in a woman who was previously menstruating. The most common etiology of secondary amenorrhea in the reproductive-age woman is pregnancy.

To elucidate the mechanisms of amenorrhea, one must understand how the reproductive axis works. The hypothalamus, at the level of the median eminence, produces gonadotropin-releasing hormone (GnRH) in a pulsatile fashion. This pulsing of GnRH is critical to achieve the pulsatile release of leutizing hormone (LH) and follicle-stimulating hormone (FSH) from the pituitary. The FSH causes folliculogenesis and resultant increased estradiol secretion, which in turn leads to the proliferation of the endometrial lining. A midcycle LH surge results in ovulation and progesterone secretion. A fall in progesterone levels is responsible for synchronous shedding of the endometrial lining and cyclical menses (Figure 41.1).

PRIMARY AMENORRHEA

The etiology of primary amenorrhea may be an abnormality occurring in any place along the reproductive axis as described in Table 41.1. Anatomical abnormalities in a phenotypic woman who has not menstruated must be ruled out first. These problems include congenital blockage of the outflow tract by imperforate hymen or vaginal septum, and congenital absence of portions of the outflow tract including the uterus or vagina.

Chromosomal anomalies can include a 45XO genotype (Turner syndrome), wherein gonadal dysgenesis due to follicle atresia prior to puberty results in a failure of endogenous estrogen production and lack of secondary sexual characteristics. Women with this syndrome have short stature, typical shield chest, and ovaries that are merely streaks. These streak ovaries should be removed upon diagnosis, as they have a high rate of malignancy. In cases of testicular feminization, the individual is genetically male with 46XY chromosomes but is insensitive to androgens. Therefore, the external phenotype is female but the uterus is absent. These phenotypic women often have large breasts, smooth skin due to lack of testosterone response in the skin, and testes located either in the pelvis or inguinal

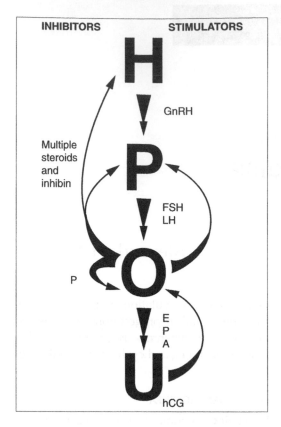

Figure 41.1 The hypothalamic–pituitary–ovarian axis

Table 41.1 Etiologies of Primary Amenorrhea

Outflow tract abnormalities
   Imperforate hymen
   Transverse vaginal septum
   Vaginal agenesis
      Vaginal atresia
      Testicular feminization
   Uterine agenesis with vaginal dysgenesis
      Rokitansky–Kuster–Hauser syndrome
End-organ disorders
   Ovarian agenesis
      Gonadal agenesis 46,XX
      Swyer syndrome—gonadal agenesis 46,XY
   Ovarian failure
      Enzymatic defects leading to decreased steroid biosynthesis
      Savage syndrome—ovary fails to respond to FSH and LH
      Turner syndrome
Central disorders
   Hypothalamic
      Local tumor compression
      Trauma
      Tuberculosis
      Sarcoidosis
      Irradiation
      Kallman syndrome—congenital absence of GnRH
   Pituitary
      Damage from surgery or radiation therapy
      Hemosiderosis deposition of iron in pituitary

ligament. Removal of the gonads should be performed after puberty to allow these individuals to reach normal adult stature; these gonads have a low likelihood of becoming malignant in the pubertal years as compared with the dysgenic gonads of Turner syndrome. Central disorders can also cause primary amenorrhea (see Table 41.1).

Figure 41.2 depicts the work-up for primary amenorrhea.

SECONDARY AMENORRHEA

The work-up of secondary amenorrhea is more complicated than that for primary amenorrhea (Figure 41.3). Central etiologies of secondary amenorrhea include systemic diseases such as hypothyroidism, hyperthyroidism, Cushing's disease, renal failure, hepatic disorders, diabetes, and congenital adrenal hyperplasia, among others. Medications that can lead to central amenorrhea include those that can elevate prolactin levels; excess prolactin interferes with GnRH pulsatility from the hypothalamus.

These agents include psychotropics, anesthetics, antihypertensives, and some antiemetics. A history of galactorrhea (discharge from the nipple) may accompany hyperprolactinemia. The patient's diet and exercise patterns may also play a role in amenorrhea. For example, anorexic patients and frequent exercisers who have very low body fat often have disturbances in the pulsatility of GnRH release from the hypothalamus. In addition, the high endorphin levels

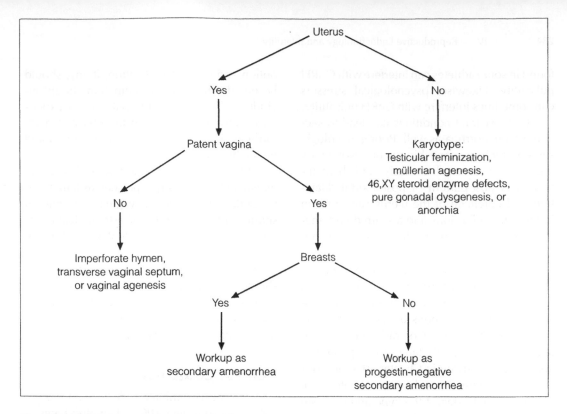

Figure 41.2 Work-up of primary amenorrhea

Source: Callahan TL, Caughey AB, Heffner LJ. Blueprints in obstetrics and gynecology. Malden, MA: Blackwell Science, 1998:135.

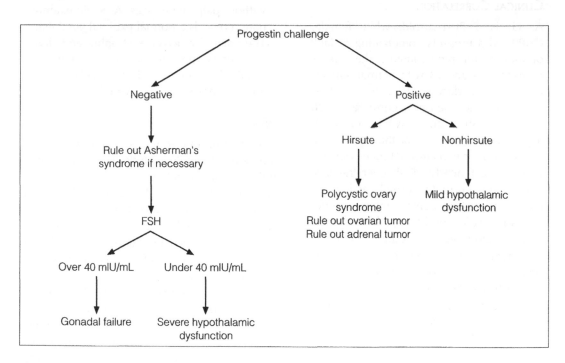

Figure 41.3 Work-up of secondary amenorrhea

Source: Callahan TL, Caughey AB, Heffner LJ. Blueprints in obstetrics and gynecology. Malden, MA: Blackwell Science, 1998:139.

found in some athletes can interfere with GnRH pulsatility. Likewise, psychological stressors can sometimes interfere with GnRH pulsatility.

Outflow tract conditions can lead to secondary amenorrhea as well. Prior gynecologic surgery such as cone biopsy or cryotherapy may cause cervical stenosis and hematometria. A post-partum or post-abortal dilatation and curettage of the uterus can result in intrauterine adhesions and a scarred endometrium that is unresponsive to hormones, a condition known as Asherman syndrome.

Ovarian etiologies of secondary amenorrhea include premature ovarian failure, which may either be physiologic or result from exposure to certain infections or medical therapy such as chemotherapy or radiation. Anovulation may be attributable to hyperandrogenism, as discussed in Chapter 40. Questions regarding excess body hair or symptoms of virilization will suggest the hyperandrogenism that may accompany polycystic ovaries, congenital adrenal hyperplasia, Cushing's disease, and certain adrenal or ovarian tumors.

CLINICAL CORRELATION

A. G. is a 20-year-old, white female, G0P0, who presents complaining of lack of menses for nine months. She reports menarche at age 13 with normal appearance of secondary sexual characteristics. In the past, her menses occurred every 28 to 30 days. She is currently a junior in college and is a member of the track team. She runs approximately 10 miles per day and has lost nearly 20 lb over the past year. She is currently sexually active and uses condoms for contraception. She denies any medical problems, takes no medications, and does not use any illicit drugs. She denies galactorrhea or excess body hair. A. B. does complain of occasional hot flushes and has dyspareunia secondary to vaginal dryness. Her greatest concern at this time focuses on her ability to have children in the future.

The patient's height, weight, blood pressure, and general habitus are important initial measurements in the work-up. The hair distri-

bution and signs of virilization, if any, should be noted. The breast examination should include asking whether the patient has experienced any discharge from the breasts (galactorrhea). The abdominal examination should highlight any masses.

The pelvic examination should discover whether clitoromegaly is present, as it may signal androgen excess. The vaginal examination should note the degree of estrogenization of the mucosa and any potential anatomical causes of amenorrhea. In addition, the presence of a cervix and any cervical stenosis should be documented. A bimanual/rectovaginal examination is performed to document the presence and characteristics of the uterus and identify any adnexal masses.

CLINICAL CORRELATION

On physical examination, A. G. measures 5 ft, 5 in, and weighs 100 lb. Her blood pressure is normal. Her neck is supple without thyroid nodules or goiter. The breasts are Tanner Stage 5 and there is no galactorrhea. Her abdomen is soft, flat, and nontender without palpable masses. A pelvic examination reveals a normal external genitalia. The vaginal mucosa is atrophic and dry. The cervix appears normal. The uterus is small, firm, anteverted, and mobile. No adnexal masses are discovered.

WORK-UP

The work-up to discover a central etiology of amenorrhea should include those factors that influence the function of the hypothalamus and the pituitary gland (Figure 41.4). Serum TSH and prolactin levels are measured to screen for thyroid dysfunction and hyperprolactinemia, respectively. An elevated prolactin level warrants an MRI of the head to rule out a pituitary adenoma.

The ovary is responsible for the coordinated production of estrogen and progesterone during the cycle. The patient's endogenous estrogen status is evaluated by giving her a progesterone challenge test consisting of 10 mg medroxyprogesterone acetate orally for 10 days. Withdrawal bleeding within 2 to 7 days after cessation of progesterone documents that

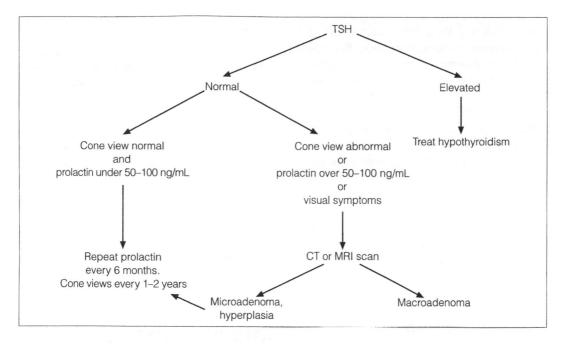

Figure 41.4   Work-up of amenorrhea with galactorrhea and prolactinemia

Source: Callahan TL, Caughey AB, Heffner LJ. Blueprints in obstetrics and gynecology. Malden, MA: Blackwell Science, 1998:138.

the ovary is producing estrogen and that the patient has an intact outflow tract. The diagnosis in a patient with a positive progesterone challenge (withdrawal bleeding present) is anovulation and the work-up is complete. A lack of withdrawal suggests either inadequate production of estrogen or an anomaly or absence of the outflow tract. If the patient takes estrogen for 25 days (for example, conjugated estrogen 1.25 mg/day) with 10 mg medroxyprogesterone acetate concomitant on the final 10 days, she will bleed upon withdrawal from these hormones if she has an intact outflow tract.

In the woman with an intact outflow tract but no endogenous estrogen production, the pituitary gonadotropins FSH and LH should be measured. Elevated gonadotropin levels (FSH > 40 mIU/mL) indicate ovarian failure. In a woman younger than 40 years old, this failure is considered premature.

Levels of gonadotropin in the low or normal range indicate a defect at the level of the pituitary or hypothalamus. These individuals should receive an MRI of the brain to rule out

pituitary lesions, meningioma, craniopharyngioma, aneurysm, metastatic brain tumor, gumma, fat deposit, tuberculoma, empty sella, or Sheehan syndrome. Sheehan syndrome involves apoplexy of the pituitary gland due to ischemia that may occur in the peripartum period. Its symptoms reflect the absence of pituitary hormones.

A normal MRI prompts the diagnosis of hypothalamic amenorrhea, a condition that is identified by exclusion. This suppression of the normal pulsatile release of GnRH from the median eminence of the hypothalamus brings GnRH concentration to a level that no longer supports ovulation. Hypothalamic amenorrhea may occur secondary to psychological stress, low body weight, low body fat, or extreme exercise.

CLINICAL CORRELATION

A. G. has normal prolactin and TSH levels. After testing negative for pregnancy, she is given a progesterone challenge. She fails to experience withdrawal bleeding, signifying a problem with the outflow tract or lack of endogenous estrogen production. Because she has had menses in the past, the examination of the genital tract was normal, and she has not undergone a dilatation and curettage of the uterus, her physician concludes that A. G. is not making adequate amounts of estrogen. The examination with vaginal atrophy and her symptoms of hot flushes and vaginal dryness are consistent with that diagnosis. An FSH sample is drawn and the hormone level found to be very low. An MRI of the head is performed, which reveals no obvious lesions. She is diagnosed as having hypothalamic amenorrhea most likely secondary to her low body weight and excessive exercise.

Management and Treatment

If amenorrhea is caused by anovulation, the woman must be treated to prevent uterine hyperplasia or carcinoma from unopposed estrogen stimulation. If she does not desire fertility, oral contraceptives are a good option. Alternatively, medroxyprogesterone acetate can be administered every three months to promote synchronous shedding of the endometrial lining. With this regimen, patients need to use a barrier method for contraception if they are interested in preventing pregnancy. If the woman desires to become pregnant, treatment with clomiphene citrate would be worthwhile.

A patient who has entered menopause or who has developed premature ovarian failure or hypothalamic amenorrhea should be counseled on the benefits of estrogen replacement therapy. Women with gonadal dysgenesis or premature ovarian failure can be given one of the standard hormone replacement regimens used in menopause or low-dose oral contraceptives. Women with hypothalamic amenorrhea who desire to become pregnant will require either GnRH administration via a pump to simulate normal GnRH pulsing or FSH/LH agonists such as Pergonal to induce ovulation.

Specific anatomical defects should be surgically corrected. Although brain lesions may require surgical resection, pituitary adenomas can often be treated medically with bromocriptine, a dopamine agonist that inhibits prolactin release.

Clinical Correlation

A. G. is counseled regarding the importance of taking estrogen to protect her skeletal and cardiovascular system. She is encouraged to gain weight and to reduce her physical stress. She is placed on a low-dose oral contraceptive pill for estrogen replacement and to provide contraception in the event that she ovulates spontaneously.

Follow-up

Patients placed on a particular therapy should be followed at regular intervals to ensure that the therapy is working and to provide an ongoing opportunity to counsel the patient appropriately.

ABNORMAL UTERINE BLEEDING

Abnormal uterine bleeding is bleeding that occurs from the uterus at times other than those of the expected menses (Table 41.2). Menstrual bleeding results from progesterone withdrawal of an estrogen-primed endometrium. Estrogen promotes the proliferation of the endometrial glands in preparation for implantation if fertilization is to occur. Progesterone is responsible for the secretory activity of the glands and inhibition of further growth. With the withdrawal of estrogen and progesterone, the coiled arteries of the endometrium constrict, thereby leading to ischemia and later relaxation of the arteries, resulting in sloughing of the endometrium. Regular ovulation ensures cyclical normal uterine bleeding.

The normal menstrual cycle is defined by an internal cycle of 28 ± 7 days, duration of blood flow of 4 ± 2 days, and a blood loss of 40 ± 20 mL. Quantification of blood loss by the patient is subjective. Pad counts are notoriously inaccurate because of differences in how frequently women change pads and how they define a soaked pad or tampon. Blood loss can be measured from the pads if they are all collected, but this tactic is not a practical approach. Instead, the patient typically describes what is abnormal for her. In addition, symptoms or laboratory tests consistent with anemia are indicative of more severe blood loss.

Table 41.2   Etiologies of Abnormal
Uterine Bleeding

Pregnancy-related complications
  Threatened abortion
  Incomplete abortion
  Gestational trophoblastic disease
  Retain products of conception
Benign genital tract lesions
  Endometrial polyp
  Endocervical polyp
  Uterine leiomyomata
  Adenomyosis
  Endometriosis
Trauma to the lower genital tract
  Lacerations due to traumatic intercourse
  Foreign body reaction
  Intrauterine device use
Genital tract neoplasms
  Endometrial cancer
  Cervical cancer
  Hormone-producing ovarian tumor
Genital tract infections
  Vaginitis
  Cervicitis
  Endometritis
Blood dyscrasias
  Platelet abnormalities
  Von Willebrand's disease
Systemic diseases
  Thyroid dysfunction
  Obesity
  Liver disease (cirrhosis, hepatitis)
  Cushing's disease
  Hyperprolactinemia
  Congenital adrenal hyperplasia
  Renal dysfunction
Dysfunctional uterine bleeding

The following terms are used to describe various patterns of abnormal bleeding. Menorrhagia is prolonged or excessive uterine bleeding that occurs at regular intervals. Polymenorrhea refers to regular episodes of uterine bleeding that occur at intervals of less than 21 days apart. Metrorrhagia describes uterine bleeding that occurs at irregular but frequent intervals, with the amount of bleeding being variable. Intermenstrual bleeding occurs in variable amounts between regular menses. Menometrorrhagia refers to prolonged bleeding that occurs at irregular intervals.

Dysfunctional uterine bleeding generally occurs as a result of disturbances in ovulation. Disruption of the hypothalamic–pituitary–ovarian axis results in anovulation, which in turn leads to inadequate progesterone production. The resultant unopposed estrogen stimulation of the endometrium produces a fragile uterine lining that desquamates easily and asynchronously. Dysfunctional uterine bleeding is a diagnosis of exclusion, being made only after all other etiologies (such as carcinoma, pregnancy, and polyps) have been ruled out.

HISTORY AND PHYSICAL

Women at the extremes of the reproductive years are more likely to experience dysfunctional bleeding. Thirty percent of cases occur in women in their teens, and about 50% occur in perimenopausal women between 40 and 50 years old. At menarche, the hypothalamic–pituitary–ovarian axis is still somewhat immature; indeed, as many as 55% of cycles are anovulatory during the first year of menarche. Adolescent bleeding abnormalities may also point toward a blood dyscrasia, as 20% of teenagers with menorrhagia have some degree of coagulopathy.

Women nearing menopause have increased variability of cycles due to waning progesterone secretion from decreased follicular responsiveness to gonadotropin stimulation. These women are at greater risk for endometrial or cervical cancer as the etiology of the abnormal bleeding. Older women also have an increased incidence of uterine myomatas, polyps, endometriosis, and adenomyosis, all of which may contribute to abnormal bleeding.

Information on the regularity of the bleeding should be obtained from the patient, as truly dysfunctional bleeding is acyclic. Anatomical lesions such as endocervical polyps can cause intermenstrual spotting; fibroids may be responsible for severe menorrhagia. Heavy blood loss is often associated with passage of blood clots. Symptoms of ovulation should also be reviewed.

Sexual history and contraception are also critical factors. Abnormal uterine bleeding may be associated with several pregnancy complications: threatened abortion, incomplete abortion, ectopic pregnancy, gestational trophoblastic disease, and retained products of conception. Vaginitis, cervicitis, or endometritis may also occur in conjunction with such bleeding. Women using oral contraceptives may develop abnormal bleeding after incorrect pill use or breakthrough bleeding because of an atrophic uterine lining from prolonged use of such medications. Occasionally, intrauterine device use is associated with menorrhagia.

Medical problems associated with abnormal bleeding include hypothyroidism, in which levels of prolactin are elevated. Hyperthyroidism may also cause dysfunctional bleeding because of disruptions in the metabolic clearance of estrogen. In addition, liver disease may affect estrogen metabolism, leading to dysfunctional uterine bleeding (DUB). Adrenal hyperfunction such as that observed with Cushing's disease or congenital adrenal hyperplasia can lead to overproduction of androgens and progestins, resulting in anovulation and DUB.

CLINICAL CORRELATION

J. W. is a 47-year-old, married, African American woman, G4P4, who presents complaining of menorrhagia for the past three weeks. She reports a long history of regular menses until about one year ago, when she began having unpredictable episodes of extremely heavy bleeding. She describes the passage of large clots, and is afraid to leave her home for fear of starting to bleed. She denies dysmenorrhea as well as ovulatory or premenstrual symptoms. She is sexually active without contraception. Her last examination and Pap smear were one year ago and were normal. She denies any other medical problems and does not currently use any medication.

Obesity and low body fat can both contribute to DUB. Hirsutism is a reflection of hyperandrogenism that may signal abnormalities of the hypothalamic–pituitary–ovarian axis. Consequently, the thyroid should be palpated for goiters or nodules. The abdominal examination should note the presence of hepatomegaly or ovarian masses.

The pelvic examination should assess the amount of active bleeding from the cervix and the amount of blood and clot in the vaginal vault. Inspection of the vagina should identify any lesions, masses, discharge, or lacerations. The cervical examination should note any lesions as well, paying special attention to cervicitis or cervical carcinoma. The os of the cervix should be identified as either open or closed and examined to see whether any tissue is protruding through it consistent with either a tumor or products of conception. The bimanual examination should assess uterine size, consistency, and tenderness. Any adnexal masses should be analyzed, as they may be an ectopic pregnancy, endometriosis, or ovarian neoplasm. A rectal examination with stool guaiac is performed to determine whether this area is the source of the bleeding.

CLINICAL CORRELATION

J. W. is mildly overweight. Her blood pressure is normal, and she has a normal hair pattern. The thyroid examination is normal, and no masses are palpable during the abdominal examination. A pelvic examination reveals copious blood and clots in the vaginal vault. A blood clot is observed protruding through a closed cervix. J. W.'s ovaries are normal in size and nontender. The uterus is small, mobile, nontender, and anteverted. No masses are palpated on the rectal examination, and the stool guaiac is negative.

DIFFERENTIAL DIAGNOSIS

All women of reproductive age should undergo pregnancy testing when abnormal uterine bleeding is reported. The adolescent with acute bleeding should have coagulation studies done and possibly a bleeding time. In sexually active women, cervical cultures for gonorrhea, Chlamydia, and serum tests for syphilis should be performed. A prolactin level and TSH test will rule out these etiologies for abnormal bleeding. If hirsutism is present, androgen studies should be carried out.

In perimenopausal women, a sample of the endometrial cavity should be taken. This sampling can usually be done in the office with a small curette or similar instrument. Endometrial cancer must be ruled out in a woman of this age who has any bleeding abnormalities. A Pap smear should also be performed.

Ultrasound, hysterosalpingogram, and hysteroscopy are all methods of documenting polyps within the endometrial cavity, fibroids, and adenomyosis.

CLINICAL CORRELATION

J. W. has a negative serum beta-hCG. Her prolactin and TSH levels are normal. Dilatation and curettage reveal uterine tissue with the diagnosis of proliferative endometrium. No lesions are visualized on hysteroscopy.

The diagnosis in J. W. is dysfunctional uterine bleeding due to anovulation related to the perimenopause.

MANAGEMENT AND TREATMENT

Treatment of abnormal uterine bleeding depends on the etiology. Infections require appropriate antibiotic therapy. Pregnancy complications, such as retained placental tissue or incomplete abortion, may require dilatation and curettage of the uterus. Ectopic pregnancy requires medical or surgical therapy. Bleeding dyscrasias may require blood product therapy depending on the abnormality. Hypothyroidism can be corrected with thyroid replacement therapy, hyperprolactinemia can be treated with bromocriptine, and congenital adrenal hyperplasia can be treated with corticosteroids.

Women with hormone-producing ovarian neoplasms will need these lesions resected. Such lesions include granulosa cell tumors, Sertoli-Leydig cell tumors, hyperthecosis associated with ovarian tumors, thecomas, and arrhenoblastomas. Anatomical lesions such as myomatas, polyps, and adenomyosis may require surgical correction to stop bleeding.

Dysfunctional uterine bleeding due to local hormonal imbalances often responds to medical management. Heavy or prolonged bleeding may lead to a denuded endometrium that must first be treated with estrogen to stabilize the fragile unshed endometrium. Typically, oral conjugated estrogens, 2.5 mg four times per day, can be given until the bleeding stops, at which time the patient is then switched to 2.5 mg per day for 25 days. During the last 10 days of estrogen therapy, the patient also takes medroxyprogesterone acetate, 10 mg per day. When the hormone therapy ends, the patient should experience a complete synchronous shedding of the endometrial lining. Alternatively, conjugated estrogen can be administered intravenously at a dose of 25 mg every four hours until bleeding stops. This therapy is followed by medroxyprogesterone, 10 mg per day for 10 days, to allow for an organized shedding of the endometrium.

Dilatation and curettage of the uterus are rarely indicated for dysfunctional uterine bleeding. The exceptions arise when hormonal therapy is contraindicated, when hormonal therapy is unsuccessful, or when endometrial cancer needs to be ruled out.

Progesterone therapy alone may halt dysfunctional bleeding as long as the bleeding is not of long duration. Doses as high as 30 mg/day of medroxyprogesterone acetate can be used. Oral contraceptives can also be prescribed to stop the bleeding—an option that is particularly useful in the young patient. Some physicians prescribe four pills per day for seven days. In most cases, the bleeding subsides within 12 to 24 hours. Withdrawal bleeding will occur when the woman stops taking the pill, and the patient should be prepared for this event.

Options for long-term therapy of DUB include low-dose oral contraceptives, periodic or continuous medroxyprogesterone acetate, or combined estrogen/progesterone therapy. In the reproductive-age woman interested in conception, dysfunctional uterine bleeding can be treated with clomiphene citrate, which induces ovulation and results in more cyclical menses.

FOLLOW-UP

The patient should keep a menstrual calendar and return in three months to assess the success of treatment. If bleeding becomes severe in the meantime, the patient should contact her physician immediately.

SUMMARY

Amenorrhea is merely a symptom, not a diagnosis of an underlying medical problem. The work-up and evaluation of this condition should be systematic, with a thorough history and physical examination being the first steps. The treatment of amenorrhea depends on the etiology of the lack of menses, the age of the patient, and the patient's desire for fertility.

Abnormal uterine bleeding is associated with myriad causes, including hormonal and anatomical etiologies. The most likely cause of the abnormal bleeding, the work-up strategy, and the treatment will depend upon the woman's age, her medical status, and her desire for fertility.

PART V

Gynecology and Gynecologic Oncology

Gynecology
and Gynecologic
Oncology

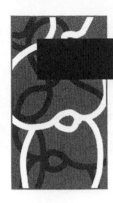

CHAPTER 42

Chronic Pelvic Pain

Brendan F. Burke

Chronic pelvic pain is any pelvic pain lasting for at least six months with or without intervals of relief. Few clinical situations will present the practitioner—and, even more importantly, the patient—with more frustrating and unrewarding results than the management of chronic pain does. Nevertheless, systematic evaluation, assessment, and education of the patient will facilitate proper management of the patient's problem.

Pain itself is a complex symptom. If the underlying cause remains untreated, however, pain can itself become a disease process. In the innervation of the pelvis and surrounding structures, the autonomic and somatic nerves respond to mechanical, chemical, and thermal irritation. Pain of uterine contractions at the time of the menses (dysmenorrhea) may be mediated by local prostaglandins; indeed, data have shown elevated levels of prostaglandins in the menstrual fluid of women with dysmenorrhea. The perceived sensation is modified by the patient's motivational state. This complex interaction helps explain why the amount of pain often does not appear consistent with the amount of tissue damage.

Pain from the uterus follows the hypogastric plexus to T11 and T12. The cervix and vagina nerve supply travel via the splanchnic nerves to S2, S3, and S4, and the lowest part of the vagina nerve supply travels via the somatic nerves (pudendal) to S2, S3, and S4. The remainder of the pelvis has a nerve supply into the lumbar or sacral plexus. Pain from pelvic organs may also be referred to a particular cutaneous region that is supplied by the same spinal cord level.

HISTORY AND PHYSICAL EXAMINATION

The historical aspect of the patient's pain is one of the most important facets of the evaluation. Obtaining the history is a dynamic process that does not end with the initial assessment. Collecting the information in the patient's own words and at an unpressured pace will help establish the proper rapport. At the initial meeting, the patient needs to be informed that assessment and management of chronic pelvic pain often requires a multidisciplinary approach involving gynecologists, general surgeons, internists, anesthesiologists, psychiatrists, and social workers.

Information about the pain's time of onset, duration, location, exacerbating or relieving factors, and character should be elicited. Temporal relationships with the menstrual cycle should be assessed. Pain that is concurrent with menses may result from endometriosis; pain that begins just after the menses may reflect pelvic inflammatory disease; and pain at midcycle may be related to ovulation.

A thorough sexual history should be obtained, including any history of sexually transmitted diseases (STDs) and sexual or other abuse. A past history of similar or other types of pain should be sought. Stress factors in the patient's life, secondary weight gain, and prior psychosomatic illness should be reviewed. Any symptoms of depression should be fully evaluated, as these may represent both the etiology of the patient's complaints and a response to her chronic pain. Social and cultural aspects of the patient's pain should be addressed as well.

The past medical and surgical histories should be obtained, with the physician undertaking a comprehensive review of systems with particular attention to the genitourinary, gastrointestinal, musculoskeletal and nervous systems. Prior and current medications should be noted, and any history of drug abuse should be elicited. The patient should be permitted to ask questions throughout the interview.

CLINICAL CORRELATION

D. G. is a 20-year-old, white female, gravida 0, who presents to the Women's Community Clinic with a chief complaint of chronic lower abdominal and pelvic pain. The pain has been present for the last two years, but now it is interfering with her ability to pursue her college studies. D. G. describes the pain as stabbing, coming at any time, yet more frequently later in the day. The pain is incapacitating, requiring bedrest. Acetaminophen and ibuprofen preparations have minimal effects in alleviating it.

D. G. has not observed any changes in her bladder or bowel habits and does not have a history of back injury. She participates three times per week in a moderate, aerobic exercise program. She has been sexually active in the past but has not had intercourse for more than two months, using condoms sporadically for contraception. Her menses occur every 30 days, and the pain is unrelated to her cycle. Her last Pap smear, taken eight months ago, was normal, as were cervical cultures for *N. gonorrhea* and *C. trachomatis*. Menarche was at 12 years of age, and D. G. became sexually active when she was 16. She was treated empirically with ceftriaxone and doxycycline three years ago when her boyfriend was diagnosed with Chlamydia

urethritis. Her review of systems and past medical, surgical, psychiatric, social, and family history are unremarkable. She is the oldest of three sisters and reports good relationships with her sisters and parents. She states that her parents have worked hard so she could go away to college and wants to do well in school.

Although the physical examination will be directed toward the abdomen and pelvis, a full examination should be performed. Abnormalities of the spine, costovertebral angle, and nervous system should be noted. Evaluation of the abdomen begins with the patient pointing to the area of pain, followed by the physician's inspection and auscultation away from the reported area of pain. If a hernia is suspected, the patient is asked to perform a valsalva maneuver. This maneuver can be repeated with the patient in the standing position. The affected area is then systematically palpated. Any guarding, rigidity, rebound tenderness, or mass is noted.

Next, attention shifts to the pelvic examination, wherein the vulva, urethra, vagina, appropriate ducts and glands, and cervix are inspected. A gentle bimanual examination should then be performed, with the clinician noting any tenderness, masses, enlargement, or thickening of tissues. If discomfort is elicited, the patient should be asked whether it mimics the pain in question. If pelvic relaxation is suspected, the patient should be asked to perform a valsalva maneuver. A rectal examination completes the evaluation.

CLINICAL CORRELATION

After the history taking is complete, the physician performs a physical examination on D. G. Her examination is normal, with a few exceptions. She appears slightly nervous, but remains cooperative throughout. Her abdominal examination is normal except for bilateral lower-quadrant tenderness without rebound or guarding. Bowel sounds are normoactive. Her vulva and vagina and cervix are normal on inspection without discharge or inflammation.

There is bilateral adnexal tenderness and enlargement. The discomfort that D. G. feels during the examination mimics the pain that she has been experiencing. No masses are noted on that rectal examination, although some tenderness was observed anteriorly. The stool guaiac is negative.

DIFFERENTIAL DIAGNOSIS

Beginning with a broad differential will help the physician avoid missing the appropriate diagnosis (Table 42.1). Systematic elimination should begin by discarding those diagnoses that are inappropriate. In those patients with organic pathology, endometriosis (discussed in Chapter 38) will be the most common diagnosis, occurring in at least 30% of patients. Adhesions—either alone or with other abnormalities—will be found in as many as one-third of all patients. Gastrointestinal etiologies are identified in approximately 20% of patients, as are urinary tract problems. In at least 10% of the patients, an underlying psychiatric illness will be diagnosed. A small percentage of patients will have myofascial syndrome as the etiology of their pain.

MANAGEMENT AND TREATMENT

Laboratory, radiologic, and procedural evaluation should progress so as to further eliminate or confirm the clinician's suspicions. Although blood work is of limited usefulness, an elevated white blood cell (WBC) count or sedimentation rate may indicate an infectious or inflammatory process. If a gynecologic etiology of the pain is suspected, cervical cultures and cytology as well as pelvic ultrasound should be utilized when indicated. Laparoscopy should be used liberally, as physical findings often will miss underlying pelvic pathology. Urine or urethral cultures, intravenous pyelogram, cystoscopy, barium enema, colonoscopy, CT scan, and radiological evaluation of the spine are other tools that may be selectively employed in the patient's evaluation. The patient should contin-

Table 42.1 Etiologies of Chronic Pelvic Pain

Gynecological
- Endometriosis
- Adenomyosis
- Leiomyoma
- Chronic pelvic inflammatory disease
  - Hydrosalpinx
  - Tubo-ovarian abscess
- Ovarian tubal mass
- Pelvic relaxation
- Ovarian remnant syndrome
- Pelvic venous congestion

Gastrointestinal
- Adhesions
- Inflammatory bowel disease
- Chronic appendicitis
- Meckel's diverticulum
- Diverticulitis
- Irritable bowel syndrome

Urological
- Urinary calculi
- Recurrent cystitis
- Interstitial cystitis
- Urethritis

Musculoskeletal
- Herniated disc
- Muscle strain
- Coccydynia

Psychiatric
- Sexual victimization
- Psychosomatic disorder
- Drug abuse
- Major depression

Other
- Nongynecologic pelvic mass/tumor

ually be informed of the progress of the evaluation. Consultation with other members of the health care team should be employed when appropriate.

CLINICAL CORRELATION

After a discussion of the differential diagnosis of chronic pelvic pain with D. G., a pelvic ultrasound is undertaken to evaluate the enlarged adnexae. Although the ultrasound identifies the presence of bilateral adnexal masses, their origin—ovarian or fallopian tube—cannot be distinguished. A decision is made to proceed with a laparoscopic evaluation. At the time of surgery, bilateral hydrosalpinges with several filmy, tubo-ovarian adhesions are noted. The physician transects these hydrosalpinges using a carbon dioxide laser. After the transection, the fimbriated ends of each fallopian tube can be visualized. The remainder of the pelvis appears normal, as does the appendix and upper abdomen (including the liver). Pelvic cultures are obtained and subsequently reported as negative. Post-operatively, D. G. is treated with seven days of antibiotics. She currently reports minimal discomfort.

Long-term management should attempt to alleviate the underlying cause of the pain, not just the symptoms. Chronic use of narcotics should be avoided. Besides traditional treatments, alternative modalities including biofeedback, transcutaneous nerve stimulation, and acupuncture have proved useful for some patients.

FOLLOW-UP

A treatment plan should be reviewed and approved by the patient. Concerns about recurrences or failures should be addressed. If referral is necessary, close follow-up of the patient will help maintain a good rapport with the patient and should enhance treatment.

CLINICAL CORRELATION

At her post-operative visit, the physician and D. G. review the findings and final culture results. They discuss chronic pelvic inflammatory disease (PID), chronic pelvic pain, future fertility, and sexually transmitted diseases. The need for potential antibiotic treatment and possible surgeries are discussed as well. D. G. demonstrates an understanding of the underlying disease process and voices appropriate concerns. She is instructed to return in six months or earlier should any problems or questions arise.

SUMMARY

The ultimate goals in the assessment and management of the patient with chronic pelvic pain are the identification of the etiology of that pain, the removal or treatment of the underlying pathology, and eventually the alleviation of the symptoms to permit the patient to carry out her activities of daily living. Many situations will require a multidisciplinary approach, which should be discussed with the patient at the initial evaluation. Acknowledging the complexity of chronic pelvic pain will aid the patient's understanding of her problem as well as validate her concerns.

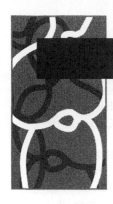

CHAPTER 43

Pelvic Relaxation and Urinary Incontinence

John J. Klutke

Fewer than half of all individuals with urinary incontinence report the problem to their caregivers. Incontinence is an enormous problem, affecting 15% to 35% of all women in the United States. Patients often do not consider the problem to be a disease, however. Instead, they may see it as an unavoidable consequence of age, as older family members may have and live with incontinence. Most women do not know that simple and effective treatments for this problem are available. The clinician can best communicate with many patients about incontinence by approaching it as a quality-of-life issue. In the quality-of-life sense, urinary incontinence is more vexing than other common, chronic diseases of older people, like osteoarthritis or diabetes.

CLINICAL CORRELATION

Since her surgery for a wrist fracture, M. M., a 70-year-old female, gravida 3, para 3, has been plagued by frequent urinary incontinence associated with a sudden, strong urge to urinate. Before surgery, she experienced urine loss with coughing or sneezing, as well as frequent urgency. In the past, she had always been able to "hold it" long enough to reach the toilet; now, however, she cannot. She also has a recent diagnosis of hypertension and coronary artery disease.

The bladder is composed of a muscular wall, known as the detrusor muscle. Urine collects in the bladder from the ureters. Normally, the bladder is quite compliant and is capable of filling to 500 to 700 mL with pressure changes of less than 15 cm of water. Bladder compliance is decreased with bladder wall inflammation or scar formation. The urethra functions as the bladder sphincter, maintaining continence as long as the intravesical pressure does not exceed the intraurethral pressure.

For bladder emptying, voluntary relaxation of the levator ani and urethral sphincter causes the bladder neck to assume a more funnel-like shape. The autonomic and somatic nervous systems act in harmony to maintain storage or empty the bladder. Consequently, the parasympathetic nerves from S2, S3, and S4 stimulate a bladder contraction. This causes the intravesical pressure to exceed the intraurethral pressure, and the bladder empties. Opposing the parasympathetic influence are the sympathetic fibers from the lumbar sympathetics. Skeletal muscles in the urethra further increase resistance with the urethra, which is innervated by the pudendal nerve and nerves of the pelvic plexus.

Urinary incontinence has several causes, each of which must be treated differently. Successful filling and storage of urine occurs when the bladder outlet is competent and the low-pressure reservoir (bladder) can store urine without contracting. Emptying occurs when a bladder contraction occurs in tandem with the opening of the unobstructed outlet. Incontinence can result from any defect in the filling or emptying phase.

Incontinence in women usually reflects a problem of the filling/storage phase, and can result from an abnormality in the bladder or the outlet. Bladder overactivity (detrusor instability) is a consequence of abnormal bladder contractions or a low-capacity bladder in which the bladder pressure rises inappropriately during filling. Patients usually complain of urgency (a strong desire to void accompanied by a fear of leakage), urge incontinence (urgency associated with loss of urine), and frequency (voiding more than seven times per day). Stress incontinence results from an incompetent bladder outlet; it is characterized by loss of urine with coughing, sneezing, lifting, laughing, walking, and other activities that increase intra-abdominal pressure (Figure 43.1). Table 43.1 lists the major characteristics of genuine stress incontinence (GSI) and detrusor instability.

Symptoms are not always reliable in pinpointing whether the bladder or the bladder outlet is defective. Because selection of an appropriate treatment depends on a precise diagnosis, urodynamic testing should be undertaken. Urodynamic testing recreates the bladder's function in a clinical laboratory. Cystometry reproduces the bladder filling and storage phase; uroflow and pressure-flow studies recreate the emptying phase. During cystometry, the bladder is filled with fluid through a bladder catheter and the bladder pressure is

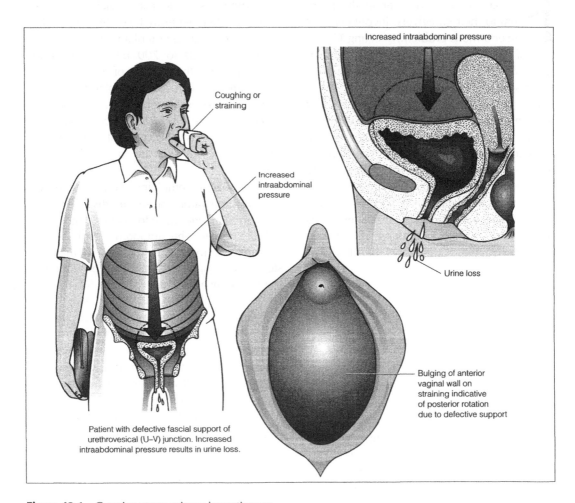

Coughing or straining

Increased intraabdominal pressure

Patient with defective fascial support of urethrovesical (U–V) junction. Increased intraabdominal pressure results in urine loss.

Increased intraabdominal pressure

Urine loss

Bulging of anterior vaginal wall on straining indicative of posterior rotation due to defective support

Figure 43.1   Genuine stress urinary incontinence

Source: Callahan TL, Caughey AB, Heffner LJ. Blueprints in obstetrics and gynecology. Malden, MA: Blackwell Science, 1998:121.

Table 43.1 Genuine Urinary Stress Incontinence Versus Detrusor Instability as Causes of Urinary Incontinence

	GENUINE URINARY STRESS INCONTINENCE	DETRUSOR INSTABILITY
Symptoms	Urine loss with increased intra-abdominal pressure such as coughing, sneezing, or laughing	Involuntary loss of urine, not associated with increased intra-abdominal pressure
Cause	Loss of normal pressure gradient between the bladder and the urethra, most commonly seen with an alteration of the angle of the urethra	Involuntary detrusor muscle contractions
Etiology	Relaxation of the paravaginal and paravesical fascia, usually secondary to aging, with loss of elasticity of the tissue and prior vaginal childbirth	Irritation of the detrusor secondary to numerous factors such as inflammation due to infection of the bladder, radiation cystitis, carcinoma in situ, chemical cystitis (chemotherapy such as Cytoxan) conditioned reflex contractions, idiopathic
Physical examination	Alteration of vesico-urethral angle (Q-tip test) possibly with a cystocele or evidence of pelvic floor relaxation	May be none or evidence of inflammation, infection, carcinoma in situ
Cystometrics	No detrusor contractions seen with patient coughing Bladder pressure exceeds urethral pressure with coughing	Detrusor contractions seen with bladder filling, associated with urethral relaxation
Treatment	Kegel exercises, pessary for support, estrogen (±), pharmacology (pseudoephedrine, phenylpro-panolamine, imipramine) Mobile bladder neck: retropubic urethropexy Immobile bladder neck: sling or collagen	Treat infections, biofeedback, bladder training, kegal exercises, pharmacology [atropine, oxybutynin (Ditropan), tricyclic antidepressants, hyoscyamine (Levsin), tolteroidene (Detrol)]

measured simultaneously until the bladder's natural capacity is reached. GSI is diagnosed if urine is lost through the urethra with stress without bladder contractions. An overactive bladder is also defined cystometrically; it is a disorder of the filling and storage phase in which the bladder contracts while the patient is attempting to inhibit it.

Uroflow testing measures the pattern of urine flow with time as the patient voids. It serves as a screening test for the more invasive pressure-flow test, in which the patient voids with pressure sensors in the bladder. Emptying problems are an unlikely cause of incontinence in women because the female urethra is short and unlikely to become obstructed. Although these tests are rarely needed, they are indicated when the patient has voiding symptoms (hesitancy, incomplete emptying); frequency, urgency, and urge incontinence after a bladder neck suspension; or elevated residual urine.

GSI is usually associated with poor bladder neck support. It is important to demonstrate this relationship, because correction of the support defect is the main effect of bladder neck suspension. If GSI is present with normal bladder neck support, a bladder neck suspension will have a high failure rate. The bladder neck support is verified with the "Q-tip test," in which a cotton swab, lubricated with local anesthetic, is introduced into the urethra to the level of the bladder neck and the patient strains (Figure 43.2). When bladder neck support is poor, the cotton swab will rotate more than 30° from its original position, or its starting position with the patient supine will be greater than 45° from the horizontal.

CLINICAL CORRELATION

M. M. returns to the clinic with a 24-hour voiding diary. The diary reproduces her history and shows no indication of polyuria. Her urinalysis is negative for blood, bacteria, or white blood cells. On physical examination, she demonstrates loss of urine with cough. Post-void residual urine was minimal. A grade II cystocele is found to be present. Her bladder neck support is poor, and a cotton swab placed in the proximal urethra rotates 90° from the horizontal when she strains.

Pelvic organ prolapse is akin to incontinence and shares its predisposing factors: age, multiparity, and connective tissue disease. Prolapse is not synonymous with incontinence, however, as many patients with large cystoceles will be perfectly continent. Patients usually complain of a prolapsing mass in the vagina, although, in cases of severe disease, they may experience altered function. The patient may not be able to defecate or void completely, and may need to reduce the bulge with her fingers to do so. Alternatively, as in M. M., the prolapse may be asymptomatic.

Prolapse is diagnosed on physical examination based on the site of the disease. If the prolapsing organ is the bowel, the prolapse is called an enterocele (Figure 43.3). A cystocele is an anterior vaginal wall defect with prolapse of the bladder into the vagina. A rectocele involves prolapse of the rectum. Vaginal vault prolapse is descent of the apex of the vagina, usually associated with uterine prolapse.

Uterine prolapse is graded according to its severity:

- Grade I describes prolapse of the cervix into the upper half of the vagina.
- Grade II involves prolapse of the cervix into the lower half of the vagina.

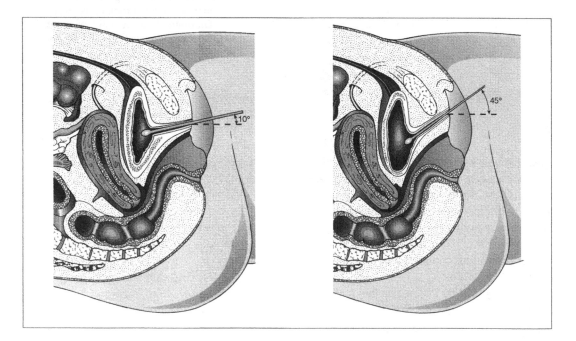

Figure 43.2   The "Q-tip" test to demonstrate alterations in the vesicle-urethral angle

Source: Callahan TL, Caughey AB, Heffner LJ. Blueprints in obstetrics and gynecology. Malden, MA: Blackwell Science, 1998:120.

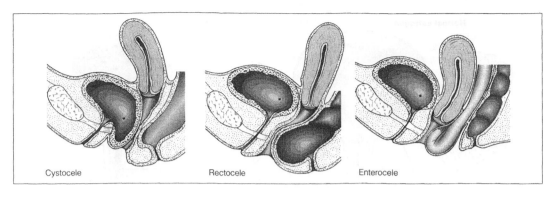

Figure 43.3 Cystocele, rectocele, and enterocele

Source: Callahan TL, Caughey AB, Heffner LJ. Blueprints in obstetrics and gynecology. Malden, MA: Blackwell Science, 1998:114.

- Grade III consists of prolapse of the cervix past the introitus.

Procidentia describes a condition in which the support of the pelvic floor is completely lost, and the uterus and vagina are everted.

CLINICAL CORRELATION

Simple therapeutic measures are instituted to aide M. M.: a bedpan is made available at home, and she begins bladder drills and Kegel exercises. M. M. declines a pessary (Figure 43.4). She is also prescribed estrogen replacement therapy and bladder relaxant medication.

When she visits her physician six weeks later, M. M. is now fully recovered from her wrist surgery and back to her normal active lifestyle. Although her urge symptoms are considerably improved, she is still incapacitated by her urinary symptoms. Cystometry is performed and verifies the diagnosis of GSI. M. M. undergoes an uncomplicated retropubic urethropexy and is dry and satisfied.

Bladder overactivity may be effectively treated with behavior modification and medical therapy. Behavior modification involves teaching the patient to void on a schedule (timed voiding) during the daytime. Every hour, on the hour, she empties her bladder, regardless of whether she has an urge to do so. In this way, the patient reestablishes central control over the bladder. If she has a strong urge, she should postpone it until the scheduled time, even if incontinence occurs. As she is able to void on her own decision—rather than according to what her bladder tells her—the interval is increased.

Medical therapy of bladder overactivity aims to control the parasympathetic cholinergic input to the bladder's smooth muscle. Anticholinergic medications such as oxybutynin, probanthine, or tolterodine can effectively block bladder contractions and increase the bladder's capacity. Estrogen receptors are present in high concentrations in the urethra, making it a target organ for this hormone. Estrogen replacement in the estrogen-deficient woman (with progestins if the uterus is present) will ameliorate urge symptoms (Figure 43.5).

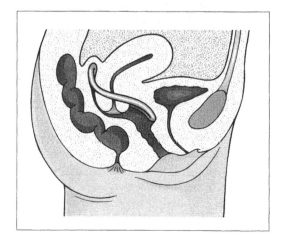

Figure 43.4 A pessary placed into the vagina

Source: Callahan TL, Caughey AB, Heffner LJ. Blueprints in obstetrics and gynecology. Malden, MA: Blackwell Science, 1998:115.

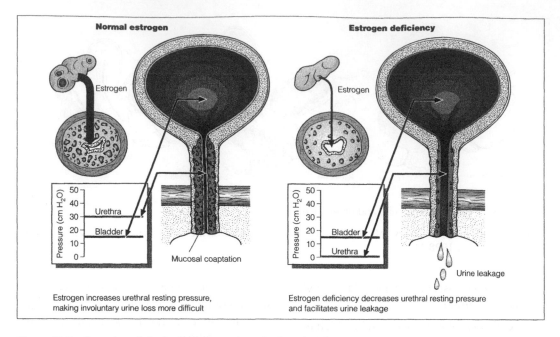

Figure 43.5   Sequelae of the lack of estrogen on the female urinary tract

Source: Callahan TL, Caughey AB, Heffner LJ. Blueprints in obstetrics and gynecology. Malden, MA: Blackwell Science, 1998:118.

Stress incontinence may be treated nonsurgically by prescribing Kegel exercises, pessaries that support the bladder neck, estrogen, and alpha-agonist medications such as Sudafed that improve tone at the bladder neck. Caution should be used when prescribing alpha-agonists, as these agents can have cardiac side effects. Kegel exercises promote continence by training the pelvic floor muscles (specifically the pubococcygeus muscle), thereby promoting their hypertrophy. Biofeedback is another nonsurgical technique that teaches the patient to do pelvic floor exercises (Kegel) more efficiently by feeding back a physiologic variable (usually electrical activity in the pelvic floor) that increases when she does the exercise properly. Approximately half of all motivated patients who are treated nonsurgically for GSI will improve to the point where no surgery is necessary.

Surgery to support the bladder neck is effective in correcting GSI in approximately 85% of all cases. With the Burch retropubic urethropexy, the surgeon corrects the poor bladder neck support associated with GSI by placing sutures in the supportive tissue alongside the urethra and bladder neck and then anchoring those sutures to the edge of the anterior pelvis at Cooper's ligament. The surgery involves an abdominal incision and retropubic dissection and requires a three- to four-day hospitalization. Complications of bladder neck suspension operations include failure to correct GSI and overcorrection (Figure 43.6). Overcorrection—which can cause de novo symptoms of urgency, urge incontinence, and frequency—can be present even if the patient is able to empty her bladder completely. Patients with severe incontinence or who experience recurrent GSI after bladder neck support will require an operation that obstructs the bladder neck. In most cases, a sling of fascia or graft material is placed around and below the bladder neck and anchored above on the pelvis.

Pelvic floor prolapse, when symptomatic, can be treated with a pessary, which is a prosthetic device that is kept in the vagina and supports the walls of the vagina. Surgery provides an effective repair and leaves a usable vagina if the patient is sexually active. Repair of a mild or moderate cystocele will usually result fortuitously from the retropubic urethropexy when performed for GSI. An anterior repair, in

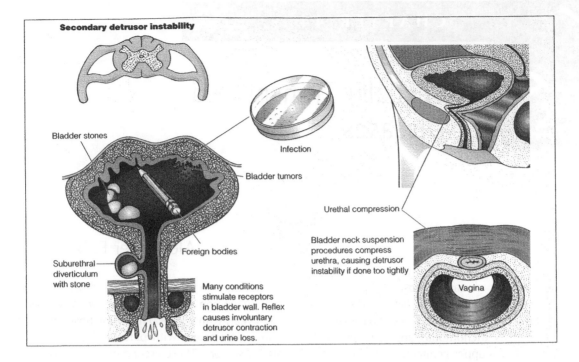

Figure 43.6 Causes of detrusor instability

Source: Callahan TL, Caughey AB, Heffner LJ. Blueprints in obstetrics and gynecology. Malden, MA: Blackwell Science, 1998:123.

which the pubocervical fascia is exposed through a vaginal dissection and plicated with sutures below the bladder and bladder neck, is the treatment of choice when the cystocele—rather than GSI—is the main problem because the patient recovers from this vaginal operation more easily. Rectocele repair involves exposing the rectovaginal fascia and plicating it along with the levator ani muscle, with sutures being placed in the midline.

Vaginal vault prolapse occasionally complicates hysterectomy. It is treated by suturing the apex of the vagina to a fixed structure in the pelvis, either the sacrospinous ligament (sacrospinous suspension, a transvaginal oper-

ation) or the periosteum overlying the sacrum (sacrocolpopexy, a transabdominal operation).

SUMMARY

Incontinence is a condition that affects many women. In general, the problem is related to the bladder or the bladder outlet. Many conditions can cause bladder contractions, and some basic screening tests should rule these sources out. Treatment should advance from simple, noninvasive measures to surgery depending on the diagnosis and the effect of the problem on the patient's quality of life.

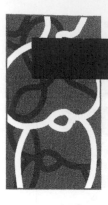

CHAPTER 44

Sexually Transmitted Diseases

Alexander F. Burnett

Infectious diseases transmitted by sexual contact are myriad in nature. They range from the simple passage of vaginal infections such as trichomonas and gardnerella, to more serious upper genital tract infections that may lead to hospitalization, surgery, or infertility, to life-threatening infections with agents that presently have no cure. Physicians should be familiar with the most common sexually transmitted diseases (STDs), their signs and symptoms, strategies for diagnosing these illnesses, appropriate therapy, and follow-up, including public health issues and partner therapy.

CLINICAL CORRELATION

L. F. is a 19-year-old, gravida 3, abortus 3, female whose last menstrual period began four days ago. She complains of severe pelvic pain of two days' duration and feeling feverish. She denies nausea, vomiting, or anorexia. Her bowel habits and urination are normal. She currently uses oral contraceptive pills for birth control and reports having intercourse over the past month with two new partners. She denies previously having pelvic infections. According to L. F., her menses this month is normal with the exception of being somewhat malodorous compared with her usual bleeding.

PELVIC INFLAMMATORY DISEASE

Pelvic inflammatory disease (PID) encompasses symptomatic infections of the upper genital tract. In the United States, more than 1 million women are treated for pelvic infections each year, with 250,000 requiring hospitalization for treatment with parenteral antibiotics and/or surgery. These ascending infections are caused by the introduction of organisms into the lower genital tract via sexual contact. The most common organisms responsible for PID are *Neisseria gonorrhoeae* and *Chlamydia trachomatis*. Also implicated are polymicrobial infections of aerobes and anaerobes originating from bowel flora.

Table 44.1 lists the risk factors for PID, most of which are related to the frequency of unprotected intercourse with multiple or new partners. The risk of all STDs can be reduced with the use of barrier methods of contraception—most notably, latex condom use.

The most frequent symptoms associated with PID are pelvic pain, vaginal discharge, and fever. The onset of symptoms occurs during or just after menses in most circumstances, as the breakdown of the endometrial lining permits transport of these bacteria from the cervix up through the uterus to the fallopian tubes and pelvis.

CLINICAL CORRELATION

Examination of L. F. reveals that she is in moderate distress. Her vital signs are as follows: temperature, 38.5 °C; pulse, 100; respiration, 18; and blood pressure, 110/70. Significant findings on physical examination include a tender abdomen that is most

Table 44.1 Risk Factors for Pelvic
Inflammatory Disease

- Age < 25
- Lower genital tract infection
  *Neisseria gonorrhoeae, Chlamydia
  trachomatis,* bacterial vaginosis
- Multiple sexual partners
  Sexual partners as high risk: lower
  socioeconomic class, engaging with
  multiple partners themselves
- Facilitated transport to the upper genital
  tract
  Iatrogenic: D&C, insertion of IUD,
  hysterosalpingogram
  Patient: disruption with menses,
  douching

sensitive to deep palpation in the lower abdomen bilaterally, no rebound, and bowel
sounds that are slightly hypoactive. She
does not have any costo-vertebral angle
tenderness. An examination of the cervix
reveals a mixed, dark, blood-purulent material discharge; cultures are taken. A
bimanual examination reveals tenderness

on movement of the cervix and bilateral
adnexal tenderness with a fullness in the
right adnexae. A recto-vaginal examination reveals a possible mass in the cul-de-
sac, although the examination is somewhat
limited by the patient's discomfort.

The signs of PID include elevated temperature, lower abdominal tenderness, mucopurulent cervical discharge, cervical motion
tenderness, bilateral adnexal tenderness, and
occasionally adnexal swelling or mass. The differential diagnosis must rule out other causes of
inflammation or infection in the pelvis, including appendicitis, diverticulitis or diverticular
abscess, and septic abortion. When the diagnosis remains unclear despite the physical
examination and laboratory findings, radiographic findings may prove helpful in cases of
a presumed tubo-ovarian abscess (TOA), diverticular abscess, or free air suggestive of perforation of a viscus. Laparoscopy may also be helpful in the diagnosis and offers an added benefit
in that the purulent contents of the pelvis can
be directly cultured (Figure 44.1). Visual criteria for laparoscopic diagnosis of PID include
hyperemia of the tubal surface, edema of the
tubal walls, and purulent exudate on the tubal
surface or coming out the fimbriae.

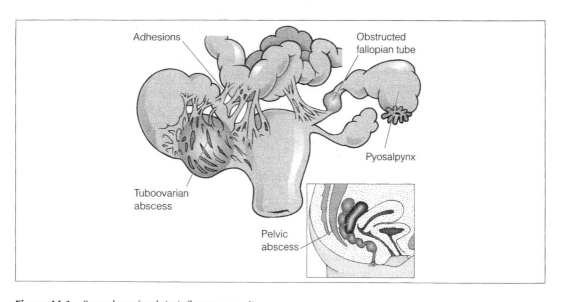

Figure 44.1 Sequelae of pelvic inflammatory disease

Source: Callahan TL, Caughey AB, Heffner LJ. Blueprints in obstetrics and gynecology. Malden, MA:
Blackwell Science, 1998:110.

The critical considerations in treating a woman with PID are to eliminate the acute sequelae of infection and to try to prevent the long-term sequelae, especially infertility and pelvic pain. More than half of women with tubal infertility have no history of PID, yet many are considered to have experienced "silent" PID. This term is used to describe infections with *Chlamydia* that have minimal signs or symptoms, such that the woman may not seek any medical care. Antibody titers to *Chlamydia* are higher in women who have tubal infertility or ectopic pregnancies when compared to those without these problems. In addition, *Chlamydia* infection is the most common STD in the United States. These data emphasize the importance of recognizing and treating even mild cases of PID.

Ideally, all women should receive parenteral antibiotics for PID to try to prevent its long-term sequelae. In reality, many women are adequately treated with outpatient regimens in terms of eliminating the acute signs and symptoms. Regimens recommended by the Centers for Disease Control and Prevention (CDC) incorporate drugs that are active against *N. gonorrhoeae* and *C. trachomatis*. Outpatient regimens typically include at least two drugs. The CDC recommends the following outpatient regimes:

- Ofloxacin 400 mg PO b.i.d. for 14 days, plus metronidazole 500 mg PO b.i.d. for 14 days
- Either ceftriaxone 250 mg IM in 1 dose, or cefoxitin 2 g IM plus probenecid 1 g PO in 1 dose, or another parenteral third-generation cephalosporin, plus doxycycline 100 mg PO b.i.d. for 14 days

Patients who do not respond to either of these regimens within 72 hours should be hospitalized and receive parenteral antibiotics.

Women who are pregnant, have a human immunodeficiency virus (HIV) infection, are afflicted with severe disease, have a pelvic abscess, or perhaps are nulligravida, or who fail to respond to outpatient regimens should receive inpatient intravenous antibiotics. This therapy should be continued for at least 24 hours after clinical improvement appears; patients may then be discharged and told to take oral antibiotics. The CDC guidelines for parenteral antibiotics include the following regimens:

- Cefoxitin 2 g IV q6h or cefotetan 2 g IV q12h, plus doxycycline 100 mg IV/PO q12h, followed by doxycycline 100 mg PO b.i.d. for 14 days total
- Clindamycin 900 mg IV q8h, plus gentamicin 2 mg/kg IV/IM loading dose, then 1.5 mg/kg maintenance dose q8h, followed by doxycycline 100 mg PO b.i.d. for 14 days total or clindamycin 450 mg PO q.i.d. for 14 days total

---

CLINICAL CORRELATION

L. F. is admitted for intravenous antibiotics and is begun on clindamycin plus gentamicin after an ultrasound reveals a 6 cm right adnexal mass consistent with a TOA. Her initial white blood cell count is 24,000/cm^3 and falls to 18,000/cm^3 after 24 hours of antibiotics. Her fevers continue, albeit with lower maximum temperatures for the next two days, and pain on deep palpation persists. A repeat ultrasound after 48 hours of antibiotics reveals the right ovary to still be 6 cm and quite tender during the examination.

TOAs—abscess formation in the pelvis secondary to PID—complicate approximately 15% of all STD cases. As their name implies, these abscesses frequently involve the fallopian tube and ovary and produce marked destruction of these organs. Appropriate management calls for intravenous antibiotics to be given initially; if no improvement occurs within 48 to 72 hours or if rupture is suspected, surgical extirpation should be considered. The inflammation present in the pelvis often makes these surgeries technically difficult, and ureteral stents placed preoperatively may be quite helpful in identifying the course of the ureters. In a young woman desiring preservation of fertility, a unilateral salpingo-oophorectomy with drainage of the pelvis should be considered to remove the abscess. After abscess removal and drainage of the pelvis, recovery is usually rapid while the woman remains on intravenous antibiotics. Occasionally, if a TOA "points" into the cul-de-sac, the abscess may be drained by culpotomy. If clinical improvement does not occur rapidly following this procedure, then surgical removal of the abscess should proceed.

In patients who undergo exploration or laparoscopy for PID or TOAs, the surgeon should explore the upper abdomen for evidence of prior infections. Adhesions may form between the liver and the anterior abdominal wall (a condition known as the Fitz-Hugh-Curtis syndrome). This syndrome indicates the existence of prior pelvic infections, and it occasionally requires lysis to alleviate right upper quadrant pain.

CLINICAL CORRELATION

After ureteral stents are placed via cystoscopy, L. F. undergoes a laparotomy. The right tube and ovary are involved in a complex abscess that is sharply removed. The left tube and ovary are hyperemic, but they do not appear otherwise involved with the infection. The uterus is grossly normal. No adhesions are observed between the liver and the anterior abdominal wall. A drain is placed into the pelvis and brought out through the skin of the anterior abdominal wall. After 24 hours, L. F. defervesces and her white blood count falls to 8000/cm^3. She is discharged from the hospital five days after surgery and told to continue taking oral antibiotics.

When a woman is identified as having PID, her partner should also be treated to prevent her reinfection. PID infections must be reported to public health officials in the United States, along with the following infectious diseases: syphilis, gonorrhea, Chlamydia, HIV/AIDS, tuberculosis, chancroid, granuloma inguinale, lymphogranuloma venereum, hepatitis A, hepatitis B, and hepatitis C.

OTHER SYSTEMIC SEXUALLY TRANSMITTED DISEASES

The other significant systemic STDs include syphilis and HIV (see Chapter 10). Syphilis is a sexually transmitted infection involving the spirochete *Treponema pallidum*.

The primary syphilis lesion has an incubation time of 10 to 90 days after infection and presents as a painless chancre in the genital or oral region that will heal on its own in 3 to 6 weeks. Serum from the lesion will demonstrate spirochetes on dark-field examination. Serologic tests for syphilis will become positive shortly after the chancre becomes evident; these tests include the Venereal Disease Research Laboratory (VDRL) test, the rapid plasma reagin (RPR) card test, and the complement fixation test. Although they are nonspecific for *Treponema,* their results are considered diagnostic if titers are high. False-positive results may occur when the woman is affected by acute fevers, collagen diseases, mononucleosis, malaria, leprosy, yaws, and lymphogranuloma. Confirmation can be obtained by a fluorescent treponemal antibody absorption test (FTS-ABS) which tests for antibodies to *Treponema.*

Secondary syphilis begins two to eight weeks after the chancre appears. This stage is characterized by cutaneous and mucous membrane lesions (typically maculo-papular rashes of the palms and soles or ulcerations on the tongue) or by condylomata of the anogenital region. Latent syphilis is asymptomatic and is diagnosed on the basis of serologic tests. Tertiary syphilis occurs when the disease has manifestations of neurologic or cardiovascular infection or gummas (generally painless granulomas) are present.

Treatment for syphilis consists of penicillin, usually given in a long-acting form. Once-daily benzathine penicillin, G 2.4 million units IM, is prescribed for primary and secondary syphilis; the dose is 2.4 million units IM per week for three weeks for latent or tertiary syphilis. Neurosyphilis requires intravenous penicillin G therapy with high doses for an extended period of time. Patients who are allergic to penicillin can be treated with oral tetracycline or doxycycline.

Identification of STDs is particularly important during pregnancy as these diseases can have disastrous sequelae on the developing fetus who is exposed during pregnancy or the newborn who is exposed during birth. Chapter 27 details the perinatal transmission and complications of gonorrhea, Chlamydia, and syphilis.

SUMMARY

Sexually transmitted diseases are common among sexually active women. Proper recognition, culture, and treatment will have a positive effect on preserving the woman's fertility. STDs have a wide variety of clinical manifestations, ranging from mild or even asymptomatic infections to life-threatening illnesses. Special recognition during pregnancy is critical to avoid profound effects on the offspring.

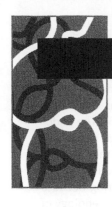

CHAPTER 45

Dysmenorrhea and Premenstrual Syndrome

Alexander F. Burnett

P ain at the time of menses and symptoms that occur around the menstrual period are frequent complaints that prompt a woman to see her gynecologist. It is important to correctly identify the difficulty, attempt to pinpoint the etiology if possible, and begin appropriate therapy for the symptoms. These syndromes can be difficult to manage and may require coordination with other health professionals in pain management or psychiatry.

CLINICAL CORRELATION

L. C. is a 20-year-old college junior who comes to her physician's office complaining of excruciating pain at the time of her menses each month. According to L. C., she has never had pain-free menses since menarche at age 13. Her periods are regular, occurring every 29 days, and she has never been pregnant. The pain lasts for four days, which is the duration of her bleeding. L. C. describes it as cramping with occasional nausea, particularly on the first day of the menses. She does not relate any changes in her mood prior to or during her menses, but notes that the pain frequently causes her to feel "edgy" during the period. She self-medicates with high-dose acetaminophen. Her past history is negative for pelvic infections, use of an intrauterine device, or pain distant from her pelvis. She currently uses condoms for contraception.

DYSMENORRHEA

Dysmenorrhea is defined as severe pelvic pain before or during menstruation. Primary dysmenorrhea does not have an identifiable organic cause and usually has its onset at the initiation of ovulatory cycles. Secondary dysmenorrhea begins later in reproductive life and results from pelvic pathology.

PRIMARY DYSMENORRHEA

Women with primary dysmenorrhea usually begin experiencing symptoms shortly after menarche. These women have regular menses, with the pain being associated with their ovulatory cycles. Uterine contractions are increased compared to those in women without dysmenorrhea. Although the exact etiology of primary dysmenorrhea is unknown, prostaglandins have been implicated as the inducing agent for these symptoms. Levels of the prostaglandins PGE_2 and PGF_2 are elevated in the serum and menstrual fluid from these women. The pain is believed to occur secondary to ischemia because of the reduction in blood flow secondary to the contractions.

Management of primary dysmenorrhea is aimed at reducing the production of prostaglandins locally. Inhibitors of prostaglandin synthesis include acetylsalicylic acid (aspirin) and nonsteroidal anti-inflammatory drugs (ibuprofen, naproxen, indoleacetic acid). Recommended doses of ibuprofen are 400 to 800 mg four times per day. Other prostaglandin inhibitors, such as mefenamic acid (Ponstel), may also block the action of prostaglandins on the target organ and may provide more effective relief of symptoms. Oral contraceptive pills provide relief to the majority of women with primary dysmenorrhea. They function by inhibiting ovulation, inhibiting prostaglandin formation, and producing a thinner endometrial lining to be shed each month.

CLINICAL CORRELATION

L. C. is given a prescription for ibuprofen, 800 mg, to be taken q.i.d. when the pain begins. She also agrees to begin a trial of oral contraceptive pills to try to reduce her discomfort. She returns to the office in three months for a refill of her prescription. She reports that her menses are shorter in duration and associated with less blood flow. The pain is significantly improved, with her last menses requiring only one or two doses of ibuprofen for relief. Her blood pressure is within normal limits, and she has not developed any other reactions to the oral contraceptives. She is given a one-year prescription and will return in 12 months for follow-up.

SECONDARY DYSMENORRHEA

CLINICAL CORRELATION

P. T. is a 34-year-old, gravida 2, para 2, female who reports increasing pain with menstruation over the last eight months. Previously, she was pain-free at the time of menses. She also states that the amount of blood passed during her period has diminished, although the duration and cyclicity of her menses remains unchanged. P. T. has had two cesarean deliveries, with the last one occurring six years ago for breech presentation. She has a history of abnormal Pap smears and moderate cervical dysplasia that was treated with cryotherapy (freezing) in the office approximately one year ago. More recently, she has noticed that the pain involves not only her pelvis but also her left mid-abdomen. She occasionally sees some dark blood in her stool at the time of her menses.

Secondary dysmenorrhea is associated with a host of potential pathologies. Its most common cause is endometriosis—that is, deposition of endometrial material in locations other than the uterine cavity (see Chapter 38). The endometrial tissue propagates and then sloughs or bleeds each cycle at the time of menses. The local irritation of blood on the peritoneal lining or adhesion formation occurring because of the bleeding is believed to be the etiology of this pain.

Cervical stenosis may be a contributing factor to the development of endometriosis. The stenotic cervix does not allow normal passage of the menstrual products, which may then pass in a retrograde fashion out the fallopian tubes and become implanted in the peritoneal cavity. Causes of cervical stenosis include prior cervical surgery, cryotherapy, or congenital defects of the cervix.

Other causes of secondary dysmenorrhea include adenomyosis (that is, deposition of endometrial glands deep in the myometrium of the uterus) and pelvic adhesive disease secondary to infections or prior surgery.

CLINICAL CORRELATION

Examination of P. T. reveals a normal abdomen without point tenderness. The pelvic examination is significant for a pinpoint cervical os that does not admit a small curette. Bimanual and recto-vaginal examinations reveal an anteverted uterus that is nontender to palpation, but moderately tender on movement. There is nodularity of the uterosacral ligaments bilaterally. Although the adnexae are nontender, they do not move when palpated.

The diagnosis in secondary dysmenorrhea often requires laparoscopy. If endometriosis is present, therapy should include fulguration or removal of endometriotic implants. Adhesions can often be lysed via laparoscopy with significant abatement of symptoms. Cervical stenosis can be relieved by dilation of the stenotic cervix, often performed under general anesthesia. Advanced endometriosis may require more extensive surgical resection or medical treatment with gonadotropin-releasing hormone (GnRH) agonists. As with primary dysmenorrhea, standard therapy will include prostaglandin inhibitors and occasionally oral contraceptive pills. Prostaglandin inhibitors may be particularly useful with a diagnosis of adenomyosis.

If all medical therapy proves unsuccessful and the woman has completed her childbearing, hysterectomy is a viable option in women with a diagnosis of adenomyosis. Women with other etiologies of dysmenorrhea, including pelvic adhesive disease and endometriosis, should be counseled that hysterectomy may not relieve their symptoms. This procedure should be undertaken only as a last resort in these patients.

CLINICAL CORRELATION

P. T. undergoes laparoscopy after progressive dilation of the cervical os. An examination of her pelvis reveals moderate endometriosis involving the utero-sacral ligaments bilaterally. A small amount of scar tissue is sharply lysed, and electrocautery is used to fulgarate the areas of endometriosis. One thick nodule of endometriosis is located on top of the lower sigmoid colon and is left in place. A sigmoidoscopy is performed when P. T. is still asleep, which reveals full thickness of endometriosis in the sigmoid colon at 17 centimeters.

After recovering from the surgery, P. T. is prescribed a GnRH agonist for six months, then placed on oral contraceptive pills. Her menses return in seven months with normal flow and minimal discomfort. She no longer has blood in her stool at the time of menses.

PREMENSTRUAL SYNDROME

CLINICAL CORRELATION

C. S. is a 34-year-old nulligravida who complains of "horrible symptoms" each month for 10 days prior to her period. During this time, she is emotionally labile, cries easily, and quickly becomes enraged. Her marital relations are extremely strained during this time, to the point where her husband is considering moving out for this period of time during each cycle. The symptoms begin to lessen rapidly on the first day of her menses and are completely gone by the end of her flow. She states she has about 2½ weeks in each month where she "feels herself."

Premenstrual syndrome (PMS) is a diagnosis based on the cyclical onset of symptomatic changes in mood and disposition that are related to the ovulatory cycle. These symptoms may reflect the presence of anxiety, depression, pain, water retention, or hypoglycemia (Table 45.1). An estimated 20% to 30% of all women have moderate to severe PMS; 1% to 10% experience debilitating symptoms. The symptoms occur during the luteal phase of the menstrual cycle and usually resolve with the onset of menses. The cyclical nature of the problem suggests that progesterone levels or estrogen-progesterone ratios may be altered in women with these complaints; however, studies have failed to show any difference in these hormone levels in women with PMS and those without the syndrome. Other theories have suggested alterations in serotonin levels, prolactin levels, hypoglycemia, or vitamin deficiencies, although none of these theories has been proven to date.

Diagnosis of PMS requires documentation of the cyclical nature of the symptoms associated with spontaneous menstrual cycles. A high percentage of women initially evaluated for PMS will have a coexisting medical or psychological disorder. Underlying psychiatric disorders sometimes revealed include bipolar disorder, anxiety, and personality disturbances. Thyroid disorders can also mimic PMS.

In the true case of PMS, the woman should be relatively symptom-free during days 4 through 12 in an idealized 28-day cycle. Symptoms should increase, particularly during the late luteal phase, when compared with the follicular phase of the cycle. To document

Table 45.1   Common Symptoms of PMS

SYMPTOM	PERCENTAGE OF WOMEN WITH PMS SHOWING SYMPTOMS
Behavioral	
Fatigue	92
Irritability	91
Labile, mood-alternating sadness and anger	81
Depression	80
Oversensitivity	69
Crying spells	65
Social withdrawal	65
Forgetfulness	56
Difficulty concentrating	47
Physical	
Abdominal bloating	90
Breast tenderness	85
Acne	71
Appetite changes and food cravings	70
Swelling of the extremities	67
Headache	60
Gastrointestinal upset	48

Source: ACOG committee opinion premenstrual syndrome number 155, April 1995. Intl J Gynecol Obstet 1995;50:80–84.

their symptoms, patients are given calendars with scales for grading levels of depression, irritability, social withdrawal, fatigue, and anxiety for each day of their cycle. In addition, they should note any sexual relations, changes in eating habits, and somatic complaints such as bloating or breast tenderness. The calendar should be kept for two months and reviewed with the physician to document the cyclicity. An absence of cyclicity or a lack of symptom-free periods during the follicular phase should direct diagnosis to other physical or psychiatric causes.

CLINICAL CORRELATION

C. S. keeps a calendar of her symptoms for the next two months. During that time, she consistently experiences depression, anxiety, and anger during the last 10 days of her cycle, accompanied by breast tenderness, bloating, and cravings for chocolate. She reports minimal symptoms for the first two weeks of her cycles, and marital relations are deemed good by the patient during this time.

Once a diagnosis is made, treatment is aimed at relieving the symptoms of PMS. Progesterone therapy has not been shown to offer any benefit for this syndrome. Diuretic therapy with spironolactone or hydrochlorothiazide can be beneficial for women with complaints of excess fluid gain. Exercise therapy is often helpful in alleviating symptoms of PMS. Changes in diet have not been of proven benefit, nor has vitamin therapy.

Medical therapies that have been shown to be helpful for PMS include fluoxetine (Prozac) given throughout the menstrual cycle, alprazolam (Xanax) given during the second half of the cycle, and GnRH agonists with add-back therapy. Surgical removal of the ovaries is not indicated for the treatment of this disorder.

CLINICAL CORRELATION

C. S. begins taking fluoxetine, 20 mg/day, throughout her menstrual cycle. By the second month of therapy, she notices a marked improvement in terms of diminished depression, fewer crying spells, and less emotional lability. She reports a decrease in her sexual desire throughout the cycle, but also notes increased sexual relations during the second half of the cycle compared with three months prior. She is given a six-month refill on the medication and will return for follow-up at the completion of that time.

SUMMARY

Pain and mood changes associated with the menstrual cycle are noted in a large percentage of women. Dysmenorrhea occurs only during the menses and can usually be improved with medications that inhibit prostaglandin production. PMS symptoms require careful diagnosis to differentiate them from other physical or psychological etiologies. Therapy is addressed to the symptoms of PMS once a correct diagnosis is made.

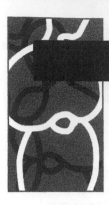

CHAPTER 46

Vulvovaginitis

Alexander F. Burnett

Disorders of the vulva and vagina are frequent complaints that prompt a visit to the gynecologist. Many common problems can be solved with over-the-counter remedies. If such a problem should persist, however, investigation by a physician is warranted. Concerns about vulvar lesions include the possibility of infection, transmission of something to a woman's sexual partner, cosmetic concerns, discomfort from pain or pruritus, and the possibility of cancer. A major difficulty associated with vulvar cancer is that it is often noticed by the patient and her physician several months before a diagnosis is made. When a new vulvar lesion is noted by the patient, biopsy diagnosis is critical.

CLINICAL CORRELATION

T. L. is a 45-year-old, G4P4, female who has noted a recent eruption of vesicles on her right lateral labia. These lesions developed two days before her visit to her physician and were associated with a flu-like syndrome. They are quite painful, particularly if some urine should touch the area when she goes to the bathroom. T. L. also notes swollen tender nodes in her right groin. She comes to the office for evaluation.

INFECTIOUS DISEASES OF THE VULVA AND VAGINA

FUNGAL INFECTIONS

Infections of the vulva and vagina may derive from overgrowth of normal flora or introduc-

tion of new agents by sexual contact. Candidiasis occurs when an overgrowth of yeast appears in the vagina and vulva. Typically, the species involved is *Candida albicans,* although *Candida glabrata* and *Candida tropicalis* are also possible pathogens. The overgrowth is often caused by precipitating factors that deplete the immune system, such as HIV infection, renal transplant with immunosuppression, or diabetes; alternatively, it may follow from alterations in the normal flora such as occurs with antibiotic therapy. Pregnancy also predisposes to a woman to candidiasis because of the presence of high local glucose levels secondary to hormonal alterations and diminished normal vaginal flora.

Typical symptoms of candidiasis include itching with redness and a curd-like white discharge. The diagnosis is made based on the typical thrush appearance of the lesion, the presence of hyphae on a potassium hydroxide slide (wet mount), an acidic vaginal pH (usually less than 4.7), or culturing of the discharge. Therapy can consist of topical agents bought over-the-counter (such as miconazole), prescription topical agents (such as terconazole), clotrimazole vaginal suppositories, or oral medication when topical agents fail (such as oral fluconazole). Recurrent candidiasis should be a sign to investigate for immunosuppression; indeed, it may be the first sign of diabetes or HIV infection.

VIRAL INFECTIONS

The most common viral infections of the vulva are caused by herpes simplex, human

Table 46.1   Vulvovaginitis

INFECTION TYPE	SYMPTOMS	CLINICAL SIGNS	DIAGNOSTIC METHOD	THERAPY
Candidiasis	Pruritus	Thick white discharge, pH 4.0–4.7	Wet prep or KOH prep (pseudohyphae)	Antifungals: topical or oral
Trichomonas	Malodorous discharge, pruritus	Frothy, yellow-green discharge, pH 5.0–7.0, "strawberry" cervix	Wet prep (mobile trichomonads)	Metronidazole
Bacterial vaginosis	Discharge, fishy odor	Thin gray discharge, pH 5.0–5.5	Wet prep, sniff test (clue cells, fishy odor)	Metronidazole, clindamycin, ampicillin
Chlamydia	Discharge	Mucopurulent discharge, cervical erosion	Culture, assay	Tetracycline, doxycycline, others
Gonorrhea	Discharge	Cervical discharge	Culture, Gram stain	Ceftriaxone, doxycycline, others
Genital herpes	Pain	Ulcerative, vulvar vesicles	Viral culture, Tzanck prep	Acyclovir
Chemical	Discharge	Erythema, may be ulcerative	History, exclusion of other causes	

Source: Adapted from LJ Copeland, ed. Textbook of gynecology. W. B. Saunders Company, 1993:506.

papillomavirus (HPV), and *Molluscum contagiosum.*

Herpesvirus is a DNA virus with two subtypes: HSV-1 and HSV-2. HSV-2 is more commonly associated with genital herpes, although either type may affect the genitalia. Genital herpes is a disease transmitted by direct sexual contact. With the primary infection, symptoms occur within three to seven days of exposure; they include painful ulcers in the genitalia with regional adenopathy, systemic malaise, and low-grade fever. Diagnosis is confirmed by viral culture from the vesicles. Alternatively, a smear may be made by scraping the epithelium of the ulcer and observing multinucleated giant cells with inclusions in the epithelium (Tzanck smear).

Therapy for herpes infections consists of antiviral therapy, either acyclovir or valacyclovir. Acyclovir may be given intravenously to treat severe primary or systemic infections, or it may be administered orally. In addition, some patients benefit from acyclovir cream applied directly to the herpetic lesion. Antiviral therapy will shorten the duration of symptoms and viral shedding. In patients with recurrent infections,

acyclovir may be used as a prophylactic measure to reduce the duration and frequency of recurrences. Typically, therapy involves 200 mg orally, five times per day, or 800 mg orally, twice per day. Suppressive therapy usually consists 400 mg, twice per day.

CLINICAL CORRELATION

T. L. is found to have an erythematous right labia majorum with multiple ulcers and a few remaining intact vesicles. A viral culture is taken from an already-opened vesicle. T. L. is given prescriptions for oral acyclovir and pain medication. She is instructed to urinate in a small amount of water in the bathtub so as to dilute the urine away from the infected area. The effected area begins to crust over in three days, and she is symptom-free within one week.

A woman who becomes pregnant and has a history of genital herpes must be followed closely due to the risk of infection to the newborn. Infants who contract herpes via the birth canal have a 50% mortality rate if untreated and a high level of neurological sequelae if they survive. One approach to managing the woman with a history of herpes who comes to the hospital in early labor is to evaluate the lower genital tract for evidence of an active outbreak. If no such evidence is found, vaginal delivery should be encouraged. In the presence of active infection or with a very recent outbreak, delivery should take place via cesarean section, although this strategy is not a 100% guarantee that the infant will not be infected.

HPV is a double-stranded DNA virus that is sexually transmitted. The clinical manifestation of viral replication is condyloma acuminata or genital warts (Figure 46.1). Many different genotypes of the virus exist, with each having a unique mucosal affinity. Most vulvar condylomas are infected with HPV type 6 or 11. Diagnosis is made by biopsy of a condyloma, which typically has the cytological appearance of a koilocyte—that is, an epithelial cell with vacuolated cytoplasm secondary to viral replication (Figure 46.2). Treatment is prompted by cosmetic or symptomatic reasons

and may be done by excision, ablation (laser, acid, chemotherapy), or immune modification (interferon). Recurrence rates for all therapies range between 15% and 25%. Studies involving both sexual partners do not document a decrease in recurrence if the male is vigorously treated. More severe manifestations of HPV infection, including genital dysplasia and carcinoma, will be covered in more detail in Chapters 49 and 50.

Molluscum contagiosum is a sexually transmitted viral infection of the genital region manifested by small papules on the skin. These papules are benign. Diagnosis is made by squeezing the contents of the papule and examining the resulting material under a microscope for the presence of characteristic cytoplasmic inclusion bodies, termed molluscum bodies. Treatment may involve curettage of the papules or destructive measures such as freezing or local acid treatment.

BACTERIAL INFECTIONS OF THE VULVA

Primary syphilis is a bacterial infection that is manifested on the vulva as a painless ulcer, called a chancre. It occurs between three weeks and 90 days after inoculation. Painless regional adenopathy may occur within one week of the appearance of the chancre. If no therapy is given, the chancre will disappear spontaneously in two to eight weeks. Diagnosis can be made by dark-field examination of fluid from the surface of the chancre, which will reveal the offending organism, *Treponema pallidum*. Secondary syphilis becomes evident approximately eight weeks after the chancre appears, being characterized by systemic symptoms such as malaise and generalized adenopathy. Skin lesions on the palms and soles are common. Occasionally, warty lesions may develop in the genitalia that coalesce to form condylomata lata, which are highly contagious lesions filled with treponemes. The various treatment regimens for syphilis are discussed in Chapter 44.

Granuloma inguinale is a bacterial infection caused by *Calymmatobacterium granulomatis*. Quite common in the Caribbean and Africa, it is rarely seen in the United States. If left untreated, this chronic destructive lesion forms granulomatous ulcers in the genital re-

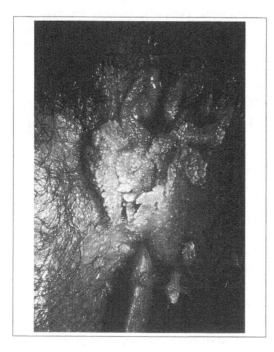

Figure 46.1 Genital warts, caused by infection with human papillomavirus

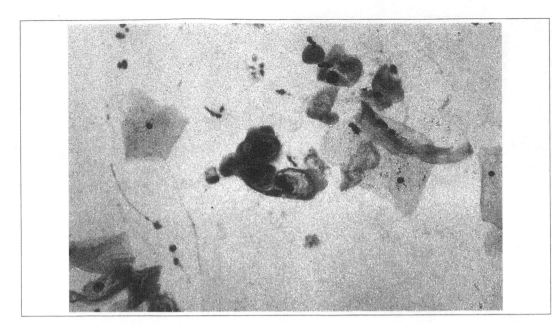

Figure 46.2 Pap smear demonstrating HPV infection. The cytoplasm is vacuolated and the cell is referred to as a koilocyte.

gion. Fibrosis and scarring are frequently seen in later stages. Tissue smears will reveal Donovan bodies—darkly staining clusters of organisms that resemble safety pins. Tetracycline is an effective antibiotic against this infection.

Chancroid is caused by infection with *Haemophilus ducreyi,* a gram-negative anaerobic bacillus. Typically, this infection causes ulcers in the genitalia with gray necrotic bases. The chancre that develops is tender, as opposed to the chancre of syphilis. Inguinal lymphadenopathy is a common finding. A smear of the lesion will reveal short, plump, gram-negative bacilli that resemble a "school of fish." Many antibiotics are effective against this infection, including trimethoprim-sulfamethoxazole and ciprofloxacin.

Chlamydia infections of the genitalia may be manifested on the vulva as lymphogranuloma venereum. This condition initially presents as a small ulcer on the vulva that resembles a herpetic ulcer. Next, the inguinal lymph nodes become swollen and tender. Long-term manifestations of this disease include edema and fibrosis of the anogenital region, which may lead to vaginal stenosis, fistula formation, or rectal stenosis. Diagnosis is based on posi-

tive serology or culture for *Chlamydia.* A variety of therapies are available to treat this infection, as described in Chapter 44.

BACTERIAL INFECTIONS OF THE VAGINA

Two infections of the vagina that frequently generate concern are *Trichomonas vaginalis* and bacterial vaginosis (BV).

Trichomonas is an infectious protozoan usually spread by sexual intercourse. The ensuing discharge is typically greenish, frothy, and foul-smelling. Erythema of the vaginal walls may be present, and patients may have pruritus over the vulva and vagina. The cervix may become quite inflamed, leading to the so-called strawberry cervix (Figure 46.3). Diagnosis is confirmed by identifying the flagellated protozoa on a normal-saline smear of the discharge (wet mount). The treatment is metronidazole, which may be given either orally or topically. *Trichomonas* infection in pregnancy has been associated with an increased incidence of premature rupture of membranes; consequently, it should be treated vigorously.

BV is a polymicrobial infection of the vagina with *Gardnerella vaginalis* and anaerobic bacteria, including *Mobiluncus* and *Bacte-*

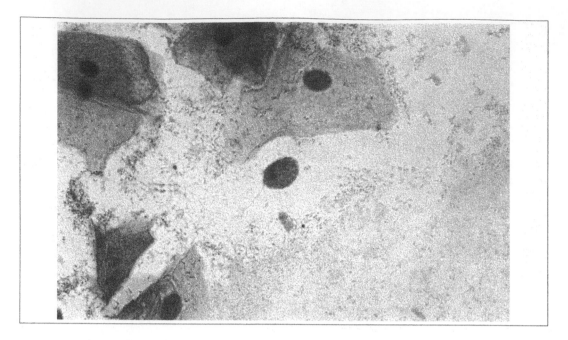

Figure 46.3   Pap smear with *Trichomonas*

Source: Courtesy of Juan Felix, MD.

roides species. In this disease, the normal lactobacilli in the vagina are replaced by these organisms. The infection is transmitted sexually. The discharge associated with BV is thin and creamy white; when a drop of 10% KOH is added to the discharge, a strong fishy (amine) odor is released. A wet mount may reveal stippling of the surface of the epithelial cells, which have a uniform granular cytoplasm and indistinct borders known as "clue cells." These alterations reflect the infection with *Gardnerella*. In addition, the pH of the vagina will be elevated above 5.0 (Figure 46.4). Oral metronidazole or clindamycin given vaginally are effective therapies against BV.

VULVAR DYSTROPHIES

CLINICAL CORRELATION

G. P. is a 53-year-old, G2P2, white female who complains of a change in the color of her vulva and intense itching for approximately four months. She denies a discharge. She has tried several over-the-counter remedies, albeit without success. She is sexually active without complaints except as related to the pruritus. On examination in the office, a large, white patch is observed over the anterior vulva. Several representative biopsies are performed.

Non-neoplastic epithelial disorders of the vulva include squamous cell hyperplasia and lichen sclerosis.

HYPERPLASIA

Hyperplasia occurs as a dermatologic reaction to some irritant. A biopsy of the area reveals thickening of the skin in response to a local irritant. Treatment is with corticosteroids.

LICHEN SCLEROSIS

Lichen sclerosis is usually associated with atrophy of the effected vulvar region. Histologically, the affected skin shows thinning and loss of the rete pegs. This disease can occur in any age group, although it is most commonly observed in post-menopausal women. Although its etiology has been proposed to be autoimmune, this relationship has not been defini-

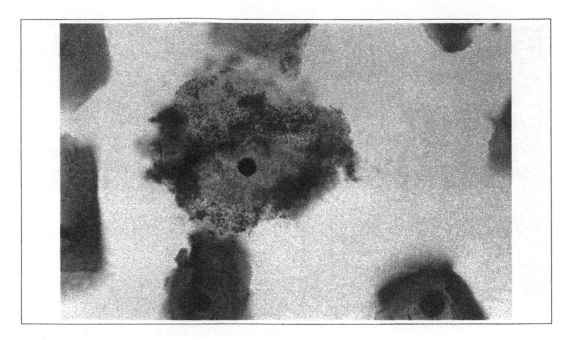

Figure 46.4 Pap smear with clue cell

Source: Courtesy of Juan Felix, MD.

tively confirmed. Some researchers have identified elevated levels of urogastrone associated with lichen sclerosis. Treatment usually consists of strong topical corticosteroids, such as clobetasol 0.1%, which quickly relieves the pruritus and slowly brings resolution of the cutaneous appearance. Many patients will need to repeat treatments periodically. Alternative therapies include topical testosterone or progesterone, although these agents do not relieve the symptoms as quickly as steroids (Figure 46.5). Vulvar cancer is associated with approximately 5% of all cases of lichen sclerosis, although it is unclear whether this relationship is causal or coincidental.

CLINICAL CORRELATION

The biopsies return as lichen sclerosis. G. P. is treated with clobetasol 0.1% cream applied two to three times per day until symptoms resolve, which takes roughly three weeks. A follow-up visit in five weeks reveals the white lesion to be greatly diminished in size. G. P. is instructed to continue with the steroid two to three times per week as maintenance therapy.

OTHER LESIONS OF THE VULVA

The Bartholin glands lie on each side of the vestibule in the postero-lateral vagina. These glands may become blocked and infected, leading to the formation of cysts or abscesses. Typically, these lesions become infected with gram-negative coliforms, although infection with *Neisseria gonorrhea* is also possible. Treatment consists of opening the abscess and allowing it to drain. In addition, the gland may be marsupialized—a technique that allows the gland to continue to drain until the infection clears. Alternatively, a small catheter (Word catheter) may be placed into the Bartholin gland to allow continued drainage. In perimenopausal and post-menopausal women, enlargement of the Bartholin gland should prompt suspicion of an adenocarcinoma of the gland and requires biopsy.

Cysts may also develop on the labia majora as fluid from the peritoneal cavity traverses down the inguinal ligament along the canal of Nuch (an embryological remnant). These hydroceles are managed by surgical removal. Other benign cysts that may develop on the vagina or vulva include leiomyomas and angiomyxomas.

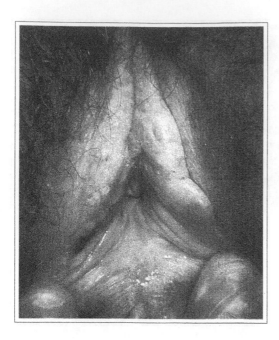

Figure 46.5 Lichen sclerosis of the vulva. This condition may occur in any age group and is characterized by thinning of the skin and pruritus.

Vulvar edema may occur from a variety of causes, including trauma, pressure, and lymphatic obstruction. Usually this condition is self-limiting, although chronic edema may require surgical resection.

Another inflammatory condition of the vulva is hidradenitis suppurativa. Hidradenitis is a chronic inflammation of the apocrine glands in the vulvar area. Over time, patients develop multiple nodules, scars, and sinuses deep in the cutaneous tissue. After infection with bacteria, these areas may become painful and foul-smelling (Figure 46.6). Several therapies aimed at reducing the activity of the apocrine glands, including isotretinoin and antiandrogens, have been successful in roughly half of patients with this condition. In addition, antibiotics may be helpful. Nevertheless, the condition typically requires surgical excision of the affected skin areas with split-thickness or myocutaneous grafting to fill the defects.

Other ulcerative conditions of the vulva include Behçet's syndrome, where herpetiform ulcers develop in the vulva, the ocular regions,

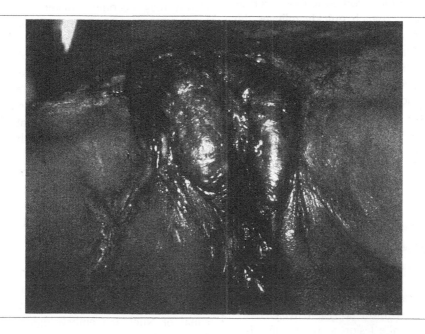

Figure 46.6   Hidradenitis suppurativa of the vulvar region. This condition is caused by an abnormality of the apocrine glands in this region. Therapy may include antibiotics, retinoic acid, and ultimately surgical resection.

and the oral cavity. Crohn's disease may sometimes affect the vulva with ulcerative granulomas.

CLINICAL CORRELATION

The biopsies return as lichen sclerosis. G. P. is treated with clobetasol 0.1% cream applied two to three times per day until symptoms resolve, which takes roughly three weeks. A follow-up visit in five weeks reveals the white lesion to be greatly diminished in size. G. P. is instructed to continue with the steroid two to three times per week as maintenance therapy.

SUMMARY

The most critical factor in determining the etiology of a vulvar lesion is the performance of a biopsy. Visual inspection alone is not accurate enough in most circumstances to determine the appropriate diagnosis and treatment. Vulvar and vaginal irritation is a common symptom for which women seek medical attention, and in most cases it can be handled successfully with simple medical therapy. The clinician must always have in the back of his or her mind, however, the possibility that a lesion might be a vulvar carcinoma.

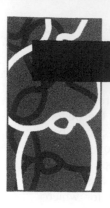

CHAPTER 47

Ectopic Pregnancy

Preston C. Sacks

A pregnancy that becomes implanted outside of the uterine cavity is referred to as an ectopic pregnancy. Although the most common site for an ectopic pregnancy is in the fallopian tube, such pregnancies can also occur in the ovary, uterine cornu, cervix uteri, or abdominal cavity (Figure 47.1). Despite recent advances in the diagnosis and treatment of ectopic pregnancies, they remain a leading cause of maternal mortality. Early diagnosis and prompt treatment can reduce both morbidity and mortality from this problem.

PATHOGENESIS OF ECTOPIC PREGNANCY

Fertilization occurs in the ampullary region of the fallopian tube within 24 hours of ovulation. The early embryo develops in this region for three to four days, reaching the blastocyst stage of development. On approximately the fifth post-ovulatory day, the embryo passes through the isthmus of the fallopian tube into the uterine cavity, where it will search for a site for implantation.

An abnormality that occurs during the transit of the embryo through the tube may cause the blastocyst to become implanted in the wall of the fallopian tube, creating an ectopic pregnancy. As the pregnancy develops, the tube will distend and eventually rupture. This distention of the tube causes the pain frequently associated with an ectopic pregnancy.

CLINICAL CORRELATION

C. B. is a 24-year-old female who presents to the office complaining of nausea and abdominal pain for the past two days. The pain is diffuse in location, intermittent in nature, and not relieved with acetaminophen. C. B. is sexually active and states that her last menstrual period began two weeks ago, but the flow was very light and lasted only two days.

DIAGNOSIS OF ECTOPIC PREGNANCY

All reproductive-age women should be questioned about their menstrual cyclicity, sexual activity, and contraceptive practices. If even a remote possibility exists that the patient may be pregnant, a pregnancy test should be performed. The most common symptoms of an ectopic pregnancy are pelvic pain and abnormal vaginal bleeding. Most women with an ectopic pregnancy, however, will not experience any symptoms until the tube is ready to rupture. The typical time for symptoms from an ampullary ectopic gestation to appear is six to eight weeks following the last normal menstrual period. The morbidity and mortality associated with ectopic pregnancy are directly related to the length of the gestation and the status of the tube (that is, whether it has ruptured). The clinician should attempt to diagnose an ectopic pregnancy early and prior to tubal rupture.

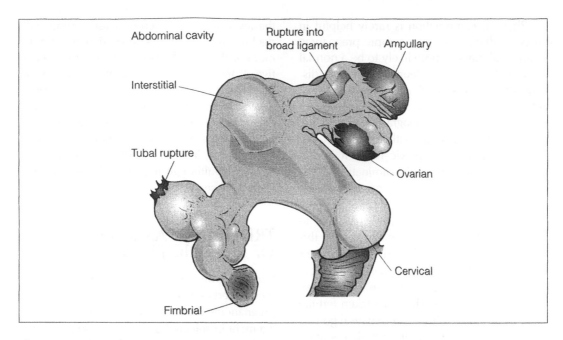

Figure 47.1   Sites of ectopic pregnancies

Source: Callahan TL, Caughey AB, Heffner LJ. Blueprints in obstetrics and gynecology. Malden, MA: Blackwell Science, 1998:11.

The incidence of ectopic pregnancy has increased steadily in recent years, mostly due to the increase in sexually transmitted diseases. Factors that increase a woman's risk of an ectopic pregnancy (Table 47.1) include the following:

- History of pelvic inflammatory disease
- Prior tubal surgery, including sterilization
- Congenital anomalies of the fallopian tube
- Use of progestin-only contraceptives

All of these factors influence the embryo's transit through the tube. Bear in mind, however, that most women with an ectopic pregnancy will not have an identifiable risk factor.

CLINICAL CORRELATION

Physical examination of C. B. is unremarkable. On pelvic examination, the uterus appears minimally enlarged, mobile, and nontender. The adnexae are neither enlarged nor tender. A qualitative pregnancy test is positive. The level of beta subunit of human chorionic gonadotropin (hCG) in the serum is 2000 mIU/mL. A transvaginal ultrasound fails to identify a gestational sac within the uterine cavity.

Table 47.1   Risk Factors for Ectopic Pregnancy

History of sexually transmitted infections or PID

Prior ectopic pregnancy

Previous tubal surgery

Prior pelvic or abdominal surgery resulting in adhesions

Endometriosis

Current use of exogenous hormones, including progesterone or estrogen

In vitro fertilization and other assisted reproduction

DES-exposed patients with congenital abnormalities

Congenital abnormalities of the fallopian tubes

Use of an IUD for birth control

Physical examination is rarely helpful in the early diagnosis of an ectopic pregnancy. An adnexal mass is more likely to be a normal ovary with a corpus luteum cyst than a distended fallopian tube. Consequently, the best method for early diagnosis of an ectopic pregnancy is sonography. Sonography is indicated in any pregnant woman with irregular bleeding, pelvic pain, or a pelvic mass. It is also helpful when the physical examination is not consistent with the expected gestational age based on the woman's last menstrual period.

The main purpose of sonography is to identify an intrauterine pregnancy. Once this type of pregnancy is confirmed, the chances of a concomitant ectopic pregnancy are very small (roughly 1 per 30,000 cases). The exception involves women who have taken fertility drugs (clomiphene citrate, menopausal gonadotropins). The incidence of multiple gestation in these women is high (5% to 15%), with that risk being accompanied by a higher possibility of concomitant ectopic pregnancy.

If sonography fails to identify an intrauterine pregnancy, three possibilities exist:

- The gestation is too early to be visualized.

- The patient has undergone a spontaneous miscarriage.

- An ectopic pregnancy is present.

The diagnosis of tubal pregnancy in a stable patient is then made by subsequent evaluation, including serial measurements of the level of beta-hCG in the serum and repeat sonography.

In normal pregnancies, the serum level of hCG doubles every 48 to 72 hours. When the level of hCG reaches 1000 mIU/mL, transvaginal sonography should reveal an intrauterine gestation greater than 90% of the time. At a level of 2000 mIU/mL, nearly all intrauterine gestations should be visible. By comparison, abdominal sonography should reveal an intrauterine pregnancy when the level of hCG is 6500 mIU/mL.

Thus it stands to reason that if the hCG reaches 1000 to 2000 mIU/mL and sonography fails to identify an intrauterine gestation, the patient has either a spontaneous miscarriage or an ectopic pregnancy. In patients with a spontaneous miscarriage (including spontaneously resolving ectopic pregnancies),

the level of hCG on serial measurements will decline. In these cases, the clinician should monitor the hCG level until it becomes negative. If the level of hCG continues to rise or plateaus, the patient likely has an ectopic pregnancy. In these cases, treatment is indicated. In ectopic gestations, the rise in hCG is generally less than that seen in normal gestations (that is, less than a doubling every 48 to 72 hours), although this condition is not universally observed.

TREATMENT AND FOLLOW-UP OF ECTOPIC PREGNANCY

Until recently, surgery was the only method recognized as an effective treatment of ectopic pregnancies. Today, however, medical management in selected patients utilizing the drug methotrexate is also available. Both options should be presented to the patient, and a treatment plan should be formulated based on the individual case.

CLINICAL CORRELATION

C. B. is counseled as to the likely diagnosis of ectopic pregnancy and treatment options. A laparoscopy is performed and reveals a 3 × 2 cm dilation of the left fallopian tube. The patient does not have any active bleeding in the pelvis, and the right fallopian tube appears normal. A left salpingectomy is performed. C. B. is discharged to go home three hours later. She will return to the office in one week for follow-up.

Surgery consists of removing the ectopic pregnancy and/or the damaged fallopian tube (Figure 47.2). In a hemodynamically stable patient, a laparoscopy is performed to evaluate the pelvis and to confirm the presence and location of the ectopic pregnancy. It is very important to evaluate the unaffected fallopian tube before arriving at a treatment decision. If the unaffected tube appears normal (normal caliber, normal-appearing fimbriae, no adhesions), then the prognosis for a subsequent intrauterine pregnancy is excellent. In these cases, removal of the entire tube containing

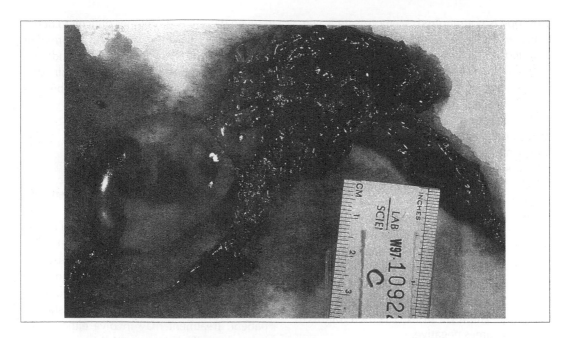

Figure 47.2 Ectopic gestation. This pregnancy was extruded as an intact gestational sac from the distal fallopian tube. The patient presented with severe pain in the lower pelvis, a positive pregnancy test, and a mass in the adnexae on ultrasound with a falling hemoglobin level.

the ectopic pregnancy is the best choice. This approach reduces the likelihood that the patient will have a repeat ectopic pregnancy in the same tube as well as her chance of a persistent ectopic pregnancy.

If the contralateral fallopian tube is abnormal, the prognosis for subsequent pregnancies is poor. Such women have both a reduced pregnancy rate and an increased risk of ectopic pregnancy. Many physicians will either (1) perform a linear salpingostomy and remove only the ectopic gestation or (2) use medical treatment to manage the ectopic pregnancy. Both of these options attempt to preserve the affected fallopian tube, in hopes that it will function better in the next pregnancy. Unfortunately, such abnormal tubes rarely perform well, and most of these patients will remain infertile. In vitro fertilization is particularly useful in this group of women.

When performing a linear salpingostomy, the fallopian tube is incised on the anti-mesenteric surface directly over the ectopic gestation. The pregnancy-related tissue is removed, and the implantation site coagulated to achieve hemostasis. The trophoblastic tissue is typically implanted into the muscularis layer

of the fallopian tube, which makes it difficult to achieve complete removal of this tissue without damaging the tubal mucosa and muscularis.

In roughly 10% of cases, trophoblastic tissue persists post-operatively and may cause bleeding and pain. To identify women with this problem, the level of hCG should be monitored post-operatively. If the hCG level plateaus or rises, methotrexate should be administered. Methotrexate blocks the action of dihydrofolic acid reductase, an enzyme necessary in the production of thymidylate. As a result, DNA synthesis is inhibited, and cellular replication stops. The cells most dramatically affected by a short-term use of methotrexate are the most actively dividing cells. Because trophoblastic tissue has an exceptionally high turnover rate, it is very sensitive to methotrexate.

In a hemodynamically stable patient with a confirmed ectopic pregnancy, methotrexate can be used as a primary treatment. Most protocols call for ensuring that the ectopic gestation is less than 3.5 to 4.0 cm in maximum diameter before this drug is given. The size of the gestation can be obtained by ultrasound—laparoscopy is not required. Methotrexate is generally well tolerated, and complications such as mucositis are rare. When patients who have received methotrexate treatment have been subsequently evaluated, their tubal patency rates have been high. Furthermore, the incidence of repeat ectopic pregnancies in the same fallopian tube appears equal to that seen following linear salpingostomy.

A single intramuscular dose of methotrexate (50 mg/m^2) is effective in resolving most ectopic pregnancies or cases of persistent trophoblastic tissue. Contraindications to its use include hemodynamic instability, liver or kidney dysfunction, and blood dyscrasias. Any patient who does not experience a decline in the level of hCG by at least 15% between days 4 and 7 after the injection should receive a second dose. The level of hCG is then followed until it becomes negative.

It is important to note that roughly 20% of patients receiving methotrexate will report an increase in lower abdominal pain within four to seven days. It is sometimes difficult to determine whether this increase in pain is normal or whether it represents tubal growth and rupture. The patient may need to be examined; if concerns persist, laparoscopy should be performed.

SUMMARY

The most important step in the management of ectopic pregnancy is early diagnosis. Early diagnosis reduces morbidity and mortality, and it permits the patient to consider more treatment options. Serial measurements of the level of the beta subunit of hCG in the serum combined with sonography allow for early diagnosis. In a stable patient, treatment may involve either surgery or medical therapy. If the woman is hemodynamically unstable, surgical treatment is necessary.

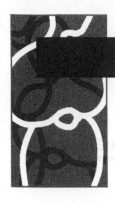

CHAPTER 48

Disorders of the Breast

William H. Hindle

Almost all women will have some breast symptoms or serious concerns about their breasts during their lifetime. Many will eventually seek medical attention for these concerns. Each woman presenting with a breast problem deserves a compassionate, thorough breast evaluation and a definite plan of management, even if the appropriate treatment is firm reassurance that no evidence of breast pathology is found. Breast cancer has the highest incidence of all the major cancers that afflict women. The mortality rate in women from breast cancer is second only to that associated with lung cancer. These facts, as well as the fear of the disfigurement caused by the treatment of breast cancer, produce profound anxiety in most women who present with breast symptoms or concerns.

Annual screening mammography beginning at age 40 is the paramount surveillance method available for detecting and diagnosing early (that is, 1 cm or less) breast cancers; such cancers have a favorable prognosis with today's treatment methods. With proper therapy, nonpalpable, mammography-detected breast cancers with no evidence of lymphovascular invasion have a 10-year, disease-free survival rate of more than 90%. In contrast, palpable breast cancers discovered by examination have a 10-year, disease-free survival rate of approximately 60% with currently available methods of treatment. Annual clinical breast examinations are nevertheless essential, because as many as 10% of palpable breast cancers are not perceived on mammography.

Breast self-examination (BSE) by a woman is useful in that she can become familiar with her breast anatomy. As a result, she may detect persistent significant changes that should be evaluated by her health care providers (Figure 48.1).

The three major breast complaints are as follows: a mass, pain, and nipple discharge. A breast-oriented history, bilateral clinical breast examination, and mammogram (for women 30 years of age and older) constitute the diagnostic triad (or triple test) for the clinical evaluation of such breast symptoms. This outpatient evaluation allows triage of benign conditions (which can be treated by primary health care providers) and lesions suspicious of malignancy (which should be expediently referred to a breast center team or a breast specialist).

The essential breast-oriented history covers the following points:

- The patient's age
- Her last menstrual period
- Breast complaints
- Family history of first-degree relatives with breast cancer
- Personal history of breast cancer
- Prior breast trauma, surgery, or treatments
- Current or past oral contraceptive therapy, estrogen replacement therapy, or hormone (estrogen and progesterone) replacement therapy

Breast Self-Exam (BSE)

Examine your breasts when they are the least tender, seven days after the start of your menstrual cycle. If you are pregnant, breastfeeding, have silicone implants or have entered menopause, you should continue to examine your breasts once a month. Breastfeeding mothers should examine their breasts when all milk has been expressed. Seek medical attention if a lump is discovered or if any changes are detected.

1. VISUAL POSITIONS: Standing

While standing in positions A,B,C and D, visually observe your breasts for changes in contour, shape, color and texture of the skin. Check nipple area for any discharge.

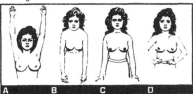

A   B   C   D

Use your left hand to examine the right breast and your right hand for your left breast. Most breast cancers occur in the upper outer area of the breast (between the underarm and nipple).

2. PALPATION POSITIONS:
Flat and Side-lying

Use the side-lying position to most effectively examine the outer half of the breast. A woman with small breasts may only need to use the flat position.

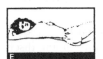

Side-lying Position (E): Lie on the side opposite the breast you are examining. Without moving your hips, rotate your shoulder back to a flat surface. This position is best for examining the outer half of the breast.

Flat Position (F): Lie down with a pillow or folded towel under the shoulder of the breast you are examining. Raise the arm of the side to be examined as shown, resting it on the flat surface. With your opposite hand, examine your breast.

Turn over for further instructions

ARLEN
MEDICAL EDUCATION PRODUCTS

Breast Self-Exam (BSE)

FEEL FOR CHANGES:

3. Area

The area to be examined includes the collarbone to the bra line and the breastbone to the underarm. Visually divide this area into vertical strips to completely cover all breast tissue. Use this as a pattern to carefully examine each section of the breast area.

4. Pads

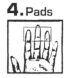

Using the pads of your three middle fingers held flat, examine your breast tissue by moving your fingers in small circular motions. Do not lift your fingers from your breast, but slide your fingers from one spot to the next.

5. Motion

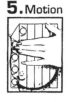

Starting with the underarm, proceed downward towards the bra line, then continue upward to the collarbone. Repeat the small circular motions applying varying degrees of pressure. Use light pressure to feel for changes below the skin surface and deeper pressure to feel for changes in the breast tissue.

Pressure

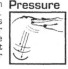

While your arm is relaxed and at your side, examine the breast tissue that extends into your underarm.

6. Nipple Discharge

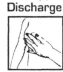

Squeeze your nipples to check for any discharge. (A discharge is normal for many women). Immediately report any breast changes to your health care professional.

This self-exam is NOT a substitute for periodic examinations or mammograms by a qualified health care professional.

© 1998 Arlen Med. Ed. (310) 820 3433

Figure 48.1   Breast self-examination

ANATOMY

Most of the breast is composed of fat. The glandular tissue spreads out from the nipple. Beginning at approximately 20 years of age, a progressive fatty replacement of the glandular tissue takes place. Lymph node drainage of the breast flows into the axillary region. The nodes are classified as either level I nodes (lateral to the insertion of the pectoralis minor muscle), level II nodes (under the insertion of the pectoralis minor muscle), or level III nodes (medial and superior to the pectoralis minor muscle).

An axillary lymph node dissection will remove both the level I and level II nodes.

A DOMINANT BREAST MASS

CLINICAL CORRELATION

A 64-year-old woman presents with the complaint of a lump in her breast that she discovered a week ago while taking a shower, although she does not perform routine BSE. The painless lump is described as hard. The patient is not on hormone replacement therapy. Her last breast examination by a physician was "years ago." She denies any prior breast treatments or surgery or family history of breast, ovarian, or colon cancer. She is in good general health, not on any medications, and physically active. Her weight is stable and within the normal range for her age.

A physical examination reveals a 3 cm, distinct, firm, dominant mass with irregular borders in the upper outer quadrant of her left breast. The mass is at the 2 o'clock position, roughly 3 cm from the areolar edge. The mass is nontender and exhibits decreased mobility within the breast tissue but is not attached to the overlying skin or the underlying chest wall. There are no associated skin changes. There is no nipple discharge. The lymph nodes are not palpable in the axillary or supraclavicular areas.

A free-hand, fine-needle aspiration (FNA) for cytology of the mass is performed and a bilateral diagnostic mammogram is ordered. The breast imaging (mammogram) reports a spiculated 3.5 cm mass in the left breast's upper outer quadrant in the position of the palpable clinically suspicious mass, highly suspicious of malignancy, BI-RADS assessment category 5. A biopsy is indicated. The FNA cytology report indicates the presence of an adenocarcinoma.

After the diagnosis is discussed with this patient (and her primary support person), she is referred to the regional breast cancer center, where she will be seen within a few days. Her prognosis and options of therapy will be discussed in detail with her and her primary support person after a comprehensive evaluation by a multispecialty team at the breast center.

A palpable dominant breast mass is a distinct, three-dimensional mass within the breast, different than any mass felt with palpation of the remainder of that breast and of the tissue in the other breast (Figure 48.2). A dominant breast mass requires definitive diagnosis by either FNA cytology with an adequate cell sample or tissue histology obtained by tissue core-needle biopsy or open surgical biopsy. The incidence of invasive breast cancer increases almost arithmetically with advancing age. In addition, the lumpy-bumpy texture of the breast that is common in many women during their reproductive years (that is, age 14 to 45) progressively decreases with age, making an abnormal mass more readily palpable.

It is humane and good medical care to arrive at the definitive diagnosis of a palpable dominant breast mass as quickly as possible. If the primary care physician is not trained and experienced in breast mass diagnosis, then the patient should be expeditiously referred to a breast specialist. Breast cancers are most commonly found in the upper outer quadrant of the breast, as this region has the largest amount of breast tissue.

Being a woman and aging are the two clinically meaningful risk factors for breast cancer. In addition, already having breast cancer in one breast and having a first-degree relative with breast cancer are moderate risk factors for breast cancer. Epidemiologic risk

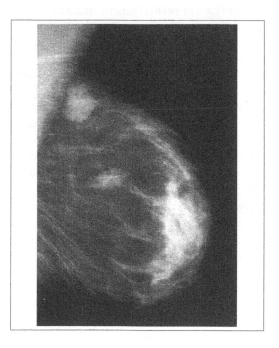

Figure 48.2 Mammogram demonstrating a dominant mass below the skin. This mass is a breast carcinoma.

Source: Courtesy of Yuri Parisky, MD.

factors for breast cancer that do not alter patient management include the following:

- Age at menarche
- Age at menopause
- Age at parity
- Diet
- Alcohol consumption
- Family history (other than first-degree relatives)
- Nulliparity
- Obesity
- Smoking

Epidemiologic data about the role of hormone therapy in breast cancer etiology are inconsistent and conflicting. At this time, current and past use of oral contraceptive therapy, estrogen replacement therapy, and hormone (estrogen and progesterone) replacement therapy are not clinically meaningful risk factors for breast cancer.

A three-generation pedigree history suggestive of an autosomal dominant pattern of breast, ovarian, or colon cancer may indicate a familial type of cancer and possibly inheritance of cancer-related genetic mutations. Two genes that may be mutated in familial breast cancer are BRCA-1 and BRCA-2. These genes presumably code for a tumor suppressor protein. When they are mutated, they are hypothesized to produce defective suppression of tumors. Women with the BRCA-1 gene have an 80% estimated lifetime risk of developing breast cancer and a 60% lifetime risk of developing ovarian cancer. The incidence of BRCA-1 mutation among women in the United States is estimated at 1 per 800 women; the incidence among women of Ashkenazi Jewish ancestry is 1 per 100 women.

Some epidemiologic studies have suggested that regular exercise, particularly in premenopausal women, may decrease the risk of breast cancer.

Stage I and II (up to 5 cm in diameter) breast cancers can be appropriately treated with breast-conserving therapy (lumpectomy, axillary lymph node dissection, and anterior chest wall irradiation) or modified radical mastectomy (Table 48.1). The long-term survival rate is the same for both options of treatment. Nevertheless, the recommendations and details of treatment should be individualized for each patient. Generally, premenopausal women with axillary lymph node involvement are given chemotherapy and post-menopausal women with similar involvement are placed on tamoxifen therapy. Recent data suggest that tamoxifen may also offer prophylactic protection against the development of breast cancer in women considered to be at high risk for this disease.

The most common histology for breast cancer is ductal carcinoma (53%), followed by mixed ductal carcinoma (28%), medullary carcinoma (6%), and lobular carcinoma (5%). A rare variant of breast cancer called inflammatory carcinoma of the breast (1% to 5%) has a particularly poor prognosis. Overall, the most critical prognostic variables remain tumor size and presence of lymph node metastases. The presence of a high concentration of estrogen receptors in the tumor generally correlates with response to hormonal therapy.

FIBROADENOMA

Fibroadenomas are the most common, benign breast neoplasms. They are not premalignant and do not increase a woman's risk of breast cancer per se.

CLINICAL CORRELATION

A 20-year-old woman presents with a palpable breast lump, which she has felt for approximately one year. Now she thinks it is getting bigger. The lump sometimes becomes painful before her menstrual periods, but the pain subsides with menstruation. She is not taking any medications. Her family and past medical histories are noncontributory.

A physical examination reveals a firm, mobile, nontender, somewhat nodular dominant mass with distinct smooth borders. There are no associated skin changes. The mass measures 2.5 cm and is located at the 3 o'clock position, 2 cm from the areolar edge, in the right breast. Except for

Table 48.1   Breast Cancer Staging

AMERICAN JOINT COMMITTEE ON CANCER TNM STAGING SYSTEM

T (TUMOR)

TX	Primary tumor cannot be assessed
T0	No evidence of primary tumor
Tis	Carcinoma in situ
T1	Tumor ≤ 2.0 cm in greater dimension
T1a	0.5 cm or less in greatest dimension
T1b	More than 0.5 cm but less than 1.0 cm in greatest dimension
T1c	More than 1.0 but less than or equal to 2.0 cm in greatest dimension
T2	Tumor > 2.0 cm, but ≤ 5.0 cm in greatest dimension
T3	Tumor > 5.0 cm in greatest dimension
T4	Tumor of any size with extension into chest wall (not including pectoralis muscles) or into the skin, or edema, skin ulceration, satellite nodules confined to the same breast, or inflammatory carcinoma

N (NODES)

NX	Regional nodes cannot be assessed
N0	No regional lymph node metastases
N1	Metastasis to ipsilateral axillary lymph node(s)
N2	Metastasis to ipsilateral axillary lypmh node(s) fixed to one another or to other structures
N3	Metastases to ipsilateral mammary lymph node(s)

M (DISTANT METASTASIS)

MX	Distant metastasis cannot be assessed
M0	No distant metastasis
M1	Distant metastasis present [includes ipsilateral supraclavicular node(s)]

AJCC STAGE GROUPING FOR BREAST CANCER

STAGE	TUMOR	NODES	METASTASIS
0	Tis	N0	M0
I	T1	N0	M0
IIa	T0,1	N1	M0
	T2	N0	M0
IIb	T2	N1	M0
	T3	N0	M0
IIIa	T0,1,2	N2	M0
	T3	N1,2	M0
IIIb	T4	Any N	M0
	Any T	N3	M0
IV	Any T	Any N	M1

diffuse lumpiness throughout both breasts, there are no other abnormalities by clinical breast examination.

An FNA procedure for cytology is performed and subsequently reported as fibroadenoma.

In the preceding case, as an alternative to FNA, tissue core-needle biopsy or open surgical excision biopsy can be used to establish a histologic diagnosis of fibroadenoma. Unless the clinical impression is invasive breast cancer, diagnostic mammography is not indicated in the breast evaluation of women younger than 30 years of age.

Once a definitive diagnosis of fibroadenoma has been made, the treatment options are elective excision or continued follow-up with annual, clinical breast examinations. The patient should be instructed in the technique of effective BSE and encouraged to perform BSE after her menstrual period every month. If the fibroadenoma continues to grow or becomes symptomatic, then she should return to her physician promptly for reevaluation.

The fibroadenoma can be excised at any time, if the patient so desires. During the perimenopausal years, fibroadenomas usually decrease in size and often become nonpalpable. An atrophic post-menopausal fibroadenoma can calcify and produce a characteristic "popcorn" pattern that is readily apparent on a mammogram.

CYSTS

Nonpalpable microcysts within the breast parenchyma are normal (physiologic) for women during the reproductive years. A small cyst can enlarge and become palpable (macrocyst) (Figure 48.3). Simple cysts are not premalignant and do not increase a woman's risk of breast cancer per se. Breast cysts are lined by benign ductal epithelium that may undergo apocrine metaplasia.

CLINICAL CORRELATION

A 42-year-old woman presents to her primary care physician with a history of a pal-

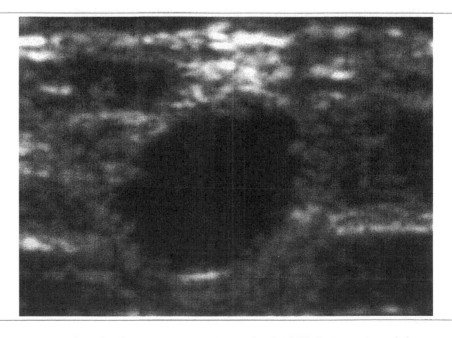

Figure 48.3   Sonography of a breast cyst appearing to be fluid-filled. Aspiration of the cyst revealed straw-colored fluid with complete resolution of the cyst.

Source: Courtesy of Yuri Parisky, MD.

pable lump in her right breast. She has been aware of the lump for a year but had been too busy to come in for medical evaluation. The lump seems to get bigger temporarily before the onset of her menstrual period and is painful at these times. Otherwise, it does not seem to be enlarging. She saw another physician elsewhere a week ago while on a trip. That physician ordered a mammogram, which confirmed the presence of a distinct mass. The radiologist recommended an ultrasound, which subsequently showed a well-defined anechoic spherical mass which increased through transmission, distal acoustic enhancement, and posterior wall bright-up, typical of a simple cyst. When the cyst was aspirated with ultrasound guidance, approximately 5 cm³ of cloudy yellow fluid was obtained. By ultrasound, it appeared that all of the cyst fluid had been aspirated. No palpable mass remained after the aspiration. The radiologist discarded the cyst fluid after showing it to the patient.

At her current visit to the physician, a physical examination reveals no palpable dominant mass or ecchymosis of the right breast. There is a bandage over the cyst aspiration site. Diffuse, fine, nodular lumpiness is observed throughout both breasts, but no abnormalities are noted by clinical breast examination. No one in the patient's family has a history of breast cancer, although her mother had experienced lumpiness and breast tenderness for years before she reached menopause.

In the preceding case, if the patient's primary care physician had been the one to see the patient initially, he or she could have performed an FNA procedure in the office that would have confirmed the diagnosis of a cyst, and the cyst could have been aspirated at the same time. Intracystic neoplasms are rare. If the aspirated cyst fluid is frank blood (not just fluid tinged with blood, which could result from the aspiration itself), if a residual palpable mass persists after the aspiration, or if the cyst refills within three months, the lesion should be evaluated by a breast specialist and a biopsy considered. Cytology of cyst fluid is not cost-effective and does not assist in the clinical management of a breast cyst.

A palpable macrocyst can be diagnosed and therapeutically managed in the outpatient (office) setting by the patient's primary care physician. Diagnostic mammography is not mandatory, although in the preceding case the woman should undergo an annual screening mammography. While ultrasound is not necessary for a palpable cyst that can be aspirated, it is just as reliable in the breast as it is in the ovary for distinguishing a cyst from a solid mass. Mammography does not reliably make this differentiation.

CLINICAL CORRELATION

After reevaluation in three months to verify that the cyst has not re-formed, the follow-up is routine, with an annual clinical breast examination and screening mammography following the established age guidelines. The patient should be encouraged to perform BSE and to return to her physician promptly if she notices any persistent changes in her breasts.

A breast cyst, like other tension cysts, can feel hard upon palpation. A cyst is usually round with smooth borders. Cysts are mobile and do not have associated skin changes. They can be painful or tender. Although cysts tend to subside with menopause, they can recur (become palpable) when an estrogen-deficient woman begins estrogen replacement therapy. Asymptomatic cysts do not require treatment.

PAIN (MASTALGIA)

Most women experience mastalgia during their reproductive years. The intensity of this pain in the breast varies from vague "heaviness" to acute pain. Many women with cyclic mastalgia consult their primary care physician because they are worried that the pain is a sign of a serious breast problem, such as cancer. Cyclic breast pain without an associated palpable mass is rarely a sign of breast cancer and tends to subside during the perimenopausal years.

CLINICAL CORRELATION

A 27-year-old woman presents with breast pain. She has been aware of the pain for more than a year. The pain increases prior to menstruation. She is worried that something is wrong with her breasts. She does BSE intermittently and says, "It all feels lumpy to me."

Her mother had similar premenstrual breast pains. Her mother also had a breast biopsy, which proved to be benign. Her grandmother was diagnosed with invasive breast cancer at age 57. The remainder of her family history and her past medical history is noncontributory.

A physical examination reveals diffuse tenderness throughout both of the patient's breasts. The tenderness is more pronounced in the upper outer quadrants. There is diffuse nodularity (lumpy-bumpy) throughout her breasts. Palpation does not identify a dominant mass.

Two questions are essential in taking the history of a woman with mastalgia:

1. Is the pain cyclic or noncyclic (constant or intermittent)?

2. Is the pain diffuse or localized?

Cyclic mastalgia may be unilateral, although the neuroendocrine explanation of one-sided breast pain remains unknown. This condition is an exaggeration of the normal response of the breast tissue to the hormonal changes during the menstrual cycle. Diffuse cyclic mastalgia is not caused by intrinsic breast pathology. In contrast, localized cyclic breast pain may be associated with a cyst or fibroadenoma.

Probably more than 75% of women presenting with breast pain—particularly cyclic mastalgia—can be effectively reassured that no evidence of breast cancer is present. Such reassurance is usually appropriate and successful treatment. On the other hand, some women with mastalgia will require symptomatic pain management, such as the use of nonsteroidal analgesia intermittently as necessary. Less than 5% of women presenting with cyclic mastalgia will require pharmacologic

hormonal therapy. Even after more than six months of therapy, however, mastalgia will return in the majority of women after their treatment is discontinued.

What a woman perceives as noncyclic, localized "breast pain" is usually caused by nonbreast etiologies of the anterior chest wall—for example, achalasia, cervical radiculitis, cervical spondylosis (at C6–C7), cervical rib, cholelithiasis, coronary artery disease, costal chondritis (Tietze syndrome), herpes zoster (shingles), hiatal hernia, infected epidermal inclusion cyst (in the skin), myalgia, neuralgia, phantom pain, pleurisy, psychological pain, trauma, and tuberculosis. These diagnoses require specific treatment.

Cyclic mastalgia can be controlled in as many as 80% of cases with medications that suppress the normal physiologic, hormonal variations associated with ovulation. Double-blind studies (conducted mostly in Europe) have shown bromocriptine, danazol, GnRH, low-dose birth control pills, and tamoxifen to be effective therapies. Danazol is the only medicine approved by the U.S. Food and Drug Administration (FDA) for the treatment of mastalgia. All of these medications are less effective in the treatment of noncyclic mastalgia.

Hormone and other laboratory tests are not indicated in the evaluation of mastalgia. Women 30 years of age and older should have a diagnostic mammogram. As with all breast symptoms and problems, if a palpable dominant mass is present, the urgent definitive diagnosis of the mass is paramount.

NIPPLE DISCHARGE

During their reproductive years, most women can elicit (with repeated squeezing) some discharge from their nipples. Nipple discharge—particularly bilateral milky discharge—is often pregnancy-related. Some mothers who are breast-feeding their infants even experience bloody nipple discharge. Pregnancy-related nipple discharge is rarely a sign of intrinsic breast pathology. Non-pregnancy-related, bilateral, spontaneous milky nipple discharge is usually a form of galactorrhea and is not caused by intrinsic breast pathology.

A 35-year-old woman presents with unilateral nipple discharge that she noticed when she was squeezing her nipples, as she had been instructed to do for her BSE. This discharge alarms her, because her aunt was recently diagnosed with breast cancer. The patient has no other breast symptoms and has not felt a distinct lump in her breast.

A physical examination reveals bilateral, serous nipple discharge from multiple duct openings on her nipples when the areolae are massaged toward the nipple. Palpation does not identify a dominant mass, nor does a bilateral clinical breast examination detect any other abnormalities.

The patient is instructed not to repeatedly squeeze her nipple as part of her BSE (or at any other times) and to return promptly if she experiences spontaneous nipple discharge.

Spontaneous nipple discharge is pathologic and requires evaluation. Intraductal papillomas are associated with spontaneous, unilateral nipple discharge from a single duct opening on the nipple. The color of the nipple discharge associated with intraductal papillomas varies from clear watery, to serous, to serosanguineous, to grossly bloody. At the Breast Diagnostic Center (Women's and Children's Hospital, Los Angeles, California), 4% of the women presenting to this consultative clinic gave nipple discharge as their primary complaint. Upon questioning, three-fourths of these patients admitted having elicited the nipple discharge themselves and did not have spontaneous nipple discharge. Thus pathologic, spontaneous nipple discharge is uncommon, accounting for only 1% of new patients seen at the Breast Diagnostic Center.

When a woman is having spontaneous, unilateral nipple discharge from a single duct opening on the nipple, a ductogram (galactogram) will usually demonstrate an intraductal lesion. The breast surgeon can then excise the involved duct through a small (2 cm or less) circumareolar incision.

Periductal mastitis (mammary duct ectasia) produces dark, often almost black, nipple discharge from multiple duct openings on the nipple and is usually bilateral. This problem usually arises in women of perimenopausal age. Periductal mastitis is not a bacterial infection, so antibiotics are not an effective treatment. If the woman cannot tolerate the discharge, then surgical ligation or excision of the ducts below the nipple is the only known method of eradicating it.

NONPALPABLE BREAST LESIONS

Mammography is the only proven and effective technique for breast cancer screening of nonpalpable lesions (Figure 48.4). A radiologist can perceive a stellate mass, a circumscribed lesion, microcalcifications, an asymmetric density, an architectural distortion, and skin changes in a mammogram. Although many of these abnormalities are benign, all of them nevertheless require a compete breast imaging evaluation. The most common mammographic finding of invasive ductal carcinoma is a spiculated (stellate) mass. Clustered, irregular, dense, linear microcalcifications are the most common findings of ductal carcinoma in situ, but their identification does not rule out microinvasive carcinoma. A comparison with prior mammograms is highly desirable, as it aids in identifying a new or enlarging lesion and assists the physician in evaluating a potential malignancy.

A mammogram is a form of medical consultation. The physician ordering the mammogram should supply the radiologist with the essential clinical data (breast-oriented history) and note the problem suspected and the location of the area of clinical concern. The radiologist should be authorized to complete the imaging evaluation. The mammographic diagnosis and recommendations are the responsibility of the radiologist, and these findings should be clearly conveyed in the written mammogram report. The American College of Radiologists' Breast Imaging Reporting and Data System (BI-RADS) should be used in reporting the findings. Physicians who order mammograms should be familiar with the

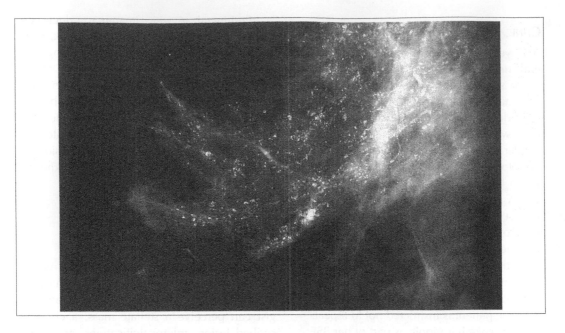

Figure 48.4   Mammogram demonstrating microcalcifications in a breast without palpable lesions. This patient had ductal carcinoma in situ.

Source: Courtesy of Yuri Parisky, MD.

BI-RADS lexicon—particularly the breast imaging assessment categories. These categories are defined as following:

0: needs additional imaging evaluation.

1: negative.

2: benign finding.

3: probably benign finding—short-interval follow-up suggested.

4: suspicious abnormality—biopsy should be considered.

5: highly suggestive of malignancy—appropriate action should be taken.

The radiologist should be contacted directly if the ordering physician has doubts about the mammographic diagnosis or recommendations. The patient must be informed about the results as well.

A negative mammogram does not rule out breast cancer. Regardless of the mammographic findings or lack thereof, a palpable, dominant breast mass must be definitively diagnosed by either FNA cytology or histology obtained by tissue core-needle or open surgical biopsy. Fat necrosis of the breast may be particularly difficult to differentiate from ma-

lignancy on mammography, because of the presence of a solid nodule and calcifications.

A woman's primary care physician is responsible for ordering her mammography following the currently established guidelines. Furthermore, the physician is responsible for obtaining the mammogram report (or documenting why the mammogram has not been performed) and for tracking the follow-up of the mammographic recommendations (or documenting why the recommendations have not been carried out).

PAGET'S DISEASE OF THE BREAST

Paget's disease of the breast accounts for less than 5% of all breast cancer. It is characterized by an eczematoid lesion of the nipple/areolar region. In approximately 50% of cases, an underlying invasive carcinoma of the breast will be present, often (though not always) with a palpable mass. If the problem is limited to Paget's disease only, surgical resection is curative. If an underlying carcinoma is found, the patient's prognosis is affected by the tumor size and her lymph node status. It is important that women with an eczematoid rash on their nipple/areola receive prompt attention to rule out an invasive cancer.

SUMMARY

Breast disease affects a high percentage of women. Most women have a tremendous fear of breast cancer. The obstetrician/gynecologist must be familiar with recommendations for routine mammograms, clinical breast examinations, and self breast examinations. Cystic lesions can be handled by the gynecologist in the office; most such lesions are benign. Lesions that appear suspicious on mammogram, that the patient palpates but the gynecologist cannot, or that are palpable but not seen on mammogram should be referred to the appropriate specialist for prompt attention.

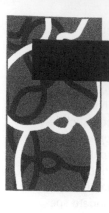

CHAPTER 49

Vulvar and Vaginal Neoplasms

Jeffrey F. Hines

VULVAR NEOPLASMS

A variety of benign and malignant neoplasms may occur on the vulva. Malignant tumors of the vulva are uncommon, however, accounting for only 3% to 5% of all female genital tract malignancies and approximately 1% of all malignancies in women. Unfortunately, improper evaluation of vulvar symptoms by health care providers delays diagnosis and treatment of many vulvar lesions, including vulvar cancers. Careful and early evaluation, including a pelvic examination and biopsy of lesions for histologic confirmation, is essential for prompt diagnosis.

CLINICAL CORRELATION

J. T. is a 67-year-old, menopausal, gravida 1, para 1, white female on hormone replacement therapy who returns to the clinic for reevaluation of chronic vulvar pruritus. She has been seen off and on during the past six months with complaints of recurring vulvar itching and now reports the presence of a vulvar lump. She has been treated with a variety of topical steroids and antifungals, but has not received any relief from these therapies.

J. T.'s past medical history is significant for hypertension and obesity. Her medications include an antihypertensive, estrogen, and progesterone. Her last Pap smear, clinical breast examination, and screening mammogram were all normal as of 10 months ago. She does not consume alcohol and does not smoke cigarettes.

The patient's physical examination is unremarkable down to the pelvis. A 1 cm, firm, right inguinal lymph node is palpable. No other groin adenopathy is appreciated. A speculum examination of the vagina and cervix is unremarkable. A repeat Pap smear is performed. Careful examination of the external genitalia reveals a 2 cm, raised, warty mass on the right labia majora. No other lesions are observed. Bimanual and rectovaginal examinations reveal a small, anteverted uterus and no palpable adnexa. The stool is hemoccult-negative. A biopsy of the vulvar mass, including some of the normal-appearing skin that borders the mass, and a biopsy of the enlarged lymph node are obtained.

A histologic evaluation of both specimens reveals invasive squamous cell cancer consistent with a vulvar primary.

APPROACH TO MANAGEMENT AND TREATMENT

The differential diagnosis of vulvar neoplasms requires an extensive investigation (Table 49.1). Patients are rarely asymptomatic and will usually complain of a palpable lump or mass or have a long history of pruritus. Careful visual inspection, palpation, and possible colposcopic evaluation of the vulva in women presenting with such symptoms is of paramount concern. Biopsy of any suspicious le-

Table 49.1 Common Vulvar Neoplasms

Benign neoplasms

Vulvar intraepithelial neoplasia (VIN) to include Bowen's disease and Bowenoid papulosis

- Extramammary Paget's disease
- Hidradenoma
- Syringoma
- Condyloma acuminata
- Fibroma
- Lipoma
- Leiomyoma
- Endometriosis
- Epidermoid inclusion cyst
- Bartholin's duct cyst

Malignant neoplasms

- Squamous cell cancer
- Malignant melanoma
- Adenocarcinoma
- Leiomyosarcoma
- Rhabdomyosarcoma
- Histiocytosis X
- Basal cell carcinoma
- Verrucous carcinoma
- Metastatic neoplasms
- Bartholin's gland carcinoma

women, with the mean age of diagnosis being 65 years. Women usually present with vulvar pruritus and an eczematoid lesion with irregular borders (Figure 49.1). Unlike its counterpart in the breast, which is usually associated with an underlying ductal carcinoma, vulvar Paget's disease is associated with an underlying adenocarcinoma in only approximately 20% of patients. Synchronous cancers of the bladder, colon, rectum, breast, and gallbladder have been described in approximately 30% of patients. The treatment of choice for extramammary Paget's disease is vulvar excision to include the underlying dermis. Histologically, pathognomonic, large, pale, Paget's cells are found adjacent to the basal epidermal layer and adnexal structures. Local recurrence of Paget's disease is common, likely reflecting inadequately excised surgical margins. This recurrence arises because Paget's disease can extend well beyond the visible gross lesion.

Intraepithelial neoplasia and carcinoma in situ (Bowen's disease) appear on the vulva as either pigmented or white, plaque-like lesions (Figure 49.2). Many of these lesions are associated with human papillomavirus (HPV) infec-

sion, mass, lump, or ulcer is warranted to confirm a diagnosis. Visual diagnosis is unreliable.

Benign neoplasms of the vulva can occur in women of all ages. Bartholin's duct cysts require incision and marsupialization or catheter drainage if they become infected or symptomatically enlarged. The occurrence of such cysts in perimenopausal and post-menopausal women may require excision to exclude the diagnosis of cancer. In contrast, epidermoid inclusion cysts occur frequently on the labia majora. Such cysts arise from the pilosebaceous apparatus, occur in clusters, and rarely have a diameter exceeding 2 cm. Unless infected, they are not problematic.

Extramammary Paget's disease of the vulva is an intraepithelial adenocarcinoma in situ. Paget's disease typically strikes white

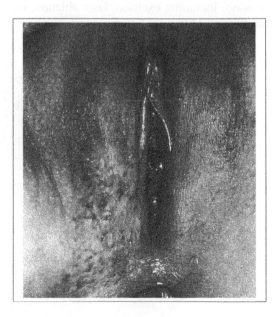

Figure 49.1 Paget's disease of the vulva. This condition presents as an eczematoid rash in the vulva. It may be associated with an underlying adenocarcinoma in the vulva or with adenocarcinoma in other areas, such as the rectum or breast.

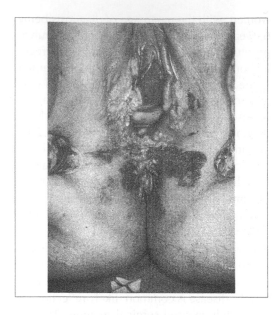

Figure 49.2   Bowenoid dysplasia—that is, widespread, pigmented, vulvar dysplasia

Source: Morrow CP, Curtin JP, ed. Synopsis of gynecologic oncology, 5th ed. Philadelphia: Churchill Livingstone, 1998:25.

tion. After careful colposcopic evaluation and biopsy, these lesions can be treated in a variety of ways, including excision, laser ablation, or application of topical 5-fluorouracil.

Bowenoid papulosis is a similar clinical entity that affects young women. The lesions associated with this disease are velvety red in nature. Bowenoid papulosis is histologically indistinguishable from carcinoma in situ and is treated with excisional biopsy or laser ablation. Other benign vulvar neoplasms include hidradenoma, syringoma, schwannoma, fibroma, leiomyoma, and endometriosis.

Approximately 85% of all malignancies of the vulva have a squamous origin (Figure 49.3). Most squamous cancers of the vulva occur on the labia majora, but the labia minora, perineum, and clitoris may also be primary sites. Typically, women with vulvar cancer present with a mass or lump. Other potential symptoms include pruritus, pain, bleeding, ulceration, and discharge. A careful palpation of the groin nodes is essential in such cases. Inspection and palpation of the entire vulva—including the mons pubis, inner thighs, perineum, vagina, urethra, and perianal areas—must be accomplished. A biopsy must be used to histologically confirm the diagnosis. A bimanual examination, rectovaginal examination, and cervical cytology are necessary to the work-up as well. A chest X ray should be taken and routine blood tests performed. Mammography and endoscopic evaluation of the bladder or colon are

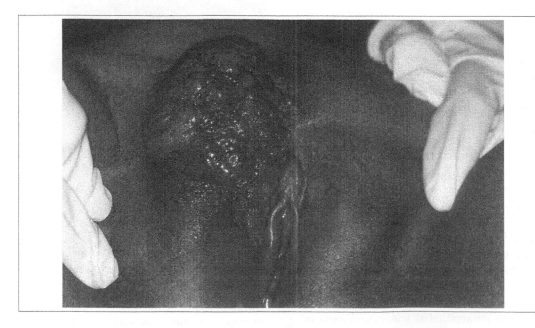

Figure 49.3   Squamous cell carcinoma of the vulva

undertaken as warranted by the other findings. In addition, imaging studies such as computed tomography (CT) and magnetic resonance imaging (MRI) may prove useful in selected cases of advanced disease.

Squamous cancer of the vulva spreads primarily by local extension to the urethra, vagina, rectum, or pubic bone; by lymphatic drainage to regional lymph nodes; and by hematogenous embolization to distant sites like the liver and lung. The incidence of lymph node metastasis for all stages of vulvar cancer is approximately 30%. In the majority of cases, lymphatic metastases spread to the superficial inguinal lymph nodes, the femoral lymph nodes, and finally to the pelvic lymph nodes. Of particular importance is the sentinel lymph node of Cloquet, which is located beneath the inguinal ligament and is the most cephalad of the femoral nodes. Staging of vulvar cancer requires a surgical procedure (Table 49.2).

Treatment for vulvar malignancies must be customized for the individual patient. The treatment modality selected must effectively address treatment of the vulvar primary site, treatment of the lymph nodes, and possible reconstructive treatment of the vulvo-vagina. Early squamous vulvar cancer can be treated surgically with radical local excision with margins of at least 1 to 2 cm; radical vulvectomy is recommended for larger or midline lesions. In such cases, the dissection is made to the level of the inferior fascia of the urogenital diaphragm. Dissection of the lymph nodes will depend upon the size of the primary tumor, distance of the primary tumor from the midline, and depth of invasion.

Advanced stage III and IV vulvar cancers may be treated with a combination of chemotherapy, radiation, and surgery. Post-operative groin and pelvic lymph node radiation is indicated for women with multiple, histologically

Table 49.2 International Federation of Gynecology and Obstetrics (FIGO) Staging for Vulvar Cancer

FIGO STAGE	TNM	CLINICAL/PATHOLOGIC FINDINGS
Stage 0	T_{is}	Carcinoma in situ, intraepithelial carcinoma.
Stage I	$T_1N_0M_0$	Lesions 2 cm or less in size confined to the vulva or perineum. No nodal metastasis.
Stage Ia		Lesions 2 cm or less in size confined to the vulva or perineum and with stromal invasion no greater than 1 mm. No nodal metastasis.
Stage Ib		Lesions 2 cm or less in size confined to the vulva or perineum and with stromal invasion greater than 1 mm. No nodal metastasis.
Stage II	$T_2N_0M_0$	Tumor confined to the vulva and/or perineum, >2 cm in greatest dimension, no nodal metastases.
Stage III	$T_3N_0M_0$	Tumor of any size with
	$T_3N_1M_0$	1. Adjacent spread to the lower urethra or the anus.
	$T_1N_1M_0$	2. Unilateral regional lymp node metastasis.
	$T_2N_1M_0$	
Stage IVa	$T_1N_2M_0$	Tumor invades any of the following:
	$T_2N_2M_0$	Upper urethra, bladder mucosa, rectal mucosa, pelvic bone, or bilateral regional node metastasis.
	$T_3N_2M_0$	
	T_4 any N M_0	
Stage IVb	Any T, any N M_1	Any distant metastasis including pelvic lymph nodes.

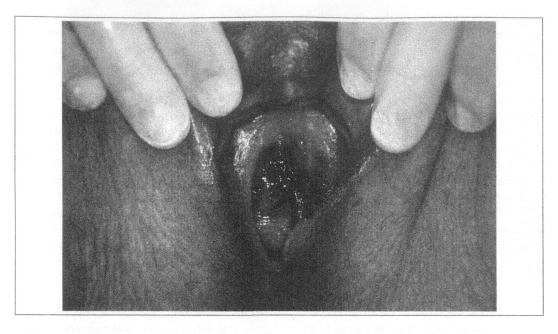

Figure 49.4   Melanoma of the vulvo-vaginal region

positive lymph nodes. Patients with one positive lymph node generally do not require postoperative radiation.

Other vulvar cancers include Bartholin's gland adenocarcinoma, sarcomas, and melanomas. These diseases are generally treated with radical vulvectomy and inguinal-femoral lymphadenectomy (Figure 49.4). Basal cell cancers of the vulva behave similarly to their counterparts on other skin surfaces. That is, they are nonmetastasizing, are locally aggressive, and require wide, local excision as therapy. One variant of squamous cell cancer of the vulva—verrucous carcinoma—resembles a large condyloma. It rarely metastasizes, is locally aggressive, and is prone to local recurrences. Verrucous cancer is treated with wide local excision. Note, however, that radiation therapy of these tumors has induced malignant transformation in some series and should therefore be avoided. Metastatic tumors to the vulva must always be considered in the differential diagnosis of vulvar cancer.

VAGINAL NEOPLASMS

Neoplasms of the vagina encompass a variety of embryologic remnants, benign masses, and primary and metastatic malignancies. As is the case with tumors of the vulva, taking a careful history in addition to inspecting, palpating, and biopsing suspicious lesions will ensure accurate and prompt diagnosis of these lesions.

CLINICAL CORRELATION

M. F. is a 31-year-old, nulligravida, African American female referred to a gynecologist by her family medicine physician for evaluation of an abnormally appearing cervix and a vaginal mass. Her past medical and surgical history are unremarkable, and she uses combination oral contraceptives for birth control. She does, however, report that her mother took a medication while pregnant with her to help prevent miscarriage. A review of M. F.'s systems is positive for metrorrhagia.

The physical examination is unremarkable down to the pelvis. Examination of the external genitalia is normal. An inspection of the vagina reveals a 2 cm mass on the anterolateral vaginal wall in the middle third of the vagina. A columnar-appearing surface appears to occupy the entire exocervix. No other gross abnormalities are evident. A repeat cervical cytology is performed. The bimanual and rectovaginal examinations are unremarkable. The stool is hemoccult-negative. Colposcopic evaluation of M. F.'s cervix reveals coarse punctation and mosaicism; consequently, a directed biopsy and endocervical curettage are performed. Additionally, a biopsy of the vaginal mass is performed.

The repeat Pap smear and directed cervical biopsy confirm severe dysplasia. The endocervical curettage shows benign endocervical tissue. Biopsy of the vaginal mass reveals clear cell adenocarcinoma. M. F. is able to confirm that her mother used diethylstilbestrol (DES) during pregnancy.

APPROACH TO MANAGEMENT AND TREATMENT

Epidermoid cysts are the most commonly noted benign tumor of the vagina. They are generally 1 to 2 cm in diameter, located in the distal vagina in the superficial mucosa, and most often the result of birth trauma. Gartner's duct cysts are mesonephric derivatives that are usually small, asymptomatic, and anterolaterally located. Other benign vaginal neoplasms include fibroepithelial polyps, endometriosis, leiomyoma, intraepithelial neoplasia, hamartoma, and adenosis (Table 49.3). Such lesions are confirmed by biopsy and then treated with local excision or ablative procedures.

Primary malignant tumors of the vagina are rare, accounting for only 1% to 2% of all gynecologic malignancies (Figure 49.5). Although the majority of vaginal malignancies are squamous cell cancers, other histologic types include melanoma, endodermal sinus tumor, sarcoma botryoides, leiomyosarcoma, and DES-related clear cell adenocarcinoma. The majority of vaginal malignancies are metastatic, usually spreading from the cervix or vulva.

The histologic type found appears to vary with the age of the patient. Endodermal sinus tumors of the vagina occur primarily in infant girls. The most common vaginal tumor of adolescence is sarcoma botryoides. DES-related clear cell adenocarcinoma is most commonly observed in the reproductive years. Finally, squamous cell carcinoma is most prevalent in the seventh decade of life.

Table 49.3 Common Vaginal Neoplasms

Benign neoplasms
- Vagina intraepithelial neoplasia (VAIN)
- Epidermoid inclusion cyst
- Gartner's duct cyst
- Fibroepithelial polyp
- Vaginal polyp
- Hamartoma
- Leiomyoma
- Endometriosis
- Condyloma acuminata

Malignant neoplasms
- Squamous cell cancer
- Malignant melanoma
- Clear cell adenocarcinoma
- Sarcoma botryoides (embryonal rhabdomyosarcoma)
- Endodermal sinus tumor (yolk sac tumor)
- Metastatic neoplasms
- Leiomyosarcoma
- Fibrosarcoma
- Angiosarcoma

In the majority of cases, squamous cell cancer of the vagina occurs in the upper third of the vagina. It presents as infiltrative, ulcerative, or exophytic lesions that require biopsy for confirmation. Such cancers spread primarily by direct extension into the bladder, rectum, and pelvic side wall and via the lymphatics. The lower third of the vagina drains to the inguino-femoral lymphatics, much like the vulva does. The upper two-thirds of the vagina drains to the pelvic lymph nodes, similar to the way that the cervix does. Hematogenous embolization is usually seen with advanced disease.

Vaginal cancers are staged clinically (Table 49.4). A primary malignancy of the cervix must be excluded. The clinical staging evaluation for patients includes a pelvic examination, cervical cytology, biopsy of suspicious vaginal lesions, chest X ray, and routine blood tests. Cystoscopic evaluation of the bladder and endoscopic evaluation of the colon are

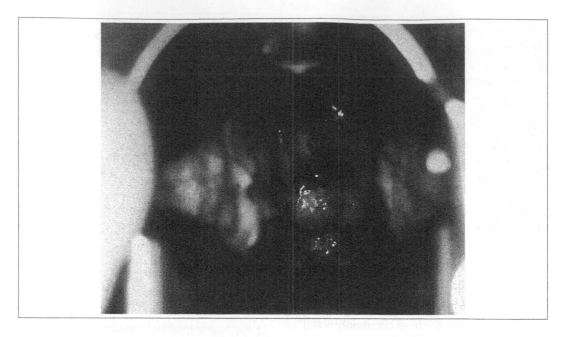

Figure 49.5   Primary vaginal carcinoma

performed as warranted by the patient's symptoms. A pelvic examination under anesthesia is sometimes indicated when the findings are difficult or equivocal. Although not a part of formal clinical staging process, diagnostic imaging techniques such as CT and MRI may assist in developing the treatment plan.

Radiation therapy is the mainstay of ther-

Table 49.4	FIGO Clinical Staging System for Vaginal Cancer
Stage 0	Carcinoma in situ; intraepithelial carcinoma
Stage I	Tumor confined to the vaginal mucosa
Stage II	Submucosal infiltration into parametrium, not extending to pelvic wall
Stage IIA	Subvaginal infiltration, not into parametrium
Stage IIB	Parametrial infiltration, not extending to pelvic wall
Stage III	Tumor extending to pelvic wall
Stage IV	Tumor extension to bladder or rectum or metastasis outside true pelvis

apy for vaginal cancers. For squamous and clear cell adenocarcinomas, approximately 5000 cGy of teletherapy is first delivered to shrink the tumor. It is followed by intracavitary implants, with or without interstitial implants placed directly into the tumor. Some proximal, stage I squamous cell cancers and adenocarcinomas of the vagina can be treated with radical hysterectomy, radical upper vaginectomy, and pelvic lymphadenectomy. Endodermal sinus tumors and sarcoma botryoides are generally treated with a combination of chemotherapy, radiation, and conservative surgery.

In utero DES exposure to the female fetus has been associated with a variety of structural, neoplastic, and non-neoplastic anomalies of the genital tract. In particular, uterine and cervical abnormalities (cervical hood, cockscomb cervix, cervical dysplasia, uterine septa) have been described. Vaginal adenosis (columnar epithelium or its products in the vagina) occurs in 30% of such women. Clear cell adenocarcinoma of the cervix and vagina has been linked to daughters exposed to DES in utero at a frequency of less than 1 per 1000 exposed. Evaluation of young women exposed in utero to DES should begin no later than age 14, with cervical cytology, colposcopy, and directed biopsy being performed. Treatment of

DES-related adenocarcinoma of the vagina primarily consists of radiation, except for some proximal vaginal lesions.

SUMMARY

Carcinomas of the vulva and vagina account for a small percentage of gynecologic cancers. They generally occur in the elderly population, although preinvasive disease is common in reproductive-age women. Complaints of pruritus, a mass, or abnormal bleeding in the lower genital region demand evaluation and, if a lesion is present, biopsy for diagnosis. The visual examination of lesions in this area is often misleading, which makes it a paramount concern to determine the lesion's histological identify before initiating therapy. Treatment for cancers of the vulva and vagina continues to be refined, with the goal of maintaining cosmesis and sexual function of these areas.

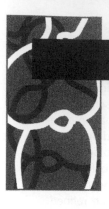

CHAPTER 50

Disorders of
the Cervix

James L. Moore and Alexander F. Burnett

Disorders of the cervix are commonly encountered in the practice of obstetrics and gynecology. Cervical cancer is the second most common malignancy among women throughout the world, although Papanicolaou smear screening has greatly reduced its incidence in developed countries.

The Pap smear is an effective screening test for a number of reasons. It is relatively inexpensive, is reproducible across a variety of laboratories, and requires little technical expertise to perform. The test's positive predictive value is increased because of the high prevalence of cervical disorders. Perhaps most importantly, the Pap smear can detect clinically silent premalignant disease (cervical dysplasia) at a time when it can be effectively treated in the outpatient setting. For this reason, implementation of cervical screening programs in industrialized nations has brought about a decrease in the incidence of cervical cancer. The American College of Obstetricians and Gynecologists currently recommends that annual screening begin at age 18, or sooner if a patient has been sexually active.

CLINICAL CORRELATION

A. B. is a 21-year-old, nulligravida, college student who presents for a routine annual examination. Her past history is unremarkable. She is sexually active in serial monogamous relationships and currently uses combination oral contraceptive pills for birth control. She has no history of sexually transmitted disease, genital warts, or abnormal Pap smears. She denies having any of the known human immunodeficiency virus (HIV) risk factors.

On the pelvic examination, no lesions are seen on the external genitalia. The vaginal vault has no discharge. The cervix is nulliparous and grossly normal. A cervical smear for cytology is obtained by using an endocervical brush first, followed by an exocervical spatula. On bimanual examination, the uterus is midplane, mobile, nontender, and of normal size. No adnexal masses or tenderness is present. The rectovaginal examination is unremarkable.

Two weeks following A. B.'s visit to the clinic, her Pap smear reports a high-grade, squamous intraepithelial lesion. A. B. is contacted and asked to return for further discussion and evaluation.

The process of obtaining a cervical smear for cytologic evaluation begins with identification of the external cervical os. A large cotton swab is used to clean the cervix of any mucus, blood, or debris. Next, the endocervical brush is inserted into the cervical canal and rotated to obtain the endocervical specimen. A wooden spatula is then placed on the cervix and rotated 720° to sample the ectocervix. The smears are immediately placed on a glass slide and sprayed with an aerosolized fixative for cytologic preservation.

Pap smear results are categorized by the Bethesda System of classification, which was adopted in 1988. Under this system, the cytologic interpretation is reported along with a descriptive diagnosis (Table 50.1). In addition, the report may include a statement about the adequacy of the specimen—for example, whether it contains exocervical and endocervical cells for evaluation. Pap smears that reveal dysplasia or worse findings, and those with atypical cells occurring repeatedly or in patients in whom follow-up may be a problem, require further evaluation.

Table 50.2 lists a number of causes, both benign and malignant, for an abnormal Pap smear. The thinning of the cervico-vaginal epithelium with menopause can cause abnormal-appearing cells on the smear. Likewise, any local inflammatory process, such as cervicitis or vaginitis, can alter the appearance of exfoliated cells in the cervical smear. Conditions of cervical healing and repair—for example, after a vaginal delivery—are still other causes for abnormal cytology. Human papillomavirus (HPV) infection, even in the absence of a dysplastic lesion, can cause changes detectable on

Table 50.2 Causes of Abnormal Pap Smears

- Cervical dysplasia
- Invasive cervical cancer
- Genital epithelial atrophy
- Cervicitis
- Cervical epithelial repair
- HPV infection
- Other pelvic neoplasia
- Air-drying artifact
- Excessive blood

the Pap smear. Finally, other genital neoplasias (endometrial, fallopian tube, ovarian) may sometimes display exfoliated neoplastic cells on cervical smears.

If the smear is allowed to dry prior to cytologic fixing, an air-drying artifact may conceal dysplastic changes. Likewise, excessively bloody smears may obscure cellular detail. Such smears should be repeated.

As is demonstrated in the preceding case, cervical dysplasia is an asymptomatic and clinically silent disease. In fact, most dysplastic lesions on the cervix are not detectable with routine visual inspection. As a consequence, the next step in evaluating an abnormal Pap smear involves careful examination with a binocular magnifying instrument called a colposcope.

Table 50.1 The Bethesda System of Reporting Pap Smears

- Statement of Specimen Adequacy
- Descriptive Diagnosis
  - Within normal limits
  - Infection
  - Reactive and reparative changes
  - Epithelial cell abnormalities
    - Atypical squamous cells of undetermined significance
    - Low-grade squamous intraepithelial lesion: includes HPV, HPV with mild dysplasia, or mild dysplasia alone
    - High-grade squamous intraepithelial lesion: includes moderate or severe dysplasia/carcinoma in situ
    - Squamous cell carcinoma
    - Atypical glandular cells of undetermined significance
    - Adenocarcinoma
- Hormonal Evaluation

CLINICAL CORRELATION

Upon her return to the clinic, various causes of abnormal Pap smears, including dysplasia, are discussed with A. B. The need for further evaluation with colposcopy and cervical biopsy as well as possible treatment options are addressed. The patient is informed that the Pap smear is not diagnostic, but merely a screen, and that the diagnosis of dysplasia or cancer is made by cervical biopsy.

A repeat examination of A. B.'s cervix reveals no gross lesion. A 15× colposcope is used to magnify the cervical portio for better visualization. The cervix is bathed with a dilute 3% acetic acid solution with a large cotton swab. After two minutes, the cervix is again visualized through the colposcope. A readily apparent patch of aceto-white epithelium is observed at the 2 o'clock position of the cervix, extending from the transformation zone to the cervical portio. Closer inspection reveals fine punctate vessels in the raised epithelial patch. The borders of this lesion are sharply defined, and the entire lesion is seen. The colposcopic examination does not reveal any other suspicious findings. The transformation zone is completely visualized.

A directed biopsy of the lesion is accomplished, followed by curettage of the endocervical canal. Hemostasis is achieved by directed application of silver nitrate.

In the preceding case, closer inspection with the colposcope permitted better definition of the etiology of the abnormal Pap smear. The dilute acetic acid caused cytoplasmic changes in the nonkeratinized cervical epithelium. Normal surface cells will show no change after application of acetic acid, whereas dysplastic cells will become a white color. These patches of dysplasia, known as "aceto-white," indicate an area of concern that should be inspected more closely. The abnormal submucosal vascular pattern, easily seen through the magnification of the colposcope, is yet another indication of dysplasia. Vascular patterns may show pinpoint punctation or a mosaic tile-like pattern. Such patterns are associated with more advanced cervical dysplasia than aceto-white changes alone.

Any colposcopically abnormal area should be biopsied. Colposcopic findings are carefully described and mapped in the patient's medical record prior to biopsy.

The colposcopic examination, including biopsies, generally takes about 10 minutes. Once it is completed, biopsies are obtained and a scraping of the endocervical canal is performed to evaluate that portion of the cervix that is not visible to the colposcopist.

The epithelium that is at greatest risk for cervical dysplasia is the area of the transformation zone between the glandular endocervical epithelium and the squamous ectocervical epithelium (Figure 50.1). If the entire transformation zone cannot be seen, the colposcopy is termed "inadequate" and surgical excision of the transformation zone may be necessary to complete the evaluation of the abnormal Pap smear.

CLINICAL CORRELATION

The final pathology of the cervical biopsy confirms a high-grade cervical dysplasia, known as cervical intraepithelial neoplasia III (CIN III). The endocervical curettage is unremarkable. Treatment options are discussed with A. B., and she elects to undergo office-based treatment consisting of a loop electro-excisional procedure (LEEP) as definitive therapy. This procedure is accomplished without difficulty using local anesthesia, and the final pathology of the LEEP specimen shows a completely excised CIN III lesion with negative margins and a negative post-LEEP endocervical curettage.

Cervical dysplasia is a disorder characterized histologically by a loss of ordered epithelial maturation, resulting clinically in unrestrained cellular proliferation. Dysplastic lesions are classified according to the amount of epithelial thickness that the abnormal cells occupy. Mild dysplasia (CIN I) has only minimal involvement of the epithelium, whereas moderate and severe dysplasia (CIN II and CIN III, respectively) are characterized by greater epithelial involvement (Figure 50.2). A higher-

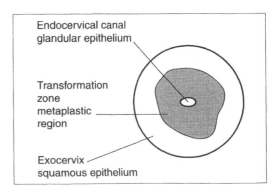

Endocervical canal
glandular epithelium

Transformation
zone
metaplastic
region

Exocervix
squamous epithelium

Figure 50.1   The transformation zone of the exocervix

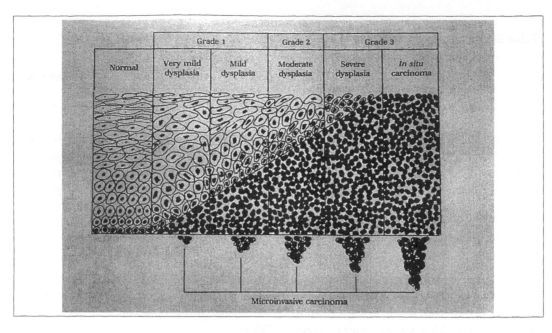

Figure 50.2   Cervical dysplasia

Source: Kurman R, ed. Blaustein's pathology of the female genital tract, 3rd ed. New York: Springer-Verlag, 1987:193.

grade dysplasia carries a more significant risk of malignant transformation than does a lower-grade dysplasia, which often resolves spontaneously. Treatment options for cervical dysplasia (as discussed in Chapter 4) include laser vaporization, LEEP excision, acid destruction, cryotherapy, and surgical excision. Because of the likelihood of spontaneous regression and the very small risk of progression, patients who can be relied on to complete follow-up care may be managed conservatively if they have CIN I or HPV changes. Higher-grade lesions (CIN II or CIN III) or patients who may be unreliable for follow-up should receive immediate treatment.

Risk factors for cervical dysplasia mirror those for invasive cervical cancer (Table 50.3). Having multiple sexual partners is a clear risk factor, as are a number of other sexual factors: Age at first intercourse, history of sexually transmitted diseases, and oral contraceptive use are all associated with cervical dysplasia. The presence of genital warts (condyloma accuminata) indicates infection with HPV. Such infections, which are also a marker of sexual activity, commonly affect the cervix as well. The overwhelming majority of cervical dys-

plasia occurs in association with HPV infection. In addition, some subtypes of the virus are associated with aggressive preinvasive lesions and cervical cancer. Diseases leading to immunosuppression—particularly infection with HIV and suppression for organ transplant—are also risk factors for cervical disease.

CERVICAL CARCINOMA

Cervical carcinoma is the third most common gynecologic malignancy in the United States, with approximately 16,000 cases occurring an-

Table 50.3   Risk Factors for Cervical Dysplasia and Carcinoma

- Multiple sexual partners
- History of sexually transmitted diseases
- Early age at first sexual intercourse
- Oral contraceptive use
- Prior cervical dysplasia
- Genital warts (HPV infection)
- Immunosuppression

Table 50.4   Oncogenic Potential of Various HPV Types—Typing Results of Cervical Dysplasias and Cancers

	LOW-GRADE SIL	HIGH-GRADE SIL	CANCER
Low risk	20.0%	3.8%	1.9%
HPV 6, 11, 42, 43, 45			
Intermediate risk	16.7%	24.0%	10.5%
HPV 31, 33, 35, 51, 52, 58			
High risk—HPV 16	16.1%	47.0%	47.0%
High risk—HPV 18	3.9%	4.9%	23.5%

Source: Lorincz et al, Obstet Gynecol 1992;328:79.

nually. Like cervical dysplasia, it is frequently a disease of reproductive-age women and has a strong association with sexual activity. In addition, cigarette smoking is a risk factor for cervical cancer. The disease is characterized along a continuum ranging from mild dysplasia to moderate dysplasia to severe dysplasia/carcinoma in situ to invasive cancer. Patients may regress to normal status anywhere along this continuum prior to the development of invasive cancer.

The development of cervical cancer is clearly associated with HPV infection. Both epidemiologic studies and HPV DNA studies indicate that a very high percentage of cancers involve HPV DNA. There seems to be a tendency for certain types of HPV to be associated with preinvasive disease and other types to be associated with cancer (Table 50.4). The HPV types associated with low-grade lesions such as condylomas (HPV types 6 and 11) are rarely, if ever, associated with cervical carcinoma.

Table 50.5 lists the most frequently encountered symptoms when patients present for treatment. Most commonly, women will complain of abnormal vaginal bleeding or discharge. Pain in cervical cancer is generally associated with advanced disease. The diagnosis is confirmed by biopsy of a cervical lesion. When a lesion is present, a biopsy—rather than a Pap smear—is required for the diagnosis. Office biopsy of a gross lesion is appropriate, and conization of the cervix is not performed when a gross lesion is present. Most frequently, carci-

noma of the cervix is squamous cell in origin, with adenocarcinoma and adenosquamous carcinoma being observed less often (Figure 50.3).

CLINICAL CORRELATION

T. L. is a 34-year-old, gravida 4, para 4, female with a chief complaint of excess vaginal bleeding. She states that her menses has increased in length from 5 days every month to 7 to 10 days and now occurs every two weeks. She particularly is distressed at the amount of bleeding that she experiences just after intercourse. Her past history is significant for coitarche at age 14 with 12 lifetime partners. She has been married and monogamous for the past 14 years. She has a history of two episodes of

Table 50.5   Symptoms of Cervical Cancer

SYMPTOM	PERCENTAGE OF WOMEN
Post-menopausal bleeding	46%
Irregular menses	20%
Postcoital bleeding	10%
Vaginal discharge	9%
Pain	6%
None	8%

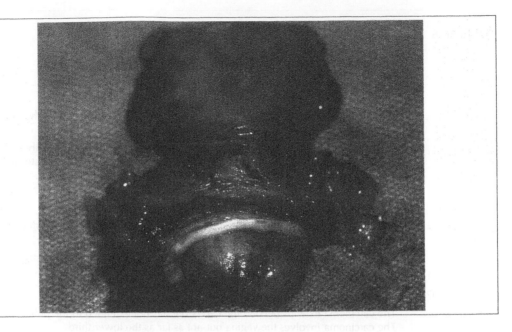

Figure 50.3 Stage Ib1 squamous cell carcinoma of the cervix. This picture shows a radical hysterectomy specimen with the parametria removed along with the uterus. Note that the ovaries are not removed as a routine part of this surgery unless warranted for other indications.

gonorrhea treated as a teenager. She currently smokes and has undergone a tubal ligation for birth control.

On examination, T. L. appears to be healthy and has no peripheral lymphadenopathy. Examination of her cervix reveals a 3 cm fungating mass off the anterior cervix, which is friable and grossly appears to be a cancer. A biopsy is performed. Bimanual and rectovaginal examinations confirm the existence of this mass, which is located on the exocervix. The cervix is mobile with no evidence of nodularity or tumor in the parametria or on the vagina. The biopsy results indicate the presence of poorly differentiated squamous cell carcinoma.

Staging of cervical cancer is clinical—that is, the stage is determined by pelvic examination, radiographic studies, and investigation of the bladder and rectum with cystoscopy and proctoscopy when necessary. Table 50.6 explains the staging system employed.

Typically, cervical cancer spreads by di-

rect extension and lymphatic routes (Figure 50.4). The lymphatic extension generally follows a contiguous path, with the pelvic lymph nodes being affected first, followed by nodes higher up the aortic chain. Hematogenous spread of this cancer is rare in early-stage disease, but may be found in more advanced cases.

Treatment for early-stage cervical cancer can involve either surgery or radiation, with both modalities showing similar survival rates. Once the woman is beyond stage IIa, treatment is limited to radiation and occasionally chemotherapy. Surgical therapy for an invasive cervical cancer involves performing an extended or radical hysterectomy, which removes the parametrial tissue on the lateral aspect of the cervix along with the uterus. This tissue contains the ureter and uterine vessels, which must be dissected prior to cutting the parametria, a process that adds significantly to the operative difficulty of the procedure (Table 50.7).

In addition, the lymph nodes that drain the cervix (the pelvic and para-aortic lymph nodes) are removed in toto with the dissection

Table 50.6   International Federation of Gynecology and Obstetrics Staging for Carcinoma of the Cervix Uteri

STAGE	CLINICAL/PATHOLOGIC FINDINGS
Stage 0	Carcinoma in situ, intraepithelial carcinoma.
Stage I	The carcinoma is strictly confined to the cervix (extension to the corpus should be disregarded).
Stage Ia	Invasive cancer identified only microscopically. All gross lesions even with superficial invasion are stage Ib cancers. Invasion is limited to measured stromal invasion with maximum depth of 5 mm and no wider than 7 mm.*
Stage Ia1	Measured invasion of stroma no greater than 3 mm in depth and no wider than 7 mm.
Stage Ia2	Measured invasion of stroma greater than 3 mm and no greater than 5 mm and no wider than 7 mm.
Stage Ib	Clinical lesions confined to the cervix or preclinical lesions greater than stage Ia.
Stage Ib1	Clinical lesions no greater than 4 cm in size.
Stage Ib2	Clinical lesions greater than 4 cm in size.
Stage II	The carcinoma extends beyond the cervix but has not extended to the pelvic wall. The carcinoma involves the vagina but not as far as the lower third.
Stage IIa	No obvious parametrial involvement.
Stage IIb	Obvious parametrial involvement.
Stage III	The carcinoma has extended to the pelvic wall. On rectal examination, there is no cancer-free space between the tumor and the pelvic wall. The tumor involves the lower third of the vagina. All cases with hydronephrosis or nonfunctioning kidney are included unless they are known to be due to other causes.
Stage IIIa	No extension to the pelvic wall.
Stage IIIb	Extension to the pelvic wall and/or hydronephrosis or nonfunctioning kidney.
Stage IV	The carcinoma has extended beyond the true pelvis or has clinically involved the mucosa of the bladder or rectum. A bullous edema as such does not permit a case to be allotted to stage IV.
Stage IVa	Spread of the growth to adjacent organs.
Stage IVb	Spread to distant organs.

*The depth of invasion should not be more than 5 mm taken from the base of the epithelium, either surface or glandular, from which it originates. Vascular space involvement, either venous or lymphatic, should not alter the staging.

Source: From American College of Obstetricians and Gynecologists. Prolog: gynecologic oncology and surgery, 3rd ed. Washington, DC, 1996:183.

(Figure 50.5). The ovaries are very rarely involved with cervical cancer; consequently, oophorectomy is not a routine part of surgery for cervical cancer.

CLINICAL CORRELATION

T. L. undergoes a chest radiograph and intravenous pyelogram, both of which are normal. The examination is consistent with a stage Ib squamous cell carcinoma of the cervix. T. L. is referred to a gynecologic oncologist, who discusses the treatment options with her. Because of its ability to preserve ovarian function and the potential for less vaginal scarring, the patient opts for surgery over radiation. She

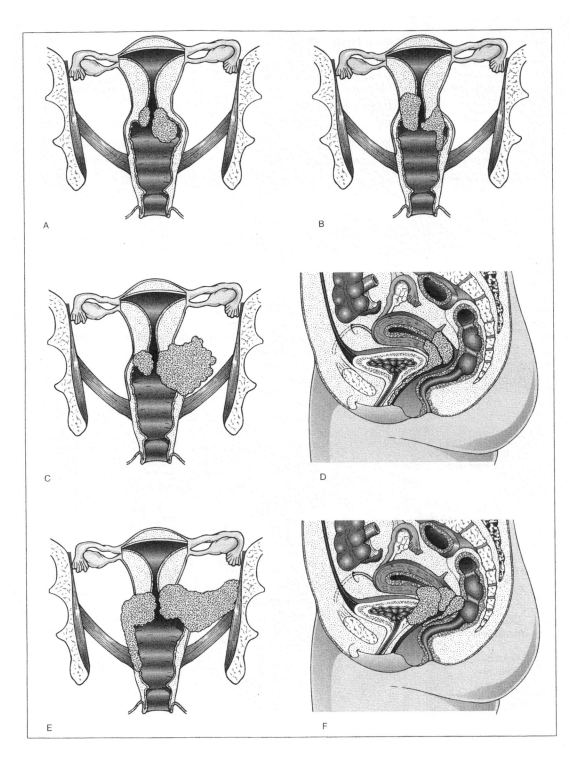

Figure 50.4 FIGO classification of carcinoma of the cervix. (A) Stage IB: carcinoma continued to the cervix, exophytic. (B) Stage IIA: carcinoma extends into the upper vagina or fornix. (C) Stage IIB: carcinoma extends into the parametrium but does not extend to pelvic wall. (D) Stage IIIA: carcinoma involves the anterior vaginal wall, extending to the lower one third. (E) Stage IIIB: the parametrium is infiltrated and the carcinoma extends to the pelvic wall. (F) Stage IVA: the bladder base or rectum is involved.

Source: Callahan TL, Caughey AB, Heffner LJ. Blueprints in obstetrics and gynecology. Malden, MA: Blackwell Science, 1998:183.

Table 50.7   Types of Abdominal Hysterectomy

	TYPE I (SIMPLE)	TYPE III (RADICAL)
Vaginal cuff removed	Rim	Upper one-third to one-half
Bladder	Partially mobilized	Mobilized
Rectum	RV septum partially mobilized	RV septum mobilized
Ureters	Not mobilized	Completely dissected to bladder
Cardinal ligaments	Resected medial to ureters	Resected at pelvic side wall
Uterosacral ligaments	Resected at level of cervix	Resected at post-pelvic insertion

Source: Adapted from Hoskins WJ, Perez CA, Young RC, ed. Principles and practice of gynecologic oncology, 2nd ed. Philadelphia: Lippincott-Raven, 1996:808.

undergoes a radical hysterectomy with bilateral pelvic and para-aortic lymphadenectomy without incidence. Her final pathology reveals a cancer limited to the anterior cervix with negative surgical margins and negative lymph nodes.

Survival in cervical cancer is most dependent on the stage of the cancer and the presence of lymphatic spread. For patients with early-stage disease who experience a recurrence after surgery, salvage therapy may involve radiation. For some women who experience a recurrence after undergoing radi-

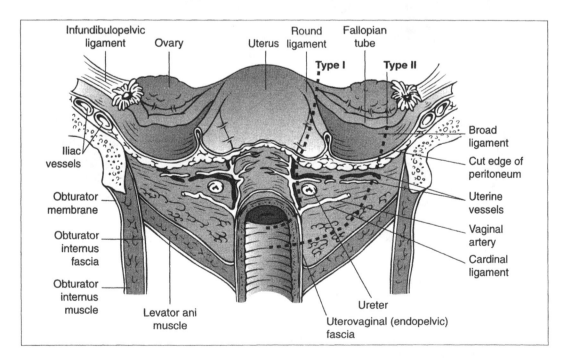

Figure 50.5   Two types of hysterectomies. Type I (simple hysterectomy) removes only the uterus and cervix. Type III (radical hysterectomy) removes the Cardinal ligament and the upper portion of the vagina and is performed for early-stage cervical cancer.

Source: Danforth's obstetrics and gynecology, 7th ed. Philadelphia: J. B. Lippincott, 1994:4.

ation therapy, salvage therapy with ultra-radical surgery may be an option. Chemotherapy for cervical cancer is generally a palliative treatment; cures with this modality occur very rarely.

SUMMARY

Cervical cancer represents a success story in terms of cancer screening, thanks to the effectiveness of the Pap smear. Nevertheless, despite the availability of this valuable diagnostic tool, many woman fail to seek out the appropriate screening. Rarely, the smear may fail to detect an existing lesion. It remains imperative to biopsy lesions when they are present. The majority of preinvasive lesions can be managed safely in the physician's office with outpatient procedures. Invasive carcinoma of the cervix should be referred to the specialist in gynecologic oncology.

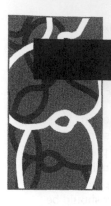

CHAPTER 51

Uterine Leiomyoma

Ronald K. Potkul

The most common gynecologic neoplasm is the uterine leiomyoma, more commonly known as a uterine myoma. Such neoplasms are also known as fibroid tumors, although this term is a misnomer. Although they sometimes exhibit fibrous degeneration, these tumors are not composed of fibrous tissue.

Approximately 25% of all Caucasian women and 50% of all African American women will develop uterine leiomyomas during their reproductive life. The leiomyoma may cause symptoms such as bleeding, pain, and pelvic pressure, or it may remain asymptomatic. It is important to distinguish between this benign entity and other pelvic masses that require more urgent intervention.

HISTORY AND PHYSICAL EXAMINATION

Despite sometimes being extremely large, the majority of uterine leiomyomas remain asymptomatic. This silent nature probably reflects the slow growth associated with most of these tumors, which allows the body to become accustomed to them. Nevertheless, one of every three women with uterine leiomyomata will eventually experience some form of pelvic pain. This pain often takes the form of dysmenorrhea (painful menses), which is postulated to occur secondary to the increased prostaglandin release by the leiomyoma. More acute, severe pain can be experienced with degeneration of leiomyoma. The extreme case of red carneous infarction occurs during pregnancy in approximately 5% to 10% of all gravida women with leiomyomas.

Approximately one in three women will experience abnormal bleeding with leiomyomas. The most common symptom is menorrhagia (heavy menses), although intermenstrual spotting may occur as well. Because leiomyomas can grow slowly, the patient may become accustomed to the heavier flow. For this reason, it is important to quantify the amount of bleeding she is experiencing by obtaining a good menstrual history including number of days of bleeding, number of sanitary pads/tampons per day, and other measurements.

A patient may also complain of pregnancy-like pressure symptoms secondary to the larger uterine mass displacing other pelvic organs. For example, she may report an increased abdominal girth in the lower abdomen. She may complain of urinary frequency and urgency or, less likely, rectal pressure. Other important details in a good history would include the interval since the patient's last gynecologic examination and the findings at that examination. A physician needs to be more concerned about the patient whose last gynecologic examination was normal but now has a larger pelvic mass; this finding suggests that the mass is not a benign uterine leiomyomata, but rather a uterine or ovarian malignancy.

Other important details to elicit from the patient are history of oral contraceptive or post-menopausal estrogen use. The growth of myomas can be stimulated by estrogen.

CLINICAL CORRELATION

D. S. is a 41-year-old, African American female, G2P2, who presents with a chief complaint of heavy menstrual bleeding. Her last menstrual period was two weeks ago. She indicates that she has been bleeding for seven days and used a box of pads for the first two to three days of her menses. In the past, her periods would last four to five days. They have always been regular, and she denies any intramenstrual or postcoital bleeding. D. S. reports mild dysmenorrhea, which has increased over the last three to four years; she takes ibuprofen on an as-needed basis to counter this problem. She complains of urinary urgency not associated with dysuria. D. S. has been taking oral contraceptive pills for approximately one year. She does recall being told by a gynecologist approximately five years ago that her uterus had some small fibroids. Her review of systems, past medical, surgical, social, and family history are unremarkable.

The physical examination will be directed toward the abdomen and pelvis. The abdominal examination should determine whether ascites are present. The diagnosis of leiomyoma is usually confirmed by finding an enlarged, firm, regular uterus on bimanual examination. It is important to characterize the mass in respect to size, shape, mobility, and contour. The discrimination between a large leiomyoma and a large ovarian tumor may prove difficult, however. If pregnancy has been excluded, sometimes placing a metal sound into the uterine cavity will help distinguish a large uterus from a large ovarian mass. The mobility of the pelvic mass and the ability of the mass to move either independently or with the uterus may be helpful diagnostically. A rectal examination should always be part of a pelvic examination that seeks to evaluate nodularity in the cul-de-sac as a possible sign of a malignant process.

CLINICAL CORRELATION

Upon completion of the history, a physical examination is performed on D. S. With a few exceptions, her examination is normal. Her abdomen was soft and non-tender, with a solid mass being palpated almost to the umbilicus. No fluid wave in the abdomen can be appreciated. The pelvic examination reveals normal external genitalia. Her vagina is pink without any lesions. The cervix is somewhat difficult to assess secondary to its very anterior location. The uterus appears to be irregularly enlarged, reaching approximately 12 cm in size, but it is freely mobile. The adnexae cannot be reviewed because of the large, central mass. The rectal examination is confirmatory and the stool guaiac is negative for occult blood.

DIFFERENTIAL DIAGNOSIS

Although uterine leiomyomata are the most common gynecologic neoplasms, other conditions needed to be excluded during the differential diagnosis (Table 51.1). In a reproductive-age patient, pregnancy is the most common cause of a pelvic mass and must always be excluded. Ovarian malignancies that require immediate surgical attention also must be ruled out. In addition, the physician must be aware of nongynecologic conditions associated with the gastrointestinal or urinary tract that can present as pelvic masses.

MANAGEMENT AND TREATMENT

Although the majority of leiomyomas may be diagnosed by pelvic examination, difficult cases will benefit from ultrasound examination. Leiomyomas have characteristic findings on ultrasound that can prove helpful in confirming a uterine origin for the mass (Figure 51.1). The use of computed tomography (CT)

Table 51.1   Differential Diagnosis of Uterine Mass

Uterine Origin
- Pregnancy

  Intrauterine

  Ectopic (cornual pregnancy)
- Leiomyoma
- Uterine carcinoma
- Uterine sarcoma

  Leiomyosarcoma

  Mixed malignant mesodermal tumor

  Endometrial stromal sarcoma

Adnexal Origin
- Fallopian tube

  Hydrosalpinx

  Carcinoma
- Ovarian

  Ovarian torsion

  Tubo-ovarian abscess

  Ectopic gestation (tubal pregnancy, ovarian pregnancy)

  Functional cyst (follicle, corpus luteum)

  Neoplasm (see Chapter 54)

    Benign

    Borderline

    Malignant
- Para-tubal cyst or neoplasm

Nongynecologic
- Gastrointestinal

  Abscess

    Appendix

    Diverticular

  Malignancy

    Colon

    Small intestine

    Mesentary

  Inflammatory

    Crohn's disease
- Genitourinary

  Distended bladder

  Bladder tumor

  Ureteral tumor

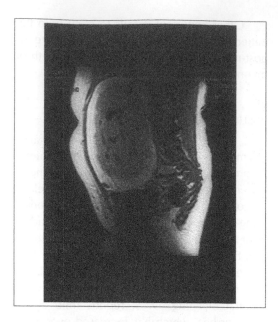

Figure 51.1   MRI demonstrating a large, myomatous uterus

and magnetic resonance imaging (MRI) may help in differentiating a benign uterine leiomyoma from a malignant uterine sarcoma. Likewise, MRI can be particularly useful in evaluating the pregnant patient because it does not use ionizing radiation.

The management of patients with small asymptomatic leiomyomas is conservative, because they invariably are benign. It is appropriate to reexamine the patients in approximately six months to assess the rate of growth. Rapidly enlarging leiomyomas in premenopausal women are usually removed, even though their malignant potential is low. Patients on oral contraceptive pills should consider stopping the medications because they may stimulate growth. A leiomyoma in a post-menopausal woman that is increasing in size needs surgical exploration to rule out a leiomyosarcoma, as benign leiomyomas usually decrease in size in conjunction with decreasing estrogen levels during the menopause.

Patients with abnormal bleeding should be investigated to rule out concurrent pathology such as endometrial hyperplasia or carcinoma. This exclusion is usually accomplished by an office endometrial biopsy. The surgical approach of hysterectomy versus myomectomy is usually determined by the patient's desire for future childbearing. The indications for myomectomy include symptomatic vaginal bleeding, pelvic pressure symptoms, pelvic pain, recurrent spontaneous abortions, and otherwise unexplained infertility. The contraindication to a myomectomy is malignancy. The value of a myomectomy in the woman who has completed childbearing is questionable. In addition, the patient must be counseled that myomectomies are associated with a 25% risk of recurrent leiomyomas. When a myomectomy is performed, particularly for the maintenance of fertility, it should be noted whether entry is made into the endometrial cavity. Depending on the extent of dissection and location of the myomectomy, the physician may choose to deliver the woman only by cesarean delivery should she become pregnant, as significant injury to the uterine muscle may predispose her to uterine rupture during labor. The indications for hysterectomy are essentially the same as those for myomectomy; hysterectomy is also the treatment of choice for presumed leiomyosarcoma.

Small leiomyomas that grow into the endometrial cavity may occasionally be managed by a hysteroscopic technique, wherein an instrument is introduced through the cervix into the endometrial cavity. The myoma is then resected under direct visualization (Figure 51.2).

Leiomyomas may be treated medically with GnRH analogues that place the patient in a menopausal state. This therapy may decrease the size of the leiomyoma by 40% to 90% in a significant number of patients. Unfortunately, with the termination of the therapy, the leiomyomas usually regrow to their pretreatment size within six months. Preoperative GnRH agonist therapy may curtail the blood loss at the time of myomectomy or hysterectomy and may decrease the size of a leiomyoma to the extent that vaginal hysterectomy becomes an option. In addition, GnRH agonists may help in stopping bleeding during the preoperative period, permitting surgery to proceed with less likelihood of transfusion (Figure 51.3).

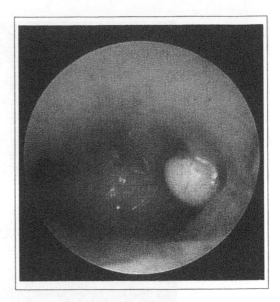

Figure 51.2 Hysteroscopy demonstrating a small myoma into the cavity of the endometrium

CLINICAL CORRELATION

After D. S. and her physician discuss the differential diagnosis of the presumed leiomyoma, a pelvic ultrasound is obtained that reveals an irregular, enlarged uterine mass with normal-appearing ovaries bilaterally. The patient desires no further childbearing and a decision is made to undertake a hysterectomy rather than a myomectomy. Because of D. S.'s increased parity and the mobility of her uterus, she is treated with four months of a GnRH agonist, which brings about a reduction of the uterine size to approximately an eight weeks gestation. She then undergoes an uneventful transvaginal hysterectomy. The ovaries are visualized and appear normal.

FOLLOW-UP

If a myomectomy is chosen, the patient needs to be followed at intervals to evaluate the recurrence of her leiomyomas. After hysterectomy, patients still need interval evaluation for cytology of the vagina and manual examination of the ovaries.

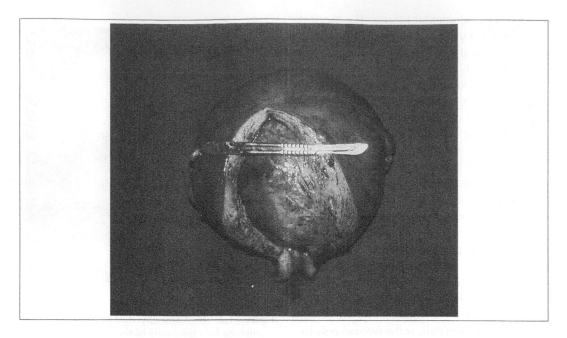

Figure 51.3   Hysterectomy specimen demonstrating a large myoma

SUMMARY

Uterine leiomyomas are the most common gynecologic neoplasms. It is important to differentiate them from other conditions that require immediate attention. Surgical treatment—either myomectomy or hysterectomy—is usually based on the patient's symptoms and takes into account her desires regarding future fertility.

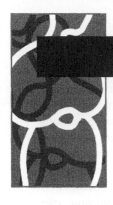

CHAPTER 52

Malignant Disorders of the Uterus

Kevin R. Brader

Malignancy may arise from any of the histologic components of the uterine corpus, including the epithelial lining or endometrium, the supportive or stromal cells, the vascular/lymphatic channels, and the smooth muscle. The latter three forms are classified as sarcomas, because they arise from cells of mesodermal origin. Malignancy arising from the epithelial lining or endometrium—known as a carcinoma—represents the overwhelming majority of uterine malignancies.

Uterine sarcomas are rare, accounting for only 3% of all malignancies of the uterine corpus. They are managed similarly to endometrial carcinoma, although their overall prognosis is much worse on a stage-for-stage basis. Unlike with carcinomas of the endometrium, no clear-cut risk factors for uterine sarcomas have been identified. Because of the rarity of these malignancies, this chapter will focus on carcinoma of the endometrium.

Carcinoma of the endometrium (endometrial cancer) is the most common gynecologic malignancy in the United States and the fourth most common malignancy among women. An estimated 36,000 new cases of endometrial cancer were diagnosed in the United States in 1999, with approximately 6300 patients dying of this disease. Endometrial cancer arises from the endometrial glands and follows a characteristic pattern of spread: invasion of the underlying myometrium, lymphatic/vascular invasion, regional pelvic organ and lymph node metastases, and distant metastases. This type of cancer causes abnormal vaginal bleeding early in its course, resulting in 70% of cases being diagnosed when the tumor is at Stage I (confined to the uterus). Because of this early diagnosis, the five-year survival for all stages of endometrial cancer is 80%. Certain patients are at especially high risk for developing carcinoma of the endometrium—patients with an exposure to high levels of either endogenous or exogenous, unopposed (by progestins) estrogen.

Central to the early diagnosis and appropriate treatment of the patient with endometrial cancer is an understanding of the disease process and the timely evaluation of patients with abnormal uterine bleeding.

CLINICAL CORRELATION

J. K. is a 53-year-old, gravida 0, obese, white female whose last menstrual period was approximately three years ago. She presents to her family practitioner complaining of uterine bleeding similar to a period. The patient reports that her last pelvic examination was approximately eight years ago. Her menstrual history is notable for menarche at age 14, with a history of irregular, sometimes heavy bleeding throughout her premenopausal life. She had attempted to conceive at an earlier point in her life but was unsuccessful. J. K. has no history of prior oral contraceptive use or hormone therapy. She has not been sexually active for nearly 25 years.

She notes that her periods ceased at approximately age 50, and she has had no uterine bleeding until the recent episode. She denies hot flashes or any other menopausal symptoms. Her only medical problem is chronic hypertension, for which she is takes an ACE inhibitor. She has never used tobacco or alcohol.

RISK FACTORS FOR CARCINOMA OF THE ENDOMETRIUM

As noted earlier, the most important risk factor for endometrial cancer is a prolonged exposure to unopposed estrogen (Table 52.1). Estrogen induces proliferation of the endometrium, which is a normal part of the proliferative phase of the menstrual cycle. In a patient with normal ovulatory function, ovulation results in the formation of the corpus luteum, which produces progesterone. Progesterone downregulates both estrogen and progesterone receptors and antagonizes the proliferative effect of estrogen. Cyclic exposure of the endome-trium to estrogen and progesterone results in regular sloughing of the endometrium or menses. Without either cyclic exposure to progesterone (as occurs in the normal menstrual cycle or with oral contraceptive use) or continuous exposure to a progestin (as occurs with most forms of combination hormone replacement therapy), estrogen promotes the unopposed proliferation of the endometrium. Endometrial hyperplasia results. Continued exposure can result in hyperplasia with cellular atypia (a precursor lesion of endometrial cancer), ultimately leading to invasive cancer.

Several conditions can result in high levels of unopposed estrogen, including persistent anovulatory states, obesity (both of which result in increased levels of endogenous estrogen), nulliparity, late menopause, estrogen-secreting tumors, and estrogen replacement therapy without progestins. Conditions that reduce estrogen exposure appear to be protective, including oral contraceptive use (which suppresses endogenous estrogen production and downregulates endometrial estrogen receptors), smoking, multiparity, and early menopause. Other, less well-understood risk factors for endometrial cancer include diabetes mellitus and hypertension. A small percentage of women with endometrial cancer do not have high estrogen levels, so uterine bleeding in a post-menopausal patient with no risk factors should not be ignored.

Although endometrial cancer is associated with particular molecular abnormalities (for example, *k-ras* mutations) in some patients, the influence of these factors on the pathogenesis of this disease is unknown. Some women appear to have a genetic predisposition toward endometrial cancer, though these patients represent only a small fraction of those who ultimately develop this disease. This condition has been identified as a component of some family cancer syndromes, and women with a history of breast, colon, or ovarian cancer are at increased risk for developing endometrial cancer.

Table 52.1 Risk Factors for Endometrial Cancer

FACTOR	RELATIVE RISK
Overweight (lb)	1.9–11
20–50	3
>50	9
Parous vs nulliparous	0.1–0.9
Late menopause (>52 years)	1.7–2.4
Diabetes	1.3–2.7
Radiation therapy	8.0
Exogenous estrogen use	1.6–12.0
Oral contraceptive use	
Sequential	0.9–7.3
Combined	0.1–1.0
Hypertension	1.2–2.1

Source: Adapted from Morrow CP. Synopsis of gynecologic oncology, 5th ed. Philadelphia: Churchill Livingstone, 1998.

SYMPTOMS

Endometrial cancer is characterized by one of the most reliable, early symptoms of any malignancy: abnormal uterine bleeding. This symptom may take the form of post-menopausal bleeding or abnormal premenopausal bleeding. Any post-menopausal patient who reports uterine bleeding—no matter how small the amount—must be evaluated. This evaluation should take the form of an office endometrial biopsy and endocervical curettage (ECC). If this procedure cannot be performed in the office or insufficient tissue is obtained, a fractional dilation and curettage (D&C) should be carried out in the operating room. It should be noted that, although almost all post-menopausal patients with endometrial cancer have bleeding, the majority of post-menopausal patients with bleeding will not have cancer. Approximately one-third will have bleeding from endometrial atrophy, and another one-third will have bleeding caused by a breakdown of a disordered, nonmalignant or hyperplastic, proliferative endometrium. Only 15% of post-menopausal bleeding results from endometrial cancer.

The premenopausal patient with endometrial cancer may be more difficult to identify. These patients typically have intermenstrual bleeding (metrorrhagia) or increasingly heavy periods (menorrhagia). The diagnosis is often delayed because these symptoms are attributed to "hormonal imbalances" or perimenopausal menstrual abnormalities. Given the ease of performing an endometrial biopsy, a high index of suspicion for endometrial cancer should be maintained for these patients. When the etiology is in doubt, a biopsy should be performed.

CLINICAL CORRELATION

Upon physical examination, J. K.'s blood pressure is 150/95. Her weight is 185 lb. Her general physical examination is unremarkable. On the pelvic examination, no blood is found in her vaginal vault. A Pap smear is performed. On the bimanual examination, her uterus is slightly enlarged and no adnexal masses are palpated, although her examination is difficult due to body habitus. The family practitioner is suspicious for endometrial cancer and refers the patient to a gynecologist, who performs an endometrial biopsy and ECC. A large amount of heterogeneous tissue is obtained during the endometrial biopsy. A

pathologic review of the biopsy demonstrates the presence of an endometrioid adenocarcinoma, grade 2, and a negative ECC. When the Pap smear is reviewed, abnormal glandular cells are identified.

PHYSICAL FINDINGS AND DIAGNOSIS

In general, the patient with endometrial cancer will have no definite physical findings. The general examination may reveal obesity and an elevated blood pressure. The cervix will usually appear normal, whereas the uterus will be of normal size or slightly enlarged. An adnexal mass may be identified if the cancer has spread to the adnexa. Advanced-stage disease may be diagnosed by the presence of an abdominal mass, ascites, or enlarged inguinal lymph nodes.

The key to making the diagnosis is the endometrial biopsy. Although the Pap smear may be abnormal, it is not a reliable finding in endometrial cancer. Only 50% of patients with endometrial cancer will have malignant cells on Pap smear. An office endometrial biopsy, such as that using a Vabra or pipelle (in which a small tube is placed into the cavity and suction applied to remove endometrial tissue), should be performed in any patient suspected of having endometrial cancer. These biopsy procedures are generally well tolerated, accurate, and technically easy to perform. An endocervical curettage should also be undertaken, either to rule out an endocervical cancer or to assess the cervix for spread of cancer from the endometrium. Occasionally, the cervical os will be too stenotic to allow a biopsy to be performed in the office, or the patient will be unable to tolerate the procedure. In such cases, the patient should be taken to the operating room for a fractional dilation and curettage (ECC, uterine sound, and D&C).

Alternatively, ultrasound can be used to assess the endometrial thickness. Although not diagnostic, endometrial cancer is highly unlikely in a patient with a thin endometrial thickness (less than 5 mm). On the other hand, a thickened endometrium (10 mm or greater)

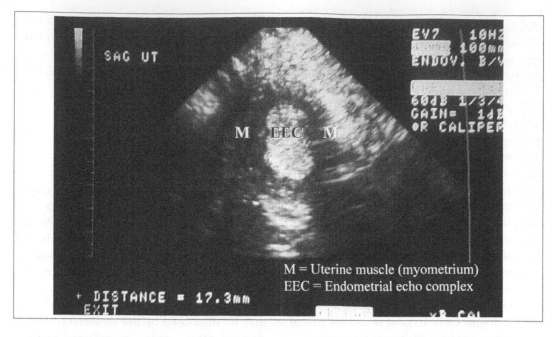

SAG UT

M   EEC   M

M = Uterine muscle (myometrium)
EEC = Endometrial echo complex

DISTANCE = 17.3mm

Figure 52.1   Ultrasound of the uterus demonstrating the myometrium (M) and endometrial echo complex (EEC). In this patient, the endometrium is abnormally thick—17.3 mm. She presented with postmenopausal bleeding.

may be seen in benign or malignant proliferations and is thus not helpful in making the diagnosis (Figure 52.1). For this reason, ultrasound should be reserved for patients who cannot undergo an office biopsy and have medical contraindications to anesthesia and a D&C. The diagnosis can be made or ruled out only by establishing a tissue diagnosis.

STAGING AND TREATMENT

Staging is the process by which a malignancy is categorized based upon its degree of spread. This categorization should be representative of the underlying disease process and have application in the treatment and diagnosis of patients with the malignancy.

Carcinoma of the endometrium was initially a clinically staged disease, which means that a stage was assigned based upon physical findings and diagnostic tests. Because the primary treatment of endometrial cancer is surgery (as described later in this chapter), evaluation of surgical specimens in endometrial cancer showed that the clinical staging system markedly understaged patients. In 1988, the International Federation of Gynecologists and Ob-

stetricians (FIGO) adopted a surgically based staging system (Table 52.2). Simplistically, this system uses the following definitions:

- Stage I disease is confined to the uterus.
- Stage II disease has spread into the cervix.
- Stage III disease has spread to other pelvic organs, to regional lymph nodes, or into the peritoneal cavity.
- Stage IV disease has directly invaded adjacent structures or spread to distant sites.

The only diagnostic test required prior to surgical staging is usually the chest X ray, which can be used to identify the presence of the rare lung metastases. A CT scan or MRI is seldom indicated, and these measures merely delay the surgical staging and increase medical costs.

CLINICAL CORRELATION

J. K. is diagnosed with endometrial cancer and undergoes a preoperative chest X ray, which is normal. As she has never received a mammogram, she undergoes this screening test as well; it is also normal.

J. K. is taken to the operating room,

Table 52.2 FIGO Surgical Staging of Endometrial Carcinoma (1988)

STAGES		EXTENSION OF DISEASE
Ia	G123	Tumor limited to endometrium
Ib	G123	Invasion of <0.5 myometrium
Ic	G123	Invasion of >0.5 myometrium
IIa	G123	Endocervical glandular involvement only
IIb	G123	Cervical stromal invasion
IIIa	G123	Tumor invades serosa and/or positive peritoneal cytology
IIIb	G123	Vaginal metastases
IIIc	G123	Metastases to pelvic and/or paraaortic lymph nodes
IVa	G123	Tumor invasion of bladder and/or bowel mucosa
IVb	G123	Distant metastases including intra-abdominal and/or inguinal lymph nodes

Source: Reproduced with permission from American College of Obstetricians and Gynecologists. Prolog: gynecologic oncology and surgery, 3rd ed. Washington, DC, 1996:182.

where an examination under anesthesia demonstrates a normal cervix and slightly enlarged uterus. Her abdomen is opened through a vertical midline incision, washings from the pelvis are taken, and the abdomen and pelvis are explored. Her uterus and ovaries appear normal, and her lymph nodes are not palpably enlarged. A total abdominal hysterectomy and bilateral salpingo-oophorectomy are performed, and the specimen is sent to pathology for frozen section analysis. A grade 2 cancer with 70% myometrial invasion is identified. The tumor fills the endometrial cavity but has not invaded the cervix. A bilateral pelvic and para-aortic lymph node sampling, and omental biopsy are performed.

J. K. has an unremarkable postoperative course and is discharged from the hospital on post-operative day 4. Her final pathology demonstrates an endometri-oid adenocarcinoma, FIGO grade 2, with 70% myometrial invasion, negative lymph nodes, washings, and biopsies. The tumor is estrogen- and progesterone-receptor-positive. Thus J. K. has a Stage Ib, grade 2, endometrioid adenocarcinoma of the endometrium.

PROGNOSIS AND ADJUVANT TREATMENT

The surgical stage of endometrial cancer is the most important prognostic factor, with surgical Stage I patients having a five-year survival rate of more than 90%. Other important considerations include the tumor grade, histologic cell type, tumor size, patient age, and tumor receptor status. Most endometrial cancers display a histology similar to the normal endometrial cell type (endometrioid). Less frequently encountered cell types—all of which are associated with a worse prognosis—are clear cell, papillary serous, and adenosquamous. A mucinous cell type, which has a histologic appearance similar to that of endocervical cells, has a prognosis similar to that of endometrioid.

Grading refers to the degree of differentiation of the tumor, with a lower grade showing a pattern more closely resembling the normal tissue. Endometrial cancer is graded based on its architectural appearance, depending upon the amount of glandular components, with less glandular areas and more solid areas representing higher-grade (more aggressive) tumors.

Depending on the patient's particular prognostic factors, additional or adjuvant treatment is often offered. Generally, patients with tumors that are confined to the endometrium or that are confined to the inner half of the myometrium are cured with no further treatment. Patients with deep myometrial invasion, a high-grade, more aggressive cell type, or any spread beyond the uterus (Stage II or higher) should receive additional treatment. Classically, this treatment plan involves pelvic radiation therapy, although chemotherapy and hormonal therapy are options as well. Radiation therapy tends to decrease the cancer's recurrence in the pelvis without improving overall survival. The benefit of chemotherapy remains unproved. Patients with widespread disease that is receptor-positive often achieve tumor regression with progestin therapy, although patients with Stage IVb disease are essentially incurable with any form of therapy.

CLINICAL CORRELATION

J. K. is referred to a radiation oncologist, who recommends whole pelvic radiation therapy and local irradiation to the vaginal cuff. In the ensuing years, she is followed at regular intervals. Three years after completing therapy, J. K. is without evidence of disease.

MESENCHYMAL TUMORS OF THE UTERUS

Carcinosarcomas and other sarcomas of the uterus account for less than 5% of all uterine corpus cancers. These rare tumors are very aggressive and recurrence—even for early-stage disease—is the rule. The malignant mixed mesodermal tumor (MMMT) or carcinosarcoma is the most common of these tumors, followed by leiomyosarcoma and (quite rare) endometrial stromal sarcoma. The tumors tend to occur in post-menopausal women, with the presenting signs typically being either vaginal bleeding or a rapidly enlarging uterus. Such cancers may develop more frequently in the patient with a history of pelvic radiation. No other clear etiologic factors have been identified. In the United States, uterine sarcomas are more common in African American women than in Caucasian women.

Standard therapy for sarcomas of the uterus consists of total abdominal hysterectomy, bilateral salpingo-oophorectomy, and pelvic washing; additional pathologic specimens, including lymph nodes, are then taken as determined by the extent of disease. These tumors tend to metastasize by both hematogenous and lymphatic spread. Because of this pattern of spread, patients are prone to recurrence with distant metastases, often located outside of the abdominal cavity. Although some physicians advocate the use of radiation in the adjuvant setting to decrease local recurrence, the overall impact of this approach on survival has not been demonstrated. Chemotherapy for these tumors has poor results. Hormonal therapy may play an important role in controlling low-grade, endometrial stromal sarcomas, as these tumors tend to have high estrogen and progesterone receptor content.

SUMMARY

Although carcinoma of the endometrium is relatively prevalent, its reliable early symptom of post-menopausal or abnormal premenopausal bleeding makes its early diagnosis possible. Thanks to this early diagnosis, overall mortality from endometrial cancer is low. Key to the management of this malignancy is the prompt and appropriate evaluation of bleeding abnormalities. Additionally, the avoidance of iatrogenic, unopposed estrogen in the post-menopausal patient with an intact uterus can significantly reduce a woman's risk of developing this disease.

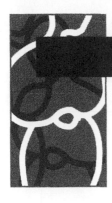

CHAPTER 53

Evaluation of the Pelvic Mass

Alexander F. Burnett

The presentation of a pelvic mass is extremely variable. Benign processes may cause torsion or rupture of an ovary with acute symptoms. In contrast, ovarian cancer may be insidious in onset and produce symptoms only late in the course of the disease. A careful evaluation, including a physical examination, radiologic studies, and serum tumor markers, is critical to attempt to detect ovarian pathology early and to discern benign conditions that may not require surgery.

CLINICAL CORRELATION

B. H. is a 42-year-old, gravida 4, para 4, female whose last menstrual period was two weeks ago. When she presents for her annual physical examination, she denies any complaints with the exception of a frequent "pressure" feeling in her lower pelvis and occasional constipation. Her periods have been regular, and she and her partner use condoms for contraception. Her past medical history is otherwise negative. After completing a speculum examination and Pap smear of the cervix, bimanual and rectovaginal examinations reveal a fixed, 8 cm mass in the posterior cul-de-sac. This mass is nontender, firm, and slightly nodular. There is no fluid wave or peripheral lymphadenopathy detectable on examination.

ETIOLOGY

Myriad etiologies of adnexal masses are possible (Table 53.1). The approach to the patient with an adnexal mass is determined in part by her characteristics. Among of the most important determinants in determining the etiology of a mass is the patient's age. Most tumors that occur in the ovaries of young, reproductive-age women are benign, with a high percentage being functional (that is, follicular cysts). As women approach menopause, the incidence of malignancy rises, with the median age of ovarian cancer in the United States being 52 years. The prepubertal girl with an adnexal mass also raises suspicion for a malignancy. Fortunately, masses in this age group are rare.

In all reproductive-age women, the suspicion of pregnancy should always be addressed. Even with seemingly regular menses and reliable contraception, a sexually active woman may become pregnant. A pelvic mass may be physiologically related to a pregnancy (corpus luteum of pregnancy) or may represent an ectopic pregnancy.

A patient may present with a surgical abdomen from a malignant or benign ovarian condition. The patient with rebound tenderness and hemodynamic instability requires exploration without further delay as part of the work-up. Any ovarian tumor may cause torsion of the adnexal vascular pedicle, thereby resulting in an acute abdomen (Table 53.2). Rupture of adnexal masses may produce hemo-

Table 53.1   Differential Diagnosis of Pelvic Mass

GYNECOLOGIC	NONGYNECOLOGIC

Functional
Follicular cyst
Corpus luteum cyst
Polycystic ovary
Pregnancy luteoma
Ovarian edema
Ovarian hyperstimulation

Infectious
Tubo-ovarian abscess

Vascular
Ovarian torsion

Endometriosis
Endometrioma

Epithelial Tumors
Serous
Mucinous
Endometrioid
Clear cell
Brenner
Mixed
Undifferentiated

1. Benign
2. Borderline (carcinoma of low malignant potential)
3. Malignant

Sex Cord–Stromal Tumors
Granulosa cell tumors
Sertoli-Leydig tumors

Germ Cell Tumors
Dysgerminoma
Endodermal sinus tumor
Embryonal carcinoma
Polyembryoma
Choriocarcinoma
Teratomas
   Immature (malignant)
   Mature
   Highly specialized
Mixed forms
Gonadoblastoma

Malignant
Colon
Appendix
Small bowel
Mesothelial tumor
Retroperitoneal tumor
Lymphoma
Metastatic

Benign
Diverticular abscess
Appendiceal abscess
Crohn's disease
Pelvic kidney

Table 53.2 Operative Findings with Adnexal Torsion

DIAGNOSIS	PERCENTAGE
Benign Neoplasm	
Dermoid	29.7
Serous tumor	9.4
Mucinous tumor	4.7
Fibroma-thecoma	3.1
Other	1.6
Serous Carcinoma	1.6
Cyst Non-neoplastic	
Para-ovarian	18.7
Corpus luteum	5.5
Serous cyst	4.7
Endometrioma	1.6
Normal Adnexa	21.1

peritoneum, chemical peritonitis, or spillage of pyogenic material from a tubo-ovarian abscess; each of these conditions has a high potential for morbidity or mortality (Figure 53.1).

Not infrequently, patients may have vague complaints when an adnexal mass is present. Detailed questioning about symptoms such as pain or pressure in the pelvis should focus on the timing of the discomfort in the menstrual cycle, particular movements or positions that elicit the most discomfort, the relationship of the pain to intercourse, and the intermittent or constant nature of the pain. Intermittent adnexal pain may reflect adnexal torsion, with off-and-on twisting of the vascular pedicle. Constitutional symptoms such as nausea or vomiting, changes in weight, changes in abdominal girth, and changes in bowel or bladder habits should be investigated in detail, as they may raise the suspicion for a malignancy.

Tumors that are found in women with pain at the time of menses may represent endometriosis, a benign condition where endometrial tissue is found in an ectopic (that is, not in the uterus) location. This tissue will respond to the hormones of the ovarian cycle with progressive proliferation and then sloughing each month. The sloughing material causes bleeding, with the blood collecting as an endometriotic cyst or causing scarring and pain in the location of the endometriosis.

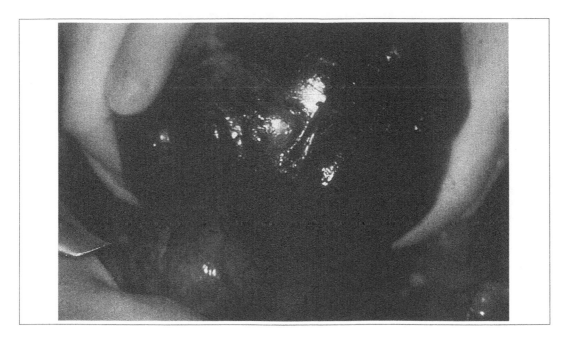

Figure 53.1 Torsion of the adnexa. An ovarian mass has twisted the vascular pedicle to the organ. The patient presented with pain of acute onset and a pelvic mass. Doppler ultrasound failed to show blood flow to the mass preoperatively.

PHYSICAL EXAMINATION

The physical examination begins with a general overview of the patient's health. Is she cachexic? Is there obvious ascites? Is she obese? Examination of the head will note whether hirsutism is present, which is suggestive of a hormonally active tumor. The chest is examined for evidence of tumors in the breasts and adenopathy in the supraclavicular region. The abdominal examination should discern whether a fluid wave is present, the mass is palpable abdominally, and tenderness or rebound is associated with the mass.

After the speculum examination, in which a Pap smear and cultures are taken if appropriate, attention turns to the manual pelvic examination. The bimanual examination notes whether cervical motion tenderness is present, the mass is contiguous with the uterus, and the mass is anterior in the pelvis. The recto-vaginal examination is the most important part of the pelvic examination, because the majority of adnexal pathology will be located in the posterior cul-de-sac. This examination characterizes the size, shape, and smoothness of the mass. Mobility and tenderness are also determined.

Finally, any other nodularity in the pelvis is noted.

The remainder of the physical examination should identify any edema of the lower extremities, which may be suggestive of lymphatic blockage in the pelvis.

RADIOLOGY

Radiologic tests used to evaluate pelvic masses include ultrasound, CT scan, and MRI.

Ultrasound has several advantages in such cases. It is relatively inexpensive and can reliably describe whether the mass is cystic or solid. Any solid component to an adnexal mass should increase the physician's suspicion of malignancy. In addition, ultrasound can identify the presence of fluid (ascites), without the use of ionizing radiation (Figure 53.2). The lack of radiation is particularly attractive whenever there is a question of pregnancy.

CT scan has an advantage in that more abdominal pathology can be detected with a single test. The role of MRI in gynecology has not been completely defined, but one can nevertheless anticipate an increase in the use of this modality in the future.

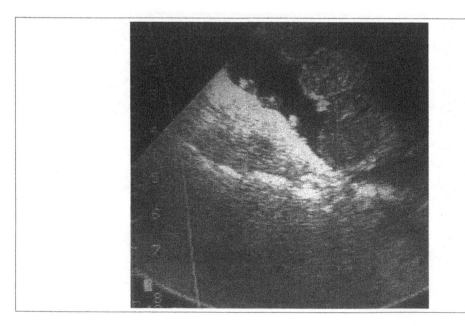

Figure 53.2   Transvaginal ultrasound of an adnexal mass. The mass is thick-walled with cystic regions in the center. Protruding into the cystic areas are papillomas. This finding is highly suggestive of ovarian carcinoma.

HORMONES

Ovarian tumors may be hormonally active. Consequently, where appropriate, symptoms of estrogen or androgen excess should be elicited. Most commonly, hormonally active tumors will be ovarian stromal neoplasms (discussed in greater detail in Chapter 54).

A benign condition that may elevate levels of circulating sex steroids is polycystic ovaries. In this common disorder, the patient is anovulatory and the ovary clonically generates estrogens and androgens. The pituitary fails to respond to the circulating estrogens with appropriate releases of follicle-stimulating hormone (FSH). Instead, FSH is continuously released such that multiple follicles develop without a dominant follicle being extruded each month. Over time, the ovaries may become enlarged with multiple cysts appearing just below the ovarian surface. Patients typically will show signs of androgen excess, such as increased hair with a male pattern distribution, occasional clitoromegaly, occasional acne, and frequent obesity.

One of the most frequently encountered ovarian neoplasms is the mature cystic teratoma, also called the dermoid cyst of the ovary.

These tumors account for 25% of all neoplasms of the ovary and are most frequently found during the reproductive years. They contain elements from all three germ cell layers (ectoderm, endoderm, and mesoderm) (Figure 53.3). Quite often, they contain a sebaceous material capable of causing a chemical peritonitis if the cyst ruptures spontaneously or is ruptured in surgery and the pelvis is not irrigated. Occasionally, mature thyroid tissue may be present in a dermoid cyst. When more than 50% of the tumor is made up of thyroid tissue, it is known as a stroma ovarii. Patients with stroma ovarii may exhibit hyperthyroidism. Malignant degeneration within a mature cystic teratoma is extremely rare, but is usually a squamous carcinoma when it occurs. Bilaterality is observed in approximately 10% to 15% of cases. Treatment with ovarian cystectomy is usually adequate.

TUMOR MARKERS

Several serum tumor markers for adnexal masses have been identified. One of the most frequently obtained markers is CA-125, an antibody for an antigen produced by coelomic epithelium, including epithelial ovarian cells.

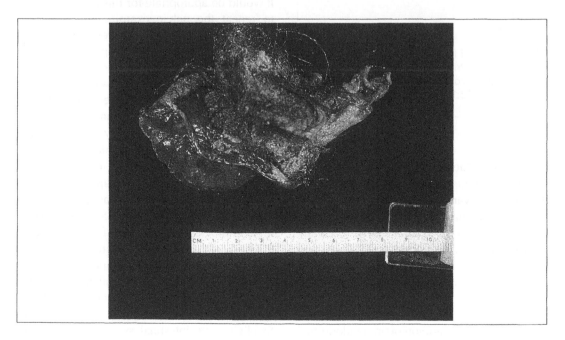

Figure 53.3 Mature cystic teratoma of the ovary (also called a dermoid cyst). Note the hair formation within the tumor.

Table 53.3   Diagnoses Associated with an Elevated CA-125 Level

Gynecologic Tumors

Epithelial ovarian cancer

Dysgerminoma

Sertoli-Leydig cell tumors

Granulosa cell tumors

Fallopian tube cancer

Endometrial cancer

Endocervical cancer

Benign Gynecologic Conditions

Leiomyomata

Endometriosis

Pelvic inflammatory disease

Adenomyosis

Pregnancy

Nongynecologic Tumors

Lung carcinoma

Pancreatic cancer

Colon cancer

Breast cancer

Nongynecologic Conditions

Pancreatitis

Cirrhosis

Laparotomy

Peritonitis

Source: Adapted from Hoskins WJ, Perez CA, Young RC, ed. Principles and practice of gynecologic oncology. Philadelphia: J. P. Lippincott, 1992:140.

The normal value for this antibody is less than 35 U/mL. Because its serum concentration is elevated in a variety of conditions, both benign and malignant (Table 53.3), CA-125 has not been proven to be an effective screening tool for ovarian cancer. If a mass is present and the CA-125 level is elevated, however, the suspicion for ovarian cancer should also be elevated.

Other markers produced by ovarian tumors include alpha-fetoprotein (endodermal sinus tumors), human chorionic gonadotropin (choriocarcinoma), lactate dehydrogenase

(dysgerminoma), and sex hormones (sex cord–stromal tumors). Each of these tests should be ordered only in the appropriate clinical setting.

CLINICAL CORRELATION

B. H. undergoes a pelvic ultrasound that reveals a 10 cm, right adnexal mass that is cystic and solid in consistency. The left adnexae appears sonographically normal. No free fluid is present. The uterus is of normal size without evidence of pathology. A CT scan is not performed. The serum concentration of CA-125 is 95 U/mL.

DIFFERENTIAL DIAGNOSIS

In the preceding case, the solid component to the mass and the elevated CA-125 level are worrisome features. B. H. would be well advised to undergo surgical exploration, with counseling informing her that surgical staging will be necessary if a malignancy is encountered.

In the reproductive-age woman with a simple cyst, particularly if it is less than 5 cm, the suspicion is high for a functional etiology. It would be appropriate for this type of patient to repeat the pelvic examination after one complete menstrual cycle, often while taking oral contraceptive pills to suppress ovulation, to see whether the cyst will resolve on its own. Persistence of even a simple cyst over several menstrual cycles warrants direct examination of that ovary. If the woman has minimal risk factors for ovarian malignancy, then she may be a candidate for initial evaluation via laparoscopy. Benign disease may often be managed completely through this approach.

A patient's differential diagnosis with an adnexal mass must account for nongynecologic etiologies as well. Most frequently, gastrointestinal pathology may mimic an adnexal mass. Diverticular abscess, appendiceal abscess, colon carcinoma, and inflammatory disease of the colon may all present as an adnexal mass. A careful bowel history should be able to elicit some intestinal symptoms, although similar complaints may be due to ovarian pathology. In addition, nongynecologic cancers may metastasize to the ovary, including breast, colon, and stomach cancers.

CLINICAL CORRELATION

B. H. undergoes surgical exploration through a midline incision. She is found to have bilateral endometriomas with extensive pelvic endometriosis. Bilaterally, ovarian cystectomies are performed with repair and preservation of the ovaries. In addition, all gross evidence of endometriosis in the pelvis is fulgurated with electrocautery. Her post-operative course is uneventful.

SUMMARY

Evaluation of a pelvic mass should be carried out in a stepwise fashion to most effectively utilize resources while best managing the patient. The history, physical examination, X-ray studies, and tumor markers will all aid the physician in making a differential diagnosis. Some pelvic masses are functional in nature (that is, related to the normal function of the ovary or ovulation) and can be watched expectantly. Even benign-appearing tumors will require surgical exploration if they persist so as to diagnose and treat neoplasia.

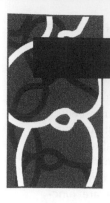

CHAPTER 54

Ovarian Cancer

Alexander F. Burnett

Carcinoma of the ovary will occur in approximately 1 in 70 women in the United States over the course of their lifetime. It is the second most common gynecologic malignancy and the fourth most common cause of cancer mortality in women, ranking behind only lung, breast, and colorectal carcinomas. Because this cancer rarely has symptoms early in its course, more than half of women affected present with stage III or IV disease. Ovarian carcinoma spreads by peritoneal seeding, lymphatic, and hematogenous routes. Symptoms that prompt a woman to seek medical care are generally related to tumor encroachment on the bowel, with subsequent diarrhea, constipation, or abdominal pain, or to an increase in abdominal girth secondary to tumor or ascites.

CLINICAL CORRELATION

B. T. is a 54-year-old, gravida 0, woman who presents to her family doctor complaining of two months of progressive gastric discomfort and a recent increase in her abdominal girth. Her past medical history is significant only for mild hypertension, which does not require medication as yet. B. T. states she is "bloated" and feels full after taking only a few bites of food. Her examination is significant for a fluid wave on abdominal examination, lack of peripheral lymphadenopathy, and a palpable fixed 8 to 10 cm mass on pelvic examination. A CT scan is ordered, as is a consultation with a gynecologic oncologist.

The etiology of ovarian cancer remains unknown. According to one theory, incessant ovulation produces a nidus of reaction on the surface of the ovary, which then triggers the development of a carcinoma. This theory is supported by data that show a decreased incidence of ovarian cancer in women who have used oral contraceptives, and an increased incidence in women who are nulligravida or have an early menarche and late menopause (Table 54.1). Alternatively, gonadotropins have been proposed to play a critical, as yet undefined, role in the etiology of ovarian cancer. In support of this theory, proponents point out that the incidence of ovarian cancer increases with increasing age. There is probably a dietary contribution to the development of ovarian cancer—the disease is most common among women in North America and Europe, where dietary fat intake is highest—although this idea remains controversial. Finally, chronic talc exposure on the perineum has been proposed as an etiology for ovarian cancer, although definitive data are lacking.

Familial ovarian cancer accounts for only a small subset of ovarian cancer patients. Approximately 3% to 5% of ovarian cancer cases are believed to have a familial contribution. There are three recognized familial entities:

Table 54.1   Risk Factors for Ovarian Cancer

RISK FACTOR	RELATIVE RISK
Positive	
Older age	3
North America, Europe	2–5
Nulligravity	2–3
Early menarche, late menopause	1.5–2
Talc exposure	1.5–2
Family history	3–4
Negative	
Oral contraceptive use	0.3–0.5
Hysterectomy	0.5–0.7

Source: Adapted from Hoskins WJ, Perez CA, Young RC, ed. Principles and practice of gynecologic oncology. Philadelphia: J. P. Lippincott, 1992:11.

- Breast–ovary familial cancers
- Lynch II syndrome with ovarian, endometrial, and nonpolyposis colorectal cancers
- Site-specific, familial ovarian cancer syndrome

These syndromes appear to be transmitted in an autosomal dominant manner with variable penetration.

So far, genetic markers associated with breast–ovarian cancer syndromes have been identified on chromosome 17 and chromosome 13; these markers are called BRCA-1 and BRCA-2, respectively. Screening for these markers is currently being performed on high-risk women in a research setting. Genetic counseling must be available to help women decide whether they qualify for testing, what the implications of a positive and negative test are, and what to do once the results of the test are known.

For a woman with one first-degree relative with ovarian cancer, her lifetime risk of developing the disease is estimated to increase from 1.5% to 3%. With two or more first-degree relatives with ovarian cancer, her lifetime risk may increase to 50%. Counseling should be provided to the patient at such a high risk regarding possible prophylactic oophorectomy at the completion of childbearing. In addition, the patient should be informed of the potential protective effect of pregnancy or prolonged oral contraceptive use.

HISTOLOGIC CLASSIFICATION

The ovary produces more varieties of tumors than any other organ (Figure 54.1). The cancers typically are derived from the epithelial cells of the ovary. Among the epithelial tumors, the serous tumors are the most commonly observed, as noted in Table 54.2. The epithelial cancers are usually bilateral and often have reached an advanced stage at the time of diagnosis. They spread by peritoneal seeding, a silent method for disseminating cancer cells. Clear cell and small cell cancers are an exception and probably confer a worse prognosis.

BORDERLINE EPITHELIAL TUMORS

Within the epithelial histologies, each tumor may present as a borderline carcinoma (also called a tumor of low malignant potential). Such tumors may grossly resemble carcinoma, including being widely disseminated over the peritoneal cavity. Nevertheless, they are histologically differentiated by complex branching papillae that are covered with stratified epithelium and a lack of stromal invasion.

The age of diagnosis for borderline tumors is between the ages of diagnosis noted with completely benign cystadenomas and cystadenocarcinomas. Seventy-five percent of such tumors are at stage I at the time of diagnosis. These tumors are treated by surgical removal. Because it is not always necessary to remove an uninvolved ovary or the uterus, occasionally fertility can be preserved. Recurrent or higher-stage borderline tumors are somewhat problematic, however, in that few data indicate that these tumors respond to either chemotherapy or radiation therapy. Occasionally, these tumors may grow and strangulate the intestines, killing the patient in a similar fashion to frank carcinomas.

Another variant of borderline tumors that is particularly difficult to treat is the mucinous

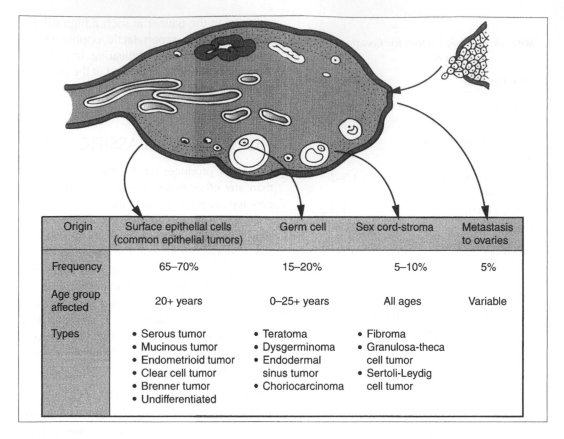

Figure 54.1   Origins of ovarian tumors

Source: Callahan TL, Caughey AB, Heffner LJ. Blueprints in obstetrics and gynecology. Malden, MA: Blackwell Science, 1998:189.

borderline tumor with associated pseudo-myxoma peritonei. In this condition, a viscous jelly collects in the peritoneal cavity and may eventually cause scarring or strangulation of the bowels.

GERM CELL TUMORS

Although germ cell tumors occur less often than borderline epithelial tumors, they are the most frequently encountered tumors in pre-pubertal and young, reproductive-age women (Figure 54.2). Some of these tumors, such as endodermal sinus tumors, may grow extremely rapidly. Prior to the advent of chemotherapy, they were almost universally fatal.

Germ cell tumors may produce a variety of unusual substances that can be measured by serologic tests and the information subse-quently used in their diagnosis and monitor-ing. Endodermal sinus tumors release alpha-fetoprotein into the bloodstream; this marker is monitored during treatment and in post-treat-ment surveillance. Choriocarcinoma of the ovary secretes human chorionic gonadotropin, with the beta subunit (beta-hCG) being moni-tored. Dysgerminomas may be associated with elevated levels of lactate dehydrogenase (LDH), specifically the fast isofraction of LDH (Figure 54.3). Mixed germ cell tumors and em-bryonal carcinomas may have elevated con-centrations of any or all of these markers. Im-mature teratomas are typically characterized by elevated levels of LDH or AFP, as described in Table 54.3.

The majority of germ cell tumors are diag-nosed while they are at an early stage and still limited to a single ovary. Therefore, with no obvious spread of tumor in a young, reproduc-tive-age woman, appropriate surgical staging includes unilateral oophorectomy with uni-

Table 54.2 Frequency of the Major Ovarian Tumors

TYPE	PERCENTAGE OF MALIGNANT OVARIAN TUMORS	PERCENTAGE THAT ARE BILATERAL
Serous	40	—
Benign (60%)	—	25
Borderline (15%)	—	30
Malignant (25%)	—	65
Mucinous	10	—
Benign (80%)	—	5
Borderline (10%)	—	10
Malignant (10%)	—	20
Endometrioid carcinoma	20	40
Undifferentiated carcinoma	10	—
Clear cell carcinoma	6	40
Granuloma cell tumor	5	5
Teratoma	—	—
Benign (96%)	—	15
Malignant (4%)	1	Rare
Metastatic	6	>50
Others	3	—

Source: Reproduced with permission from Robbins S, Cotran R, Kumar V. Pathologic basis of disease. Philadelphia: W.B. Saunders Company, 1991:1159.

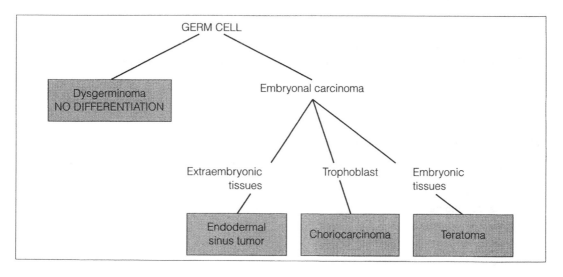

Figure 54.2 Origins of germ cell tumors of the ovary

Source: Callahan TL, Caughey AB, Heffner LJ. Blueprints in obstetrics and gynecology. Malden, MA: Blackwell Science, 1998:190.

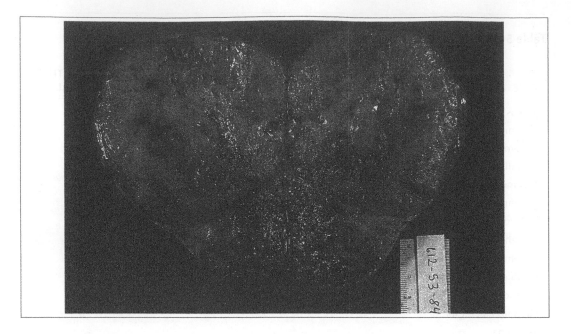

Figure 54.3   Dysgerminoma of the ovary. These tumors are usually solid and have a lobulated, "brain-like" appearance. They may produce high levels of lactate dehydrogenase.

lateral pelvic and para-aortic lymph node sampling, peritoneal washing, and careful examination of the peritoneal surfaces. If the other ovary contains a cyst, this cyst should be removed and the remaining portion of the ovary left intact. Dysgerminoma is the one germ cell tumor with a higher propensity for bilaterality—occurring in approximately 15% of cases. Therefore, if the frozen section is consistent with dysgerminoma, the contralateral ovary must be carefully examined but most often should be allowed to remain in situ.

STROMAL TUMORS

Ovarian stromal tumors are even less common than germ cell tumors. These tumors are composed of hormonally active stromal cells of the ovary. They may present rather dramatically with hirsutism and virilization from androgens, or with symptoms of estrogen excess, including bleeding from endometrial cancer. Any

Table 54.3   Serum Tumor Markers for Germ Cell Neoplasia

TUMOR	hCG	AFP	LDH	CA-125
Mixed germ cell tumor	+	+	+	+
Embryonal carcinoma	+	+	±	+
Endodermal sinus tumor	−	+	±	?
Dysgerminoma	±	−	+	+
Immature teratoma	−	±	±	+
Choriocarcinoma	+	−	±	?

Source: Reproduced with permission from Frederickson H, Wilkins-Haug L. Ob/gyn secrets. Philadelphia: Hanley and Belfus, Inc., 1991:119.

premenopausal woman who develops endometrial cancer should be examined for the possibility of a granulosa cell tumor. This type of tumor typically secretes estrogen, but may also secrete inhibin, leading to elevated values of this protein in the serum. Sertoli-Leydig cell tumors of the ovary are composed of testicular elements and may secrete androgens.

> ### CLINICAL CORRELATION
>
> B. T. undergoes a CT scan of the abdomen and pelvis, which reveals marked ascites, bilateral adnexal masses (each measuring approximately 7 cm and containing both cystic and solid areas), and a tumor cake appearing to involve the omentum over the anterior abdomen. A CA-125 sample is drawn and the concentration of this serum marker is found to 1054 U/mL (normal is less than 35 U/mL). A gynecologic oncologist examines the patient and recommends surgical exploration.

MANAGEMENT

Cancers of the ovary are surgically staged (Table 54.4). The proper staging procedure for an epithelial cancer includes total abdominal hysterectomy, bilateral salpingo-oophorectomy, omentectomy, peritoneal washings for cytology, multiple peritoneal biopsies, and, in selected cases, lymphadenectomy. As previously mentioned, germ cell tumors may be surgically managed more conservatively. The goal of any surgical procedure for carcinoma of the ovary is to remove as much tumor as possible. After tumor-reductive surgery, patients with more than a stage Ia epithelial tumor should receive chemotherapy, most commonly involving a combination of Taxol and a platinum compound. Although ovarian cancers tend to be highly responsive to chemotherapy, the long-term survival rate for advanced disease remains poor (Table 54.5).

Some types of ovarian cancer are associated with endometrial cancer. Stromal tumors

---

Table 54.4 Staging of Ovarian Carcinoma

Stage I. Growth limited to the ovaries

    Ia—one ovary involved

    Ib—both ovaries involved

    Ic—Ia or Ib and ovarian surface tumor, ruptured capsule, malignant ascites, or peritoneal cytology positive for malignant cells

Stage II. Extension of the neoplasm from the ovary to the pelvis

    IIa—extension to the uterus of fallopian tube

    IIb—extension to other pelvic tissues

    IIc—IIa or IIb and ovarian surface tumor, ruptured capsule, malignant ascites, or peritoneal cytology positive for malignant cells

Stage III. Disease extension to the abdominal cavity

    IIIa—abdominal peritoneal surfaces with microscopic metastases

    IIIb—tumor metastases < 2 cm in size

    IIIc—tumor metastases > 2 cm in size or metastatic disease in the pelvic, para-aortic, or inguinal lymph nodes

Stage IV. Distant metastatic disease

    Malignant pleural effusion

    Pulmonary parenchymal metastases

    Liver or splenic parenchymal metastases (not surface implants)

    Metastases to the supraclavicular lymph nodes or skin

Source: Reproduced with permission from American College of Obstetricians and Gynecologists. Prolog: gynecologic oncology and surgery, 3rd ed. Washington, DC, 1996:181.

Table 54.5   Survival in Ovarian Cancer

STAGE	FIVE-YEAR SURVIVAL RATE (%)
I	
a	85.3
b	69.0
c	59.0
II	
a	62.0
b	51.0
c	43.0
III	
a	31.4
b	38.0
c	18.0
IV	8.0

Source: Adapted from Morrow CP, Curtin JP. Synopsis of gynecologic oncology, 5th ed. Philadelphia: Churchill Livingstone, 1998:246.

that produce estrogen and granulosa cell tumors both have a 20% to 50% incidence of concurrent endometrial hyperplasia or carcinoma. As many as one-fourth of all endometrioid carcinomas of the ovary are associated with histologically identical endometrioid carcinomas of the uterus. In this situation, both tumors are often diagnosed at an early stage of development and represent synchronous dual primary sites rather than disease that has metastasized from one site to another.

CLINICAL CORRELATION

During B. T.'s initial surgery, her gynecologic oncologist is able to remove approximately 95% of the cancer. The surgeon performs a total abdominal hysterectomy, bilateral salpingo-oophorectomy, total omentectomy, and partial small bowel resection and reanastamosis to reduce this stage IIIC epithelial ovarian cancer to a residual tumor of less than 2 cm (Figure 54.4). After the surgery, B. T. undergoes six cycles of combination cis-platinum and Taxol chemotherapy over the next 6 months. Her CA-125 serum concentration rapidly falls to a negative level (<35 U/mL) while she is receiving treatment. At the completion of therapy, B. T. refuses a second-look procedure. She continues to do well and remains clinically free of disease.

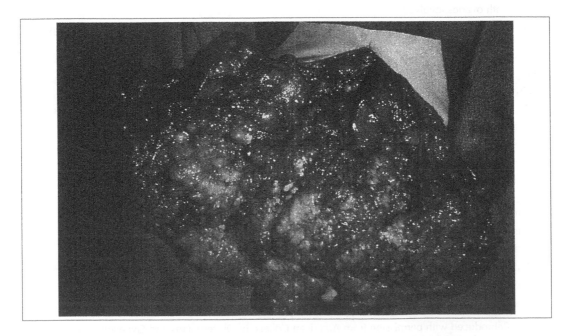

Figure 54.4   A large omentum filled with metastatic ovarian carcinoma—the so-called omental cake. This patient has at least a stage IIIc cancer, based on the disease observed in the upper abdomen.

Chemotherapy is generally given via an intravenous or intraperitoneal route in ovarian cancer. A few types of chemotherapy are occasionally given by mouth. Once initial therapy is completed, some patients opt for a second-look procedure to document pathologically that the cancer is gone. This procedure involves careful inspection of all surfaces of the peritoneal cavity, with selective biopsies being performed on areas at risk for microscopic disease. Even with a negative second-look procedure, the recurrence risk has been reported to be as high as 50%. Therefore, except in research settings, this procedure remains controversial because it has not been shown to significantly improve survival. If the second-look procedure is negative, some patients will opt for consolidation therapy with additional courses of platinum/Taxol.

Second-line therapy for ovarian cancer generally has poor efficacy, although occa-sional remissions and even cures are reported. Death in ovarian cancer usually occurs secondary to starvation, as the cancer covers the intestines and makes them ineffective in providing nutrition for the patient.

SUMMARY

Ovarian cancer is a very lethal disease in its late stages. Most patients will present with late-stage disease, however, because early disease has very few symptoms. To date, no effective screening program has been developed to detect early ovarian cancer in the general population. The treatment consists of surgical resection, followed by chemotherapy in most situations. Early-stage ovarian cancer can occasionally be treated with maintenance of fertility and preservation of an unaffected ovary, tube, and uterus.

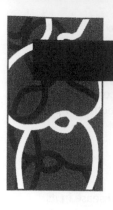

CHAPTER 55

Gestational Trophoblastic Disease

Alexander F. Burnett

Abnormalities of placental tissue represent a wide variety of illnesses, ranging from benign processes to extremely malignant tumors. These diseases of the reproductive-age woman may occur concomitant with abnormal pregnancies or they may follow ectopic pregnancies, spontaneous abortions, therapeutic abortions, or, rarely, normal gestations. Early diagnosis and treatment is critical to maintain the woman's reproductive capacity and, occasionally, to save her life. The most malignant form of gestational trophoblastic disease (GTD), choriocarcinoma, is an extremely aggressive cancer that spreads quickly via hematogenous routes. Prior to the era of chemotherapy, this cancer was almost uniformly fatal.

The most common manifestation of GTD is molar gestation, which can be complete (lacking any fetal association) or incomplete (associated with a fetus or fetal remnants). The usual presentation consists of vaginal bleeding, amenorrhea with a positive pregnancy test and no fetal heart tone, or a pregnancy with a discrepancy in gestational size of date. Frequently, the ovaries are enlarged secondary to stimulation by human chorionic gonadotropin (hCG), which forms large, bilateral theca lutein cysts.

CLINICAL CORRELATION

T. B. is a 16-year-old female whose last menstrual period was 12 weeks ago. Until this time, her menses had been regular, occurring every 28 days since age 12, and lasting 4 to 5 days. T. B. has not had any prior pregnancies. She has been sexually active but has not used birth control because she desired to have a child. She presents for her first prenatal visit. On examination, the uterus is approximately 14 weeks gestational size and fetal heart tones are absent by Doppler. Her urine pregnancy test is strongly positive. T. B. has a stable blood pressure and temperature, but her breathing is somewhat labored at a rate of 32 breaths per minute. Chest auscultation reveals course rails throughout her lung fields.

The normal purpose of placental tissue is to insinuate into the uterine blood supply and thereby provide nourishment for the growing fetus. In GTD, placental tissue is present and has the same tendency to invade blood vessels. Not infrequently, these tumors will present with hematogenous metastases, with the most frequent occurrence being found in the lungs (the first capillary system that blood leaving the uterus encounters).

Molar gestation occurs most frequently at the reproductive age extremes. A very young patient with absent fetal heart tones, enlarged uterus, and a positive pregnancy test should be suspected of having GTD. Symptoms that are suggestive of this disease include hyperemesis

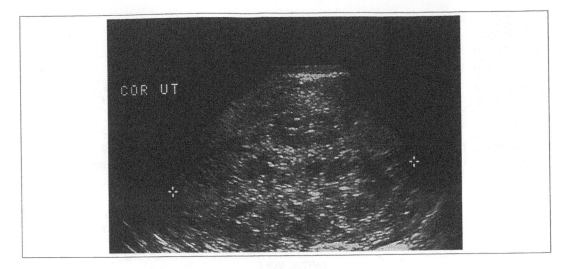

Figure 55.1   Sonogram of the uterus demonstrating a placental pattern consistent with a molar gestation

that extends beyond the first trimester and hypertension or pre-eclampsia prior to 20 weeks gestational age. Diagnosis is most readily made by ultrasound and a serum beta subunit of hCG.

Molar gestation is unique in that it has a virtually ideal tumor marker in hCG, with levels of this glycoprotein corresponding to the presence and extent of trophoblastic tissue. This marker is so specific for trophoblastic disease that persistent elevation of hCG alone may prompt the administration of chemotherapy without a histologic diagnosis. The beta subunit of hCG is monitored because of cross-reactivity of the alpha-subunit with subunits of LH, FSH, and TSH.

Ultrasound will show a typical "snowstorm" appearance to the uterine contents, like that shown in Figure 55.1; only rarely is there evidence of a viable fetus. Occasionally, the woman will have passed blood from her vagina or have grape-like vesicals, which are indicative of the abnormal hydropic villi.

CLINICAL CORRELATION

T. B. is sent for diagnostic ultrasound. A beta-hCG sample is drawn and the level is measured at 380,000 mIU/mL. Ultrasound confirms a "snowstorm" appearance to the uterine contents but no identifiable fetal parts. A chest radiograph shows bilateral infiltrates without definite masses. The remaining laboratory tests are significant for a hematocrit of 45%, a normal white blood cell count, and a normal coagulation profile. The patient is prepared for suction curettage of the uterus under general anesthesia.

With a presumptive diagnosis of GTD, the uterus should be evacuated in the most expedient manner. In most cases, suction curettage with a large-caliber curette is performed to reduce the likelihood of perforation of a thin-walled uterus. Uterine contraction is assisted with the addition of intravenous oxytocin once curettage is begun and continued post-operatively until bleeding has abated. These patients are at significant risk for blood loss due to the uterus's inability to contract adequately. Uterine contents should be sent for pathologic study.

PATHOPHYSIOLOGY

The two types of molar gestations—partial (Figure 55.2) and complete (Figure 55.3) hydatidiform moles—are believed to be of paternal origin (Table 55.1). Chromosomal studies have verified that the majority of complete moles are 46, XX, with both X chromosomes being paternally derived. Incomplete moles are gen-

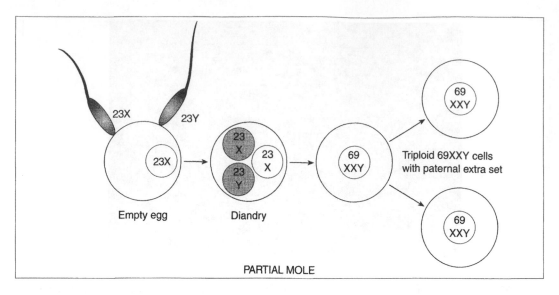

Figure 55.2   The formation of a partial mole

Source: Callahan TL, Caughey AB, Heffner LJ. Blueprints in obstetrics and gynecology. Malden, MA: Blackwell Science, 1998:195.

erally triploid—69, XXX—with the abnormal duplication of chromosomes occurring in paternally derived chromosomes. Histologically, complete moles possess villi that are edematous, lack blood vessels, and have a proliferation of trophoblastic cells surrounding them. Incomplete moles are less common and histo-logically have less swelling of the villi; fetal parts or remnants (fetal red blood cells) are also frequently present. Incomplete moles are less likely to persist or require treatment.

Follow-up after removal of a molar pregnancy is identical for both complete and incomplete moles:

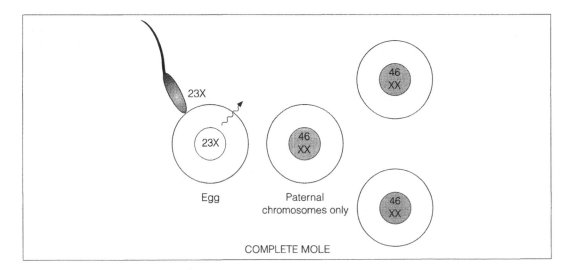

Figure 55.3   The formation of a complete mole

Source: Callahan TL, Caughey AB, Heffner LJ. Blueprints in obstetrics and gynecology. Malden, MA: Blackwell Science, 1998:194.

Table 55.1 Hydatidiform Moles

	COMPLETE	PARTIAL
Embryo	No remnants	Usually dies by 9 weeks, may survive to term
Villi	All swollen	Focal swelling
Fetal RBCs	Absent	Present
Gestational age	8–16 weeks	10–22 weeks
hCG titer	>50,000 mIU/mL	75% are <50,000 mIU/mL
Malignant potential	15%–25%	5%–10%
Karyotype	46, XX (95%)	Triploid (80%)
Size for dates		
Small	33%	65%
Large	33%	10%

1. Serum beta-hCG levels are drawn every week until they become negative; measurements are then repeated for two more weeks. The beta-hCG sampling is repeated every other week for two to three months, then checked monthly for one year.

2. Reliable contraception for one year is required. Generally it consists of oral contraceptives or depo-progesterone.

3. Following a year of negative beta-hCG levels, the patient may become pregnant again.

4. If the beta-hCG concentration rises or plateaus during follow-up, the patient has persistent GTD and needs treatment (chemotherapy). Pregnancy must also be ruled out.

Reliable contraception is critical to avoid pregnancy during the follow-up period. If the patient were to become pregnant, it would be unclear whether the rise in beta-hCG titer is due to persistent GTD or the pregnancy. The beta-hCG samples should be sent to the same laboratory for each patient to ensure consistent results. These levels can be plotted on a regression curve (Figure 55.4) to track the benign regression of hCG following molar pregnancies. Patients who significantly deviate from this curve in terms of a plateauing or rising titer require therapy.

T. B. undergoes suction curettage under general anesthesia. The procedure is well tolerated and post-operative bleeding is minimal. The pathology returns as a complete hydatidiform mole. Post-evacuation

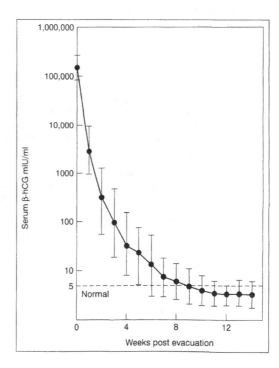

Figure 55.4 Normal regression curve of serum hCG levels after evacuation of a molar pregnancy

Source: Callahan TL, Caughey AB, Heffner LJ. Blueprints in obstetrics and gynecology. Malden, MA: Blackwell Science, 1998:197.

examinations reveal normal-size ovaries and appropriate resolution of uterine enlargement. T. B. is placed on oral contraceptive pills. Her beta-hCG titers fall to 60,000 mIU/mL immediately. Her weekly titers are 8000 mIU/mL at one week, 6000 mIU/mL at two weeks, and 4500 mIU/mL at three weeks.

PERSISTENT GESTATIONAL TROPHOBLASTIC DISEASE

When a patient is diagnosed with persistence of GTD after molar gestation, chemotherapy must be initiated. A staging work-up is performed as rapidly as possible, consisting of a chest radiograph; ultrasound to rule out intrauterine pregnancy if it is a possibility; CT or MRI of the brain (Figure 55.5), abdomen, and pelvis; complete blood count; platelet count; liver function and renal function tests; coagulation profile; and thyroid function tests.

Staging will place patients into one of three categories:

- Nonmetastatic GTD
- Metastatic, good-prognosis GTD
- Metastatic, poor-prognosis GTD

Figure 55.6 delineates the differences between good-prognosis and poor-prognosis metastatic GTD. This categorization helps the physician in deciding which treatment is best for the patient. Patients with brain metastases should begin radiation therapy to the head emergently to prevent the possible hemorrhagic sequelae from these vascular tumors. Patients with nonmetastatic or good-prognosis, metastatic GTD may initially be treated with single-agent chemotherapy, usually consisting of methotrexate or actinomycin D. Patients with poor-prognosis GTD should be treated with a multiagent regimen, usually consisting of MAC (methotrexate, actinomycin D, cyclophosphamide) or EMACO (etoposide, methotrexate, actinomycin D, cyclophosphamide, oncovin). Treatment should continue until the patient has a negative titer, with one additional treatment given for nonmetastatic and good-prognosis, metastatic GTD, and two additional treatments given for poor-prognosis,

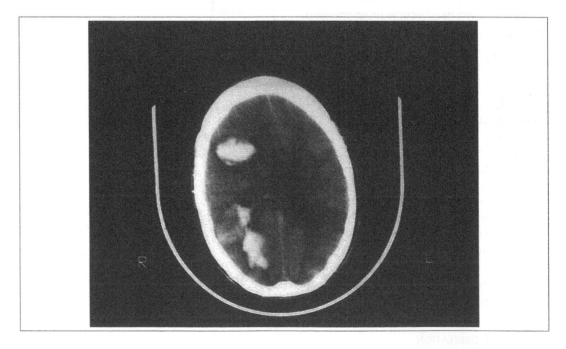

Figure 55.5   CT scan of the head of a patient with a history of GTD demonstrating a hemorrhagic lesion consistent with a metastatic focus of GTD. The patient immediately underwent whole-brain radiation and chemotherapy, but died shortly after this condition was discovered.

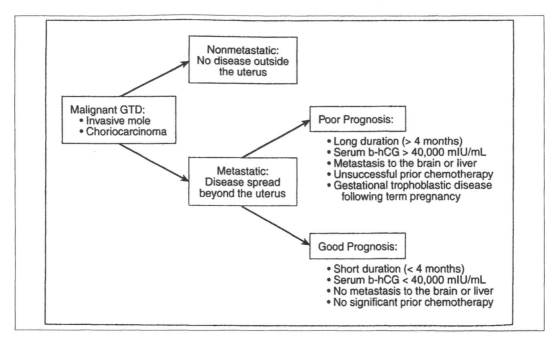

Figure 55.6   Prognostic classification of GTD

Source: Callahan TL, Caughey AB, Heffner LJ. Blueprints in obstetrics and gynecology. Malden, MA: Blackwell Science, 1998:196.

metastatic GTD after a negative beta-hCG titer is achieved.

Other treatment modalities include hysterectomy, which is employed as primary therapy in patients whose families are complete and occasionally as therapy for persistent, chemotherapy-resistant disease where the only known focus of the tumor is in the uterus. In addition, solitary, chemotherapy-resistant metastases may be surgically removed for a cure of this disease. The most common sites of metastases for GTD are the lungs, vagina, pelvis, brain, and liver.

CLINICAL CORRELATION

T. B. is diagnosed with good-prognosis, metastatic GTD on the basis of lung metastases, a beta-hCG titer of less than 40,000 mIU/mL, a lack of liver or brain metastases, a short duration of symptoms, and no prior chemotherapy. She is treated with weekly methotrexate given intramuscularly at 40 mg/m². Her beta-hCG titers rapidly fall to negative levels (less than 2 mIU/mL) in three weeks' time. She receives one additional course of chemotherapy, which is well tolerated. She is followed closely over the next year while she uses reliable contraception and has no evidence of return of her disease.

SUMMARY

Gestational trophoblastic disease, with its propensity for hematogenous spread, can mimic any other type of malignancy. Consequently, any reproductive-age woman who is undergoing a work-up for a new diagnosis of cancer should obtain a serum beta-hCG measurement to rule out this disease. When detected early and treated early, GTD is almost uniformly curable. Successful pregnancies after adequate treatment and appropriate follow-up observance period are commonplace.

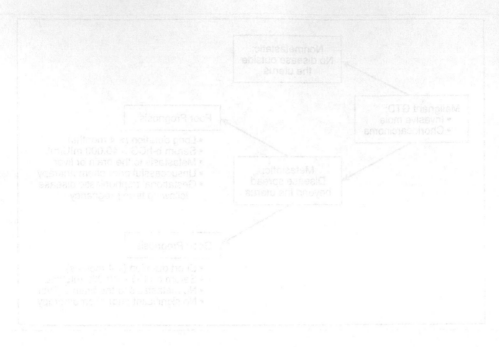

Other Issues

PART VI

Other Issues

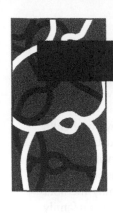

CHAPTER 56

Legal Issues in Obstetrics and Gynecology

Raquel D. Arias

The practice of obstetrics and gynecology in the United States requires an understanding of how the laws affecting medicine apply specifically to the care of women.

INFORMED CONSENT

A competent person has the right to accept or refuse medical care. She also has the right to receive information that is pertinent to making an informed decision. Three areas have been specifically mentioned by the U.S. Supreme Court as necessary to informed consent:

1. The nature of the treatment
2. The risks, benefits, and possible complications of the treatment
3. Alternatives to the treatment with their associated risks

Special requirements apply to some procedures, including sterilization, hysterectomy, experimental procedures to treat breast cancer, blood tests for HIV, and blood transfusion.

Exceptions to the doctrine of informed consent include emergency procedures, cases in which the patient requests not to be informed, and therapeutic exception. The therapeutic exception is that rare circumstance in which the physician believes that "the disclosure would so seriously upset the patient that she would not be able to dispassionately weigh the risks of refusing to undergo the recommended treatment." It seems unlikely in the current social climate that such an exception would routinely be upheld. When relying on one of these exceptions, the prudent physician should document which of these criteria apply in the given situation.

In those cases in which the patient refuses a recommended procedure, the physician has the obligation to explain the consequences of such a refusal. An "informed refusal" is also best documented in the patient's medical record.

CLINICAL CORRELATION

T. S. is a 43-year-old, gravida 2, para 2, female with a history of heavy irregular menses of two years' duration. She is known to have leiomyomata uteri that are now 18 weeks' size. Her Pap smear is normal, and her endometrial biopsy reveals a secretory endometrium. At the time of her annual examination, her gynecologist recommends a total abdominal hysterectomy. T. S. declines at that time, opting instead for iron therapy. T. S. has been a practicing Jehovah's Witness for three years. What aspects of informed consent and informed refusal need to be documented in her medical record?

In addition to the nature of the procedure in this case (a hysterectomy), T. S. needs to consider the risks of heavy bleeding in light of her religious beliefs, which preclude transfusion. Leiomyomata uteri are known to increase the risk of uncontrollable uterine bleeding. Should she continue to refuse surgery, it should be documented that the risks of uncontrolled bleeding were discussed with her and that an informed refusal was given.

CONSENT BY MINORS

The laws that authorize minors to give consent vary considerably from state to state. In California, minors who are married (or divorced), in active duty with the U.S. Armed Forces, emancipated by a court order, or are self-sufficient may give legal consent to medical treatment. Separate statutes govern the authority of minors to consent for the prevention or treatment of pregnancy, the treatment of sexually transmitted diseases, the treatment of rape, and the care of drug- or alcohol-related problems. Table 56.1 describes the various laws pertaining to mandatory delays and minors' rights to abortion in the various states.

CAPACITY TO CHOOSE

Before obtaining consent, the physician must assess whether the patient has the capacity to understand the nature of her medical problem as well as the potential consequences of her acceptance or refusal of care. The patient's ability to communicate her decision may also play a role in the decision-making process. Although a psychiatric evaluation is not always required to determine a patient's decision-making ability, input from a psychiatrist may prove useful in difficult cases. The capacity to choose may be altered by such things as drug use (prescribed or recreational), situational stress, or physical or psychiatric disorders.

If treatment is nonemergent and the patient's diminished capacity is likely to resolve, a delay in treatment is reasonable. Otherwise, consent from a legal representative, next of kin, or a court order may be obtained.

SURROGATE DECISION MAKERS

When relying on a surrogate decision maker, priority should first be given to an attorney-in-fact. If the patient has executed a durable power of attorney before losing capacity, her health care agent has an authority greater than that of any other surrogate, unless that agent's decision is inconsistent with the patient's known wishes.

When no power of attorney for health care has been executed, the next best surrogate is a court-appointed conservator. In the absence of either of the aforementioned surrogate decision makers, a close family member may authorize medical care. Relying on family members is complicated by the possibility of disagreement between equally close relatives and potential financial or emotional gain for bad outcomes.

No discussion of informed consent is complete without mentioning the forms so often associated with this decision-making process. It must be emphasized that no printed material—however complete, understandable, or "interactive"—can take the place of the discussion between patient and physician where the risks, benefits, and alternatives are explained in language with which the patient is comfortable, taking the amount of time necessary for both parties to be assured of understanding. When a form is used, it should be considered to be only an adjunct to the actual informed consent that is obtained by discussion.

The decision to use a printed form has become more popular as physicians attempt to document ever more thoroughly the extent to which complications were discussed. It would nevertheless be an error to assume that the mere signing of a document is as important as the process previously discussed. A notation in the patient's chart as to the nature and extent of the informed consent discussion is highly recommended.

ADVANCE DIRECTIVES

Advance directives are written instructions that express a patient's wishes in the event of her loss of ability to communicate or give consent. Examples of advance directions include the following:

• Durable power of attorney for health care
• A living will
• Natural Death Act declaration

Table 56.1 Abortion Laws in Various States

STATE	MANDATORY DELAY	PARENTAL CONSENT FOR MINORS
Alabama		Consent of one parent
Arkansas		Notification of both parents with 48-hour delay
Delaware		Notification of one parent or waiver, 24-hour delay for <16 years old
Georgia		Notification of one parent with 24-hour delay
Idaho	24-hour delay	Notification of parents if possible with 24-hour delay
Indiana	18-hour delay	Consent of one parent
Iowa		Notification of one parent with 48-hour delay
Kansas	24-hour delay	Notification of one parent with mandatory counseling
Kentucky		Informed consent of one parent
Louisiana	24-hour delay	Consent of one parent
Maine		Informed consent of adult family member
Maryland		Notification of one parent or doctor waiver
Massachusetts		Consent of one parent
Michigan	24-hour delay	Consent of one parent
Minnesota		Notification of both parents with 48-hour delay
Mississippi	24-hour delay	Consent of both parents
Missouri		Informed consent of one parent
Nebraska	24-hour delay	Notification of one parent with 48-hour delay
North Carolina		Consent of one parent or grandparent
North Dakota	24-hour delay	Consent of both parents
Ohio	24-hour delay	Notification of one parent with 24-hour delay
Pennsylvania	24-hour delay	Informed consent of one parent
Rhode Island		Consent of one parent
South Carolina	1-hour delay	Informed consent of one parent for <17 years old
South Dakota	24-hour delay	Notification of one parent with 48-hour delay
Utah	24-hour delay	Notification of parents if possible
Virginia		Notification of one parent with 24-hour delay
West Virginia		Notification of one parent or doctor waiver with 24-hour delay
Wisconsin	24-hour delay	Informed consent of one parent or adult family member
Wyoming		Consent of one parent with 48-hour delay

Note: 1999 information.

CONFIDENTIALITY

Both federal and state law agree that medical information may not be released to anyone other than the patient herself without the patient's written authorization. In some situations, however, disclosure of information is discretionary. These situations include communication between professionals to aid in diagnosis or treatment, or to aid in obtaining a referral. Exceptions to the general rules surrounding confidentiality may exist with regard to a minor's medical records and HIV test results.

A general medical records release does not necessarily cover the release of blood tests for HIV or the diagnosis of AIDS. In some states, this information is covered by more stringent confidentiality standards.

ABANDONMENT

The failure to provide necessary medical care to a current patient without previous adequate notice of termination constitutes patient abandonment.

A patient–physician relationship must exist before a claim of abandonment can be made. Usually, this relationship is forged during an office visit in which a history, physical assessment, and plan are made. This scenario generally establishes an obligation to continue care. In some instances, this obligation can be expected if the physician has given verbal (including telephone) assurances of care or if the physician accepts a referral of a specific patient.

Either the physician or the patient may end the therapeutic relationship. The physician may not terminate a patient based on race, color, religion, or physical disability. Nevertheless, gynecologists may refuse to treat men, pediatricians may restrict their practice to a specific age group, and other appropriate instances based on specialties may exist.

A patient may end a therapeutic relationship either by explicitly informing the physician, or by her conduct. It is prudent to make a notation in the patient's medical record describing either the patient's explicit termination of the relationship or those acts that lead one to believe that the patient has left your medical care.

such an emergency situation. If Dr. Andersen had given M. M. written notice of his termination of the therapeutic relationship, leaving her with adequate time and opportunity to find another care giver, he might then claim to no longer be her doctor.

CONTRACTUAL NATURE OF MEDICAL BENEFITS

Many, if not most, patients seen by today's obstetrician/gynecologists will have contracted with an insurance company or the federal government to pay for their medical care. The relationships between physician, patient, and health plan are codified in the contracts made by all parties. In certain well-publicized cases, the best interests of the health plan have been at odds with the perceived best interests of the patient or doctor. These cases have resulted in legislation at both the state and federal levels.

CLINICAL CORRELATION

As part of her incentive package, Dr. Davis was offered a contract that increases her proportion of the year-end bonus when she is able to discharge her obstetric patients in less than 48 hours following a vaginal delivery.

The federal legislature has found that the hospital stay following delivery should be based on the mother's health, the adequacy of home support, the confidence of the parents, the medical stability of the newborn, and the family unit's access to follow-up care. The judgment of discharge timing is held to be the responsibility of the physician in consultation with the mother.

The California legislature has specified several safeguards related to a mother's postpartum hospital stay. Under California law, if a discharge less than 48 hours following vaginal delivery or less than 96 hours after a cesarean section is considered, the following conditions should be met:

1. The health plan must cover a follow-up visit within 48 hours.

2. The physician must let the patient know that this visit is covered.

3. After assessing at least potential transportation, difficulties, and social visits, the physician must decide (with the mother's assent) where this visit will occur. Potential locations include the patient's home, the physician's office, and some other facility under contract with the health plan.

4. This visit must be made by a licensed health care provider who provides postpartum and newborn care as part of the scope of his or her practice.

5. The visit must include, but not be limited to, patient education, instruction or assistance with breast- or bottle-feeding, and any indicated maternal or neonatal assessments.

6. All of these services must be available on physician prescription without prior authorization.

7. Plans may not penalize the physician for prescribing these services.

8. Plans may not reward physicians for providing care in a manner inconsistent with the intent of the legislation.

9. Plans may not penalize mothers for taking advantage of these benefits.

10. Plans may not reward mothers for accepting less than the minimum coverage outlined above.

The subject of "gag clauses" has also been evaluated by state and federal governments—most notably, in regard to provision of information regarding pregnancy termination for women covered by Medicaid.

Generally speaking, a strong physician–patient relationship—especially for patients with acute conditions—has been held to be of therapeutic benefit and "important to the health and well-being" of participants. In California, health care plans are prohibited from restricting doctors from giving out information that may help the patient receive medically appropriate care (B.P. code 2056). In addition, plans may not include provisions in their contracts that limit the physician's ability or authority to communicate about treatment options, alternative health plans, or other coverage arrangements.

Medicare recipients are expressly protected by Operationally Policy Letter 44, which states that beneficiaries are entitled to the advice of their doctor on medically necessary treatment that may be appropriate for their condition. Thus physicians providing care to Medicare patients may not be restricted by the cost- or risk-containment strategies pursued by the patient's health plan.

FRAUD

Health care fraud is a specific federal offense. It is defined by Congress as follows:

> "Knowingly and willfully defrauding any health care benefit program or obtaining, by any means of false or fraudulent pretense, any money or property owned by or under the custody and control of any health care program." (18 U.S.C. 1347)

A physician is responsible for all activities conducted in his or her offices, including billing and maintenance of records. The U.S. Department of Health and Human Services' Office of the Inspector General issues "Fraud Alerts" that may help the physician to scrutinize contracts that may spur investigation by federal enforcement authorities.*

RISK MANAGEMENT

In certain predictable situations, the possibility of litigation is increased. These situations include injuries to the patient (whether predictable or unexpected), instances in which the patient is dissatisfied with the outcome of her disease or treatment, and unexpected death. The importance of careful record keeping cannot be overemphasized. In litigation circumstances, the plaintiff's attorney will review records for evidence of a lapse in the standard of care that resulted in the patient's injury (or presumed injury).

Careful record keeping is concise and pertinent. It is not endless, redundant (defensive), or obviously self-serving. Do not record in-

*To obtain these alerts, contact the following Web address: http://www.os.dhhs.gov/search/. Enter "fraud alert" in the search box.

teractions with attorneys or risk management activity in the medical record. On the other hand, be sure to record all complications in a straightforward manner that avoids the use of superlatives or unnecessarily colorful language.

When the patient threatens or complains, that event should be noted in a matter-of-fact tone, paying attention to how this attitude may affect compliance with the therapeutic plan. Statements regarding causation should not be prematurely placed in the medical record.

CLINICAL CORRELATION

P. P. is a 26-year-old, G2P2, female brought in by her husband with complaints of shortness of breath and chest pain. She delivered a term infant eight weeks before her presentation and was breast-feeding. Her obstetrician/gynecologist had given her a progestin-only pill the week before symptoms began. A diagnosis of deep, venous thrombosis and pulmonary embolism is made when both Doppler studies of the right leg and spinal CT of the lungs reveal evidence of a clot. P. P. is admitted for intravenous heparin therapy. The patient's husband tells the admitting doctor that his wife's problems were caused by the pill prescribed by her obstetrician/gynecologist.

The preceding scenario provides the opportunity for misinformation to be perpetuated in the medical record if the emergency room doctor includes the husband's theory of causation in this assessment. The potential for repetition to be perceived as fact may be realized, especially when the chart is reviewed by lawyers or laypersons who do not realize that progestin-only medications have not been associated with an increased risk of thrombosis.

CHILD ABUSE AND DOMESTIC VIOLENCE

Physicians have an ethical responsibility to protect their patients from foreseeable harm. This protection does not extend to ignoring abuse by the patient or her spouse to their children. The laws covering reporting requirements vary from state to state. In California, physicians who have knowledge of or observe a child in their professional capacity or within the scope of their employment whom they know or reasonably suspect has been the victim of child abuse must report this abuse. Abuse includes the following:

- Physical injury (other than accidental)
- Sexual abuse
- Unjustifiable or unlawful corporal punishment or injury
- Neglect

The reports must be made both by telephone and in writing to a county welfare department, a police or sheriff's office, or a county probation department. The telephone report must be made as soon as possible, and the written report must be made within 36 hours on standardized forms available from the child protective services agency.

Special protocols for performing physical examinations on victims of sexual assault exist for both minors and adults.

Physicians who hire practitioners licensed by the state of California must obtain a signed statement that acknowledges an understanding of their child abuse reporting obligations.

DOMESTIC VIOLENCE

Domestic violence is defined as "the infliction of or threat of physical harm against past or present adult or adolescent intimate partners." Given the prevalence of domestic violence (estimated at 25% of all U.S. households), many states have enacted laws requiring screening and reporting of evidence of domestic violence.

California's law requires that injuries resulting from partner abuse be reported to local law enforcement. Failure to report any injury caused by domestic violence is a criminal offense. The physician is required to make an immediate telephone report to police, followed by written confirmation within 48 hours. If a patient identifies herself as a victim, but is not being treated for current injuries, reporting is not mandatory but the patient should be asked to file a police report; in addition, all incidents and past injuries reported by the patient should be documented in the medical record.

Because child abuse occurs concurrently with domestic violence in an estimated 50% of cases, inquiring into the safety of children living with the patient should be made. Appropriate referrals for adult or child protective services should also be given.

SEXUAL ASSAULT

The annual incidence of sexual assault in the United States is approximately 200 per 100,000 persons. As many as 20% of women are sexually assaulted by the time they are 21 years old. Sexual assault occurs in all age, racial, and socioeconomic groups.

Rape is the act of sexual intercourse without consent. Some sources further classify rape into such categories as marital rape (sexual intercourse of a spouse without consent) and date rape (where the woman may voluntarily participate in sexual foreplay but coitus occurs, often forcibly, without her consent). In one survey, 55% of date rape victims reported that they were under the influence of alcohol when the event occurred.

The American College of Obstetricians and Gynecologists describes the psychological impact of rape as a "rape-trauma" syndrome. The acute phase of this syndrome occurs within the first few hours to days after the event and is characterized by distortion or paralysis of the woman's coping mechanisms. Physical complaints during this time may include generalized pain, pelvic pain, headache, sleep disturbances, vaginal discharge, and rectal pain. Emotional behaviors may include depression, anxiety, and mood swings. The delayed phase may occur months or years after the event and is characterized by flashbacks, nightmares, and phobias.

The physician's role in sexual assault includes both a medical and a legal obligation (Table 56.2). Most jurisdictions have a sexual assault assessment kit that is mandated for forensic purposes. Rape crisis counselors should be involved when available. Documentation of the event in the victim's words should take place in addition to taking a gynecologic history. The physical examination documents any trauma and collects samples for cultures, sam-

Table 56.2   Physician's Role in Evaluating the Victim of Sexual Assault

Medical

Obtain informed consent from the patient

Obtain accurate gynecologic history

Assess and treat physical injuries

Obtain appropriate cultures and treat any existing infections

Provide prophylactic antibiotic therapy and offer immunizations

Provide therapy to prevent unwanted conception

Offer baseline serologic tests for hepatitis B virus, human immunodeficiency virus, and syphilis

Provide counseling

Arrange for follow-up medical care and counseling

Legal

Provide accurate recording of events

Document injuries

Collect samples (pubic hair, fingernail scrapings, vaginal secretions, saliva, blood-stained clothing)

Report to authorities as required

Assure chain of evidence (orderly and unbroken progress of specimens to legal authorities)

Source: Adapted from Sexual assault. ACOG bulletin number 242, November 1997.

ples for serological testing, and forensic samples, including vaginal secretions, saliva, pubic hair, or blood-stained clothing. A Wood's lamp can be used to visualize dried semen on the patient's skin. Prophylactic antibiotic therapy for sexually transmitted diseases should be provided as well as therapy to prevent unwanted pregnancy. Minor injuries may be repaired at the time of examination. Approximately 1% of victims sustain injuries requiring hospitalization.

The legal examination documents trauma and evidence of sexual contact. This evidence should be collected as soon as possible and in a manner that preserves the integrity of the evidence in case it is needed for subsequent legal proceedings. "Rape" and "sexual assault" are legal terms and, as such, do not belong in the medical record. Instead, phrases such as "findings consistent with the use of force" are more appropriate in the medical description.

Patients should have access to appropriate counseling services, often provided by experts in the field. Follow-up should be scheduled to assess the patient's ongoing medical and psy-

chological condition. If the patient appears overwhelmed psychologically, an emergency psychiatric consult may be in order.

The physician may subsequently be subpoenaed to testify in cases that go to trial. As a medical expert, the physician is charged with describing the physical findings and allowing the legal experts to determine the legal issues in the case.

SUMMARY

Legal aspects of obstetrics and gynecology run the gamut of the obligations of the physician–patient relationship, ranging from patient's rights issues to evaluation of victims of sexual assault and physical abuse. A physician needs to be aware of the laws pertaining to issues in medicine in general, and to obstetrics and gynecology in particular, for the doctor's own state. When any doubt arises regarding specific situations, members of the legal profession should be consulted for their expertise.

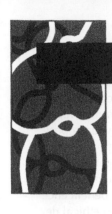

CHAPTER 57

Ethics in Obstetrics and Gynecology

Alexander F. Burnett

Ethical issues of beneficence and patient autonomy are commonly brought to the forefront in obstetrics and gynecology. Inherent in this specialty is the element of dealing at times with two lives—those of the mother and that fetus—one of whom is contained within the other and, therefore, unable to represent itself. Balancing maternal rights against fetal rights is critical in discussing interventions for fetal well-being, abortion, and interventions for maternal well-being. Many situations also involve rights as defined by law for the mother or fetus.

Other issues in this specialty include patient care in situations of death and dying, informed consent, and presentation of treatment options to the woman. Because the specialty is so closely involved with women's sexuality, ethical considerations of appropriate and inappropriate relations between physician and patient also come into play.

CLINICAL CORRELATION

P. R. is a 16-year-old, gravida 1, female at 20 weeks gestational age. Her first prenatal visit was at 16 weeks. The triple screening performed at that time returns with a high alpha-fetoprotein. A subsequent sonogram confirms a large spina bifida. The pregnancy resulted from rape by a relative, who has recently been jailed for the offense. The patient desires to terminate the pregnancy. Her parents are of a fundamental religious order that opposes termination on any grounds and refuse to allow her to end the pregnancy.

BASIC BIOETHICAL PRINCIPLES

AUTONOMY

Autonomy has been broadly defined as personal rule of the self while free from both controlling influences of others and personal limitations that prevent meaningful choice. The concept of autonomy incorporates the rights of informed consent in treatment decisions. Because of the difference in knowledge of medical matters held by the physician as opposed to that held by the patient, the physician is obliged to disclose information and ensure understanding of the various options available to the patient in a particular situation.

In obstetrics and gynecology, the issues of autonomy are sometimes broadened to encompass the society as a whole. As an example of this situation, consider a minor who becomes pregnant. She is emancipated under the law to make her own decisions regarding medical care without the necessity of parental consent. In other issues, autonomy becomes more restricted by society's perceptions of the rights of the unborn, and subsequent laws may either restrict or expand the mother's abilities to terminate pregnancy.

Central to the concept of autonomy is the belief in the patient's ability to make competent decisions on her own behalf. Competence in decisions does not imply correctness in decisions (at least from the physician's view), but rather assumes the woman's ability to rationally evaluate the information available and decide on the care that she considers in her best interest.

BENEFICENCE

Beneficence is the concept of providing benefit to the patient. A physician is required to act in a manner that attempts to provide the maximum positive effect on the patient. This concept involves more than mere avoidance of harm, but acting in a helpful way according to the patient's wishes.

PATERNALISM

Sometimes the physician may feel that the patient's decisions, while made in a competent manner, are so different from the physician's interpretations of the correct decisions, that the doctor may decide to intervene in the patient's care contrary to her stated desires. Paternalism implies that beneficence in certain circumstances can outweigh autonomy. Paternalism, it has been argued, is justified only when the harm prevented or benefit provided outweighs the loss of independence. For example, a physician may order an involuntary commitment of a mentally ill patient or one whom the physician feels is highly likely to commit suicide on the basis that the greater good is to protect the patient from her own actions.

ETHICAL DECISION MAKING

In cases where a conflict arises regarding medical care, ethical considerations may help to clarify the appropriateness of certain actions. Legality may be an issue in such situations as termination of pregnancy and the right to make autonomous decisions when pregnant regardless of age. In the case described at the beginning of this chapter, the issues from a legal perspective are fairly clear in terms of the mother's autonomy to make health care decisions that affect her pregnancy regardless of parental consent. But how far does the issue of autonomy go when considering competence on the basis of age? For instance, should a 12-year-old girl have the same autonomy over pregnancy decisions as a 17-year-old woman?

Ethics committees are often composed of a wide variety of individuals who may represent opposing viewpoints and advocacy positions. Physicians, ethicists, clergy members, lawyers, community members, parents, and patients may all participate in discussions that strive to maintain autonomy and beneficence simultaneously. The legal aspect in ethical decisions cannot be underestimated, particularly when patients are presented with nonstandard choices or heroic, unproved options. Ethics committees may even consider a cost/benefit analysis of certain procedures in an effort to protect the "greater good" of society in using limited resources.

PHYSICIAN–PATIENT RELATIONSHIP

Having established that the physician optimally desires to practice in such a way as to maintain patient autonomy with beneficence, we can also define what is appropriate and inappropriate in physician–patient relations.

CLINICAL CORRELATION

T. L. is a 24-year-old, G1P0010, female who has made several office visits during the past three months for recurrent yeast infections of the vagina. On each visit, her physician detects minimal *Candida* organisms on a potassium hydroxide prep of her vaginal discharge. T. L. dresses in an increasingly more provocative manner with each subsequent visit. On the fourth visit, after the nurse has left the room, the patient begins to cry and describes how she has had several failed relationships and is very lonely. She tells her physician, "You are the only one who really understands my problems. Thank you so much for listening to me. Before you leave, will you hug me?" Her physician awkwardly obliges but feels uncomfortable as the patient presses very firmly on the embrace.

Obstetricians/gynecologists frequently have relationships with patients that last for many years, spanning adolescence, the reproductive years, and the menopause. By the nature of the specialty, obstetricians and gynecologists are familiar with the intimate details of a woman's life, including her desires for reproduction and her sexuality. As with any specialty in medicine, physicians sometimes begin sexual relations with patients. In surveys in the United States and elsewhere, between 3% and 7% of obstetricians/gynecologists have reported beginning a sexual relationship with a patient, a rate similar to that for other specialties, such as internal medicine or psychiatry. The American Medical Association has stated that "sexual contact that occurs concurrent with the physician–patient relationship constitutes sexual misconduct." The American College of Obstetricians and Gynecologists (ACOG) further states:

> Sexual contact or a romantic relationship between a physician and a current patient is always unethical.
>
> Sexual contact or a romantic relationship between a physician and a former patient may also be unethical.

The ethical argument against a physician–patient sexual or romantic relationship is that the nature of the relationship prohibits adequate consent on the part of the patient and, therefore, violates the patient's autonomy. McCullough, a biomedical ethicist, states that "as a result of vulnerability, transference phenomena, fear in the presence of authority, and other factors, the crucial condition of voluntariness for an informed consent to a sexual relationship by the patient in most or, perhaps, virtually all cases does not exist." He further argues that, while sexual activity by the patient may be voluntary in some instances, sexual or romantic relations should be prohibited on the basis of proper physician virtues, which dictate that the physician blunt his or her self-interest and direct his or her attention and concern to the interests of the patient.

The ACOG recommends that a chaperone be present for all physical examinations, irrespective of the physician's gender. Indeed, the case mentioned earlier fails to identify the physician as being male or female, as both could be placed in such a circumstance. The chaperone can provide comfort for the patient during the examination and provides protection for the physician and patient if claims of inappropriate behavior are made.

Medical students often have difficulty initially with patient encounters that involve the sexual organs. It is worthwhile to have mentors to whom the student can express these concerns and who can model the appropriate behavior. It will take experience for the doctor in training to learn what is and is not considered appropriate behavior by patients, and what actions by patients may be construed as sexual advances. Chaperones help to lessen the likelihood that certain patients will act out their impulses, and they can protect the physician should accusations arise. The ACOG also encourages physicians to be cognizant of any instances of sexual misconduct of any health professional, and stresses that health care providers have an obligation to report such conduct to the appropriate authorities.

SUMMARY

Ethical issues play an important role in all medical decision making. Perhaps obstetrics and gynecology is more influenced by ethical considerations than other clinical specialties because it deals with issues relating to sexuality, childbirth, abortion, birth control, and death and dying. Most institutions have multidisciplinary ethics boards that review particularly complicated cases. The personal behavior of physicians should uphold basic ethical practices of providing informed consent, not intentionally harming the patient, and respecting the patient's rights in the decision-making process.

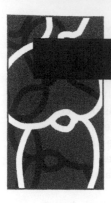

CHAPTER 58

Domestic Violence

Tina Raine

Domestic violence refers to the intentional use of force to assert power and control over an intimate partner or spouse. Violence against women takes many forms, including verbal and emotional abuse, personal and financial control, humiliation and intimidation, sexual assault, and battering. Rape and assault may occur within the confines of marriage as well, as discussed in Chapter 56. Domestic violence is pervasive, with more than 50% of all women in marriages or ongoing relationships being abused at some point. This type of attack is the most common cause of injury to women, occurring more frequently than automobile accidents, muggings, and rapes combined. Battered women also suffer more frequently from other health problems, such as substance abuse, depression, chronic somatic complaints, and suicide.

Battered women come from all ethnic, religious, and socioeconomic backgrounds. There is no "typical" victim. Pregnant women are not immune to violence either—estimates of the percentage of women who are abused during pregnancy range from 5% to 17%.

Although many battered women seek emergency medical care as a result of traumatic injuries, a large majority of these victims are seen in the outpatient primary care medical setting for routine care or for specific problems such as somatic complaints or stress-related illnesses. Consequently, primary health care providers can play a pivotal role in identifying battered women and initiating appropri-

ate care. Several studies have indicated that only a small percentage of women who present to emergency rooms or primary care outpatient settings with injuries or symptoms related to ongoing abuse are identified as such. Table 58.1 lists some common reasons why physicians fail to explore the possibility of domestic violence with their patients. Physician identification and response to domestic violence are vital, however, because these women are at risk for escalating physical violence that may ultimately result in serious injuries or death.

PATIENT HISTORY

Physical injuries are the most obvious signs of battering. Nevertheless, patients with physical injuries do not always admit to being victims of battering. Signs that injuries may have occurred as a result of battering include a time delay in presenting for injuries, inconsistent explanation for injuries, multiple injuries, or injuries in different phases of healing. When interviewing a patient with injuries, it is important to ask direct questions about the possibility of abuse. Questions such as "Did someone cause these injuries?" or "Did someone you know hit or try to injure you?" are appropriate ways to inquire how injuries were obtained. Table 58.2 presents some screening questions for eliciting an abuse history.

In the absence of physical injury, victims of abuse may be more difficult to identify; many, however, present with associated signs and

Table 58.1 Reasons Physicians Fail to Question Patients about Domestic Violence

- Misconceptions about the type of women who can be victims of domestic violence (i.e., assuming it occurs in only women from low socioeconomic backgrounds)
- Fear of offending patients or invading a patient's privacy
- Failure to confront one's own past experiences with violence or abuse
- Feeling ineffective in one's ability to intervene
- Time constraints—lack of time to address the problem

Table 58.3 Clinical Presentations That May Be Consistent with a History of Abuse

- Eating disorders
- Sleeping disorders
- Headaches
- Gastrointestinal disturbances
- Chronic pelvic pain
- Sexual dysfunction
- Recurrent vaginal discharge or itching
- Depression
- Anxiety and panic disorders
- Substance and alcohol abuse
- Attempted suicide

symptoms that can serve as clues. A history of abuse or rape as a child is more common in battered women. Likewise, a history of substance abuse, depression, or attempted suicide may be an important identifying factor. Women who are abused may make frequent visits to a primary care provider for a variety of somatic complaints. In addition, they may be escorted or "chaperoned" on their visits by their abuser. Table 58.3 lists some general and gynecological presentations that may be seen in patients who are victims of domestic violence.

CLINICAL CORRELATION

C. J. is a 40-year-old, gravida 0, white female who presents to the outpatient obstet-

Table 58.2 Screening Questions for Eliciting an Abuse History

- Are you safe at home?
- Are you afraid of your partner/husband or anyone else?
- Within the past year (or since becoming pregnant), have you been hit, slapped, kicked, or otherwise physically hurt by someone?
- Have you ever been forced to have sex with your partner/spouse?
- Are you in danger from a current or past partner?

ric/gynecologic private clinic with a chief complaint of vaginal dryness and painful intercourse. The onset of symptoms coincided with her discontinuation of estrogen replacement therapy approximately one year ago and has become progressively worse over the past six months. She states that her former gynecologist discontinued the estrogen for reasons that were unclear to her. She describes the pain during intercourse as "almost unbearable" and stated that she has intercourse only to appease her husband.

C. J. had menarche at age 12 and became sexually active when she was 18. Her last Pap smear, which was performed one year ago, was normal. The patient had a total abdominal hysterectomy and bilateral salpingo-oophorectomy 15 years ago. She reports a long history of pelvic pain and abnormal menses prior to her hysterectomy. She had recurrent episodes of vaginal hemorrhage and multiple dilations and curettage prior to her hysterectomy. She was placed on estrogen replacement therapy after her hysterectomy and continued it until one year ago. She reports having experienced hot flushes and mood swings when she initially discontinued the estrogen.

Although she denies a history of rape or child abuse, C. J. admits to a long history of emotional and verbal abuse from her husband and reports not feeling "safe" all of the time. A real estate agent, C. J. states that the couple has significant financial debt because of multiple failed business ventures initiated by her husband. She denies past or current history of physical abuse and does not feel she is in imminent danger of injury. Her review of systems, past medical, surgical, psychiatric, social, and family history are otherwise unremarkable.

PHYSICAL EXAMINATION

The physical examination should focus primarily on identifying findings related to the gynecological complaints. When a history of abuse is elicited, however, the physician should also attempt to identify any signs of emotional stress or physical trauma from abuse. During the physical examination, the woman's demeanor and affect should be monitored. Evasiveness, flat affect, hesitancy, or avoidance of eye contact may be significant findings. Physical examination may reveal signs of recent or healed injuries such as bruises or cuts.

Attention should then be directed toward the pelvic examination. Extreme anxiety or complete dissociation during the pelvic examination should be viewed with suspicion. The external genitalia should be inspected for signs of trauma. Using the speculum, the vagina and cervix should be examined for signs of trauma or sexually transmitted diseases. Patients may become hostile or refuse a rectal examination when there is a history of sexual assault. Patients should be alerted in advance of all steps and procedures of the examination. Bimanual and rectal examinations should be performed slowly and carefully, with the physician noting any tenderness or pelvic masses. All findings should be accurately and objectively documented in the medical record.

CLINICAL CORRELATION

On physical examination, C. J. is relaxed and cooperative. She weighs 135 lb and is 5

ft, 6 in, tall. Her blood pressure is 120/65. Her general examination is normal. No recent or remote bruises are apparent. Palpation of the breasts reveals no nipple discharge, skin changes, or masses. Her abdominal examination is normal without tenderness. Her pelvic examination reveals normal external genitalia. On speculum examination, the vagina is atrophic with minimal vaginal secretions. The cervix is surgically absent. The bimanual examination is normal with an absent uterus and no pelvic masses. There is minimal discomfort on rectal examination. The stool guaiac is negative.

DIFFERENTIAL DIAGNOSIS

Although C. J.'s chief complaint was sexual dysfunction, a history of domestic violence was also elicited. The latter finding may or may not be related to the initial complaint. It is important to determine whether abuse is the patient's primary problem and her other complaints are a secondary consequence. History items such as onset and duration of complaints in relation to the history of abuse will help to make this distinction.

Once it is established that a patient is a victim of domestic violence, the physician must acknowledge and further assess the problem. The doctor should consider whether underlying emotional or psychiatric problems are present. He or she should also assess the patient's own appraisal of the seriousness of the situation and her ability to take appropriate safety precautions.

MANAGEMENT

In addition to addressing the initial complaint (painful intercourse for C. J. in the case described in this chapter), the patient's management should be directed toward determining her risk for escalating abuse and helping her remain safe. The physician should try to obtain as much social history as possible. Consultation with allied health professionals in social work or counseling may prove helpful, especially when patients are embarrassed or reluctant to describe the situation in detail. The physician can play an important role in validating the problem, acknowledging the seriousness of the situation, and referring the patient to the appropriate resources.

The physician should also assess the patient's immediate safety. This analysis takes into account threats related to substance abuse, depression, homicide, or suicide. If necessary, the physician or support staff should help the patient develop a plan of action for emergency situations. Finally, the patient should be informed of additional resources available in the community, such as residential, financial, and legal support services. Any other gynecological problems that are identified should be treated as well. Follow-up appointments should be scheduled if necessary to reinforce messages and assess the patient's progress.

list of telephone numbers for social support agencies in the community.

C. J.'s symptoms of vaginal dryness and painful intercourse are most likely secondary to a hypoestrogenic state after surgical menopause and withdrawal of estrogen replacement therapy. After reviewing her past medical history for contraindications to estrogen replacement therapy, estrogen is restarted. C. J. is instructed to request her medical records from her past gynecologists. She is advised to follow up in one month to assess her status on estrogen replacement therapy and to discuss her progress in resolving the problem of abuse in her relationship with her husband.

CLINICAL CORRELATION

Information on C. J.'s family and social network is obtained, including whether others are aware of the dynamics of her relationship with her husband. The patient's immediate safety is assessed, including determining whether he has ever been volatile or possesses weapons. After a thorough discussion of her relationship with her husband, C. J. is given careful advice.

First, it is emphasized that her relationship with her husband is not normal and that her safety may be in danger. It is explained that abuse often escalates. Thus, even though her husband is not physically abusing her currently, she may be at risk for injury or even death. A possible scenario of escalating abuse is discussed, and C. J. is instructed on measures to take to ensure her ability to leave her husband in an emergency if necessary. She is given a

SUMMARY

Domestic violence is found among women from all backgrounds. Injuries as a result of domestic violence account for a significant proportion of morbidity and mortality seen in the medical setting. Physicians need to be alert to presenting signs and symptoms of abuse, and they need to pose routine questions about abuse to all women. In addition to treating injuries from abuse, physicians should offer these patients advice and support to help them end abusive relationships. This effort requires the physician to spend time and develop an understanding of the dynamics of abusive relationships. It also requires a knowledge of available community, social, and legal resources. It is important for physicians to develop a rational approach to patients who are victims of domestic violence so as to provide effective interventions in the clinical setting.

CHAPTER 1:
HISTORY OF OBSTETRICS AND GYNECOLOGY

1. Used since the time of Hippocrates as an abortifacient, Queen Anne's lace apparently works by which of the following actions?
   a. Inducing uterine contractions and expulsion of the fetus
   b. Blocking human gonadotropin production
   c. Blocking progesterone production
   d. Acting as a spermicidal agent
   e. Inhibiting prostaglandin production

2. All of the following are true statements regarding the history of barrier methods of contraception except:
   a. Vulcanization of rubber made possible the mass production of condoms as early as the late eighteenth century.
   b. Some of the earliest condoms were made from animal intestines.
   c. Primitive sponge-like devices are described by the ancient Roman physician Soranus.
   d. In ancient China and Japan, diaphragms made of oiled silk were placed in the cervix.
   e. All of the above are true.

3. Which of the following statements regarding Oliver Wendell Holmes's 1843 review of puerperal fever published in the *New England Quarterly Journal of Medicine and Surgery* is accurate?
   a. He contended that puerperal fever was caused by careless midwives, and his research supported the notion that physicians were the proper attendants at deliveries.
   b. He contended that puerperal fever was the result of an infectious agent spread from patient-to-patient by physicians and midwives.
   c. Through his research, Holmes gained widespread respect in the medical community.
   d. Both a and c.
   e. Both b and c.

4. Ignaz Semmelweis's research on puerperal fever in Austria's lying-in hospitals led to which of the following interventions that enabled a reduction in post-partum mortality from 45% to 4% in only four months?
   a. Separating patients into two wards—those delivered by physicians and those delivered by midwives
   b. Instructing physicians to wear gloves while attending at autopsies
   c. Introducing sterilization techniques at newborn deliveries
   d. Instructing medical students to wash their hands immediately after attending autopsies and prior to deliveries

5. Which of the following statements regarding use of the cesarean delivery during the Roman era is true?
   a. Julius Caesar was the first infant to survive a cesarean delivery.
   b. Pompilius enacted a Lex Regia (royal law) requiring incisional delivery of the fetuses of all pregnant women who died late in pregnancy.
   c. In the Roman era, cesarean delivery was reserved for women in positions of stature because it was considered a more sanitary method than vaginal delivery.
   d. Both a and b.
   e. Both a and c.
   f. All of the above.

6. In the Roman era, a woman might undergo 24 hours suspended upside down from a ladder followed by bedrest
   a. To reduce a uterine prolapse.
   b. To stop post-partum bleeding.
   c. To avoid a premature delivery.
   d. As a method of birth control that would act by blocking the ascent of sperm through the cervix.

Questions 7–10 Match the following contribution to the history of obstetrics and gynecology with the individual with whom it is most closely associated.
   a. James Marion Sims
   b. George Papanicolaou
   c. James Young Simpson
   d. Edward Porro

e. Edmund Piper

f. Peter Chamberlen

g. Ephraim McDowell

7. Pioneer in the use of obstetrical anesthesia

8. Inventor of forceps used to facilitate breech deliveries

9. Considered the father of modern gynecologic surgery for his contributions to the field, including innovations in the repair of vesico-vaginal fistulae

10. Developer of a screening technique credited with dramatically reducing cervical cancer mortality in the United States

CHAPTER 2:
CLINICAL ANATOMY OF THE PELVIS

1. The groin nodes receive primary lymphatic drainage from all of the following structures of the female pelvis except the:
    a. Mons.
    b. Labia minora.
    c. Labia majora.
    d. Upper two-thirds of the vagina.
    e. Clitoris.

2. Which of the following describes the normal response of the vaginal lining to the effects of estrogen?
    a. The squamous epithelium undergoes cornification.
    b. The columnar epithelium is transformed into squamous epithelium.
    c. The squamous epithelium atrophies.
    d. The squamous epithelium undergoes rapid proliferation, followed by desquamation.

3. Pain fibers from the vagina
    a. Travel with the sacral sympathetic nerve fibers and enter the spinal cord via L2–L4.
    b. Travel with the sacral sympathetic nerve fibers and enter the spinal cord via S2–S4.
    c. Travel with the sacral parasympathetic nerve fibers and enter the spinal cord via S2–S4.
    d. Travel with the sacral parasympathetic nerve fibers and enter the spinal cord via L2–L4.

4. The majority of cervical dysplasias occur at the
    a. Transition zone of the cervix.
    b. Transformation zone of the cervix.
    c. Cornification zone of the vagina.
    d. Cornification zone of the cervix.

5. All of the following statements about the Cardinal ligaments (parametria) are correct except:
    a. They traverse the inguinal canal and connect to the labia majora.
    b. They support the lower aspect of uterus, cervix, and upper vagina.
    c. They contain the ureters, uterine arteries, and lymphatic drainage of the cervix.
    d. They are covered by the broad ligaments.

6. Major blood supply to the uterus is via the
    a. Pudendal artery.
    b. Cardinal artery.
    c. Para-aortic artery.
    d. Hypogastric artery.
    e. Internal inguinal artery.

7. Fertilization of the ovum by a sperm normally occurs in the
    a. Fimbria of the fallopian tube.
    b. Isthmus of the fallopian tube.
    c. Ampullary region of the fallopian tube.
    d. Uterine cornua.
    e. Uterine trigone.
    f. Interstitium of the fallopian tube.

8. All of the following muscles form the levator ani except the
    a. Coccygeus muscle.
    b. Puborectalis muscle.
    c. Iliococcygeus muscle.
    d. Pubococcygeus muscle.

CHAPTER 3:
HISTORY AND PHYSICAL EXAMINATION

1. A female patient who has had one set of twins delivered at 34 weeks, a spontaneous abortion at 12 weeks, and two full-term infants is appropriately represented by which of the following?
    a. G5P2214
    b. G5P2215
    c. G5P2304
    d. G4P2114
    e. G4P2214

2. Pain during sexual intercourse is called
   a. Dysparesthesia.
   b. Dyscoitus.
   c. Dysuria.
   d. Dysparunuria.
   e. Dyspareunia.

3. With respect to uterine position, "version" refers to the
   a. Angle between the cervix and the uterus.
   b. Angle between the uterus and the rectum.
   c. Angle between the vagina and the uterus.
   d. Angle between the vagina and the cervical canal.

CHAPTER 4:
GYNECOLOGIC PROCEDURES

1. In most cases, the appropriate next step in the work-up of an abnormal Pap smear is
   a. Endocervical curettage.
   b. Cryosurgery or laser vaporization.
   c. Repeat Pap smear.
   d. Colposcopic examination.
   e. Loop electrosurgical excision procedure (LEEP).

2. Drawbacks associated with cryosurgery include which of the following?
   a. Cervical stenosis
   b. Contraindicated during pregnancy
   c. Infertility
   d. Permanent distortion of the cervical transformation zone
   e. Both a and b
   f. Answers a, b, and d
   g. All of the above are drawbacks associated with cryosurgery.

3. Which of the following techniques preserves tissue for pathological examination?
   a. LEEP
   b. Cone biopsy
   c. Cryosurgery
   d. Laser vaporization
   e. None of the above
   f. Both a and b
   g. Both b and d

4. Lugol's solution
   a. Is an acetic acid preparation that turns abnormal cervical epithelium white.
   b. Is an iodine solution that stains nuclear material in dysplastic cervical cells.
   c. Is an iodine solution that stains glycogen stores in abnormal cervical cells but fails to stain normal cervical cells with low glycogen contents.
   d. Is an iodine solution that stains glycogen stores in normal cervical cells but fails to stain dysplastic cells with low glycogen contents.

5. A 57-year-old woman presents to the gynecologist's office with the complaint of vaginal bleeding. She entered menopause at age 54. She reports intermittent spotting for the last three months. She has no history of blood dyscrasias or other medical problems, and she is currently taking only 1200 mg of calcium and 400 IU of vitamin D along with a multivitamin. Appropriate work-up of this woman's vaginal bleeding would likely include which of the following?
   a. A trial of oral contraceptives to stabilize the uterine lining and mitigate the bleeding
   b. Review of CBC and treatment for anemia if indicated
   c. Endometrial biopsy and pathological examination
   d. LEEP or laser vaporization

CHAPTER 5:
ANESTHESIA IN OBSTETRICS AND GYNECOLOGY

1. A patient being prepared for surgery is inadvertently administered an excess of benzodiazepine, and her respiratory effort drops precipitously. Appropriate medical management may include administration of which of the following?
   a. Naloxone
   b. Midazolam
   c. Epinephrine
   d. Flumazenil

Questions 2–8 Match the following drug with its characteristic feature.
   a. Hepatic dysfunction has been reported in conjunction with its use
   b. Used to supplement other anesthetics due to its low potency
   c. A popular local anesthetic agent useful for regional blockades
   d. Used to supplement other anesthetics due to its low MAC
   e. A nonsteroidal agent used as an alternative to opioids

f. Used during the induction phase of anesthetic administration due to its rapid onset

g. A benzodiazepine derivative often used to premedicate patients undergoing anesthesia due to its antianxiety and amnesiac properties

h. An opioid antagonist used to reverse the respiratory depression caused by opioid overdose

i. An opioid agent commonly used in anesthesiology

2. Propofol (Diprivan)

3. Fentanyl

4. Midazolam (Versed)

5. Halothane

6. Nitrous oxide (N_2O)

7. Lidocaine

8. Ketorolac (Toradol)

9. The pain associated with the first stage of labor
   a. Travels to the thoracolumbar spinal cord.
   b. Travels via the pudendal nerve to the sacral spinal cord.
   c. Is often controlled by pudendal nerve blockade.
   d. Can be relieved with paracervical blockade but possibly at the risk of fetal bradycardia.
   e. Both a and d.
   f. Both b and c.

10. An appropriate landmark for the administration of a pudendal nerve blockade includes
   a. Ischial tuberosity.
   b. Uterosacral ligament.
   c. Posterior forchette.
   d. Ischial spine.
   e. Pudendal ligament.

Chapter 6:
Obstetric and Gynecologic Sonography

1. Gestational age
   a. Is most accurately measured during the first trimester via crown-rump length (CRL).
   b. Is most accurately measured during the first trimester via biparietal diameter (BPD).
   c. Is most accurately measured during the third trimester via CRL.
   d. Is most accurately measured during the second trimester via head circumference (HC).

2. Oligohydramnios is defined as
   a. An amniotic fluid index > 25 cm.
   b. An amniotic fluid index > 8 cm.
   c. An amniotic fluid index < 5 cm.
   d. An amniotic fluid index < 8 cm.

3. Select the most accurate statement regarding sonographic techniques.
   a. Higher-frequency ultrasound probes provide increased penetration but poorer resolution than lower-frequency ultrasound probes.
   b. Higher-frequency ultrasound probes provide better resolution but at the expense of decreased penetration compared to lower-frequency probes.
   c. Higher-frequency ultrasound probes provide increased penetration and better resolution than lower-frequency ultrasound probes.

Chapter 7:
Psychosocial Aspects of Women's Care

1. The leading cause of cancer death among women is
   a. Endometrial cancer.
   b. Breast cancer.
   c. Ovarian cancer.
   d. Cervical cancer.
   e. Lung cancer.

2. Requirements for the diagnosis of fetal alcohol syndrome include
   a. Growth retardation, facial dysmorphology, and limb abnormalities.
   b. Mental retardation, facial dysmorphology, and short stature.
   c. Growth retardation, central nervous system involvement, and facial dysmorphology.
   d. Mental retardation, facial dysmorphology, and history of maternal alcohol abuse during the pregnancy.

3. The approximate incidence of fetal alcohol syndrome is
   a. 3 per 100.

b. 3 per 1000.

c. 3 per 10,000.

d. 3 per 100,000.

4. A 34-year-old G1P0 with a history of major depression is currently in her second trimester of pregnancy. She has been treated with fluoxetine (Prozac) during the pregnancy and asks whether this treatment will impact her unborn baby. You reply that

   a. The limited research that has been done on the use of fluoxetine during pregnancy has failed to find any significant effects on global IQ, language, or behavioral development.

   b. The limited research on the use of antidepressant medication during pregnancy has indicated that, as a class, monoamine oxidase inhibitors (MAOIs) are safer than the selective serotonin reuptake inhibitors (SSRIs) and she should be switched to an MAOI if possible.

   c. The limited research that has been done on the use of fluoxetine during pregnancy indicates that it often has significant effects on global IQ, language, and behavioral development.

   d. Extensive research on this subject has confirmed that use of the fluoxetine during pregnancy has no significant effects on global IQ, language, or behavioral development.

5. Post-partum depression

   a. Is a fairly common disorder arising in as many as 25% of pregnancies.

   b. Often involves an element of post-partum psychosis that is responsive to antidepressant and/or antipsychotic medication.

   c. Occurs with higher frequency among patients with a history of major depression.

   d. Occurs with equal frequency among patients with a history of major depression and those without such a history.

CHAPTER 8:
PREVENTIVE SCREENING GUIDELINES

1. Standard guidelines in the preventive care of women include

   a. Routine Pap smears beginning at menarche or by 18 years of age.

   b. Routine Pap smears beginning at menopause.

   c. Routine Pap smears beginning at coitarche or by 18 years of age.

   d. Routine Pap smears in women with a personal or family history of cervical dysplasia.

   e. Routine Pap smears in women with a history of Chlamydia, herpes, genital warts, or any other sexually transmitted disease.

2. Select the most accurate statement regarding the American Cancer Society's screening guidelines.

   a. Digital rectal examination, fecal occult blood testing, and flexible sigmoidoscopy should begin at age 50 years, and sigmoidoscopy should be repeated every five years.

   b. Digital rectal examination should begin at age 30 years, fecal occult blood testing at 40 years, and flexible sigmoidoscopy at 50 years of age, with repeat sigmoidoscopy every five years.

   c. Digital rectal examination and fecal occult blood screening should begin at age 40 years, with flexible sigmoidoscopy recommended for patients with a positive family history of colon cancer or colonic polyps.

   d. Digital rectal examination and fecal occult blood screening should begin at age 40 years, and flexible sigmoidoscopy is recommended beginning at age 50 years, with repeat examinations every five years thereafter.

3. The American Cancer Society recommends routine mammograms beginning at

   a. 35 years.

   b. 40 years.

   c. 45 years.

   d. 50 years.

   e. Perimenopause.

   f. Menopause.

CHAPTER 9:
HUMAN SEXUALITY

1. Select the response that places the Masters and Johnson phases of sexual response in order from earliest to latest.

   a. Orgasm, excitement, plateau, resolution

   b. Excitement, orgasm, plateau, resolution

   c. Excitement, plateau, orgasm, resolution

   d. Excitement, orgasm, resolution, plateau

2. Female orgasm is characterized by
   a. Elevation and retraction of the clitoris, increased labial diameter, and nipple engorgement.
   b. Lengthening of the vaginal cul-de-sac, and vaginal and uterine contractions.
   c. Elevation of the cervix and elongation and distention of the vagina.
   d. Elevation of the uterus and clitoral descent.

3. Which of the following statements accurately explains the physiologic effects of menopause on female sexual function?
   a. Loss of estrogen leads to increased cornification of the vaginal epithelium with subsequent vaginal atrophy.
   b. Increased production of androgens sometimes leads to an increase in libido.
   c. Loss of estrogen leads to decreased cornification of the vaginal epithelium with subsequent vaginal atrophy.
   d. Loss of estrogen decreases vaginal lubrication and may contribute to dyspareunia.
   e. Both a and b.
   f. Both b and c.
   g. Answers a, b, and d.
   h. Answers b, c, and d.

CHAPTER 10:
HIV IN OBSTETRICS AND GYNECOLOGY

1. A patient presents to your office and describes an episode of unprotected sex that occurred five days ago. She is concerned about HIV infection and desires testing. Along with appropriate counseling about the HIV test, the possibility of pregnancy, and the risk of other sexually transmitted diseases, you should also
   a. Explain that she is required to tell her partner the results of the test and encourage him to get tested as well.
   b. Explain that since her potential exposure occurred so recently, the test may return falsely negative and she should be retested in six weeks, maintaining safe sexual practices during the time interval between tests.
   c. Explain that since her potential exposure occurred so recently, the test may return falsely negative and she should be retested in six months, maintaining safe sexual practices during the time interval between tests.

2. Which of the following is most accurate regarding the management of pregnant women infected with HIV?
   a. Their babies should be delivered by cesarean section due to the increased risk of HIV transmission to the fetus during transit through the vaginal canal, but breast-feeding is not contraindicated.
   b. Their babies should be delivered by cesarean section, and breast-feeding is discouraged.
   c. Their babies can be delivered vaginally, and breast-feeding is recommended.
   d. Their babies can be delivered vaginally, but breast-feeding is discouraged.

3. Prompt initiation of AZT therapy after the fourteenth week of gestation in HIV-infected women with CD4 counts greater than 200/mL has resulted in
   a. Reduction of HIV transmission to the fetus to 25%.
   b. Reduction of HIV transmission to the fetus to less than 10%.
   c. Limited effect on HIV transmission rates but milder HIV disease in the unborn fetus.
   d. A high risk of birth defects but reduction of HIV transmission to the unborn fetus.

CHAPTER 11:
MATERNAL/FETAL PHYSIOLOGY

Questions 1–5 Match the following descriptions with their appropriate terms.
   a. Estrogen
   b. Progesterone
   c. Human chorionic gonadotropin (hCG)
   d. Ladin's sign
   e. Goodell's sign
   f. Chadwick's sign
   g. Linea nigra
   h. Striae
   i. Relaxin

1. Bluish discoloration of the cervix used as a clinical indicator of pregnancy

2. Responsible for ductal proliferation of the breast

3. Responsible for areolar hypertrophy of the breast

4. Term used to describe the effects of alpha-melanocyte-stimulating hormone on the midline of lower abdomen

5. Compound responsible for changes in the symphysis pubis and uterine ligaments that facilitate the birthing process

6. The increased sensitivity of the maternal respiratory center to carbon dioxide that is seen during pregnancy is most likely the result of which of the following?
   a. Increased levels of estrogen acting directly on the respiratory center
   b. Increased levels of progesterone acting directly on the respiratory center
   c. Increased levels of human chorionic gonadotropin acting directly on the respiratory center
   d. Hyperventilation resulting from reduced diaphragmatic excursion and increased uterine mass

Questions 7–10 For the physiologic parameters listed, select from the following three choices the one that best describes the direction of change associated with pregnancy.
   a. Increase
   b. Decrease
   c. No change

7. Tidal volume

8. Systemic vascular resistance

9. Plasma volume

10. Red cell volume

11. Fetal hemoglobin efficiently extracts oxygen from maternal hemoglobin because
   a. It has an oxygen dissociation curve to the left of maternal hemoglobin and binds 2,3-DPG only weakly.
   b. It has an oxygen dissociation curve to the right of maternal hemoglobin and binds 2,3-DPG only weakly.
   c. It has an oxygen dissociation curve to the left of maternal hemoglobin and binds 2,3-DPG strongly.
   d. It has an oxygen dissociation curve to the right of maternal hemoglobin and binds 2,3-DPG strongly.

12. Estriol is
   a. Derived from a hormone produced by the fetal adrenal gland.
   b. The product of placental conversion of another hormone.
   c. A component of the "triple screen" used to assess fetal well-being.
   d. Both a and b.
   e. Both b and c.
   f. Both a and c.
   g. All of the above.

CHAPTER 12:
PRECONCEPTION AND ANTEPARTUM CARE

Questions 1–5 Select the number of weeks of gestation at which each of the following procedures or tests is routinely performed. Answers may be used more than once.
   a. 5 weeks
   b. 8 weeks
   c. 12 weeks
   d. 16 weeks
   e. 20 weeks
   f. 28 weeks
   g. 36 weeks
   h. None of the above

1. Urinary hCG is detectable by home pregnancy tests.

2. Rho-GAM is administered, if indicated.

3. Triple screening test is offered.

4. Rubella vaccine is administered to nonimmune mothers.

5. Screening glucose tolerance testing is administered to patients without known risk factors for gestational diabetes.

CHAPTER 13:
GENETIC COUNSELING

1. Down syndrome is associated with
   a. Elevated maternal serum alpha-fetoprotein (MSAFP) detected during the triple screen.
   b. Depressed maternal serum alpha-fetoprotein (MSAFP) detected during the triple screen.
   c. Depressed maternal hCG detected during the triple screen.

d. Elevated maternal hCG detected during the triple screen.
e. Elevated estriol detected during the triple screen.
f. Depressed estriol detected during the triple screen.
g. Answers b, c, and f.
h. Answers b, c, and e.
i. Answers b, d, and f.
j. Answers b, d, and e.
k. Answers a, d, and f.
l. Answers a, d, and e.

2. The risk of procedure-associated miscarriage during routine amniocentesis is approximately
a. 1 in 50.
b. 1 in 100.
c. 1 in 200.
d. 1 in 300.
e. 1 in 400.
f. 1 in 500.

3. All of the following may cause an elevated maternal serum alpha-fetoprotein (MSAFP) except:
a. Multiple gestations.
b. Fetal demise.
c. Open neural tube defect.
d. Gastrointestinal atresia.
e. Renal agensis.

4. BRCA-1 and BRCA-2 are
a. Oncogenes that, if detected in a female patient, predict that she will develop breast and/or ovarian cancer some time in her life.
b. Suspected tumor suppressor genes, specific mutations which are associated with an increased risk of breast and/or ovarian cancer.
c. Suspected tumor suppressor genes that, if present, predict early-onset breast and/or ovarian cancer compared with women who do not have the genes.
d. None of the above.

CHAPTER 14:
FIRST TRIMESTER BLEEDING

1. Select the most accurate statement regarding first trimester bleeding.
a. First trimester bleeding is a common problem but rarely results in spontaneous abortion.

b. First trimester bleeding is an uncommon problem but when it occurs usually results in spontaneous abortion.
c. First trimester bleeding is a fairly common problem in obstetrics and results in spontaneous abortion in nearly one-half of all cases.
d. First trimester bleeding is an uncommon problem in obstetrics that rarely leads to pregnancy loss.

Questions 2–4 Match the following terms with their appropriate description.
a. Threatened abortion
b. Spontaneous abortion
c. Inevitable abortion
d. Missed abortion
e. Complete abortion
f. Incomplete abortion

2. The patient presents with bleeding and an open cervical os.

3. The patient presents with bleeding and a closed cervical os.

4. The patient presents with a history of bleeding two days ago; vaginal ultrasound reveals absence of a gestational sac and no fetal heart beat; the cervical os is closed.

5. Recurrent abortion is defined as a history of how many successive pregnancy losses?
a. 1
b. 2
c. 3
d. 4
e. There is no set number.

6. A woman with a history of two or more abortions who has never delivered a liveborn infant has approximately what risk of having another abortion during her next pregnancy?
a. 20%
b. 30%
c. 40%
d. 60%
e. 80%
f. near 100%

CHAPTER 15:
MULTIPLE GESTATIONS

1. Twin–twin transfusion syndrome
a. Results when vascular anastamoses be-

tween the placentas cause one twin to receive preferentially more blood supply
than the other.

b. Results when there is blood type incompatibility between the twins of a multiple gestation, causing antibody formation against
the blood type perceived as foreign.

c. Results when vascular anastamoses between the placentas fail to develop adequately.

d. Results when the placental villi develop
abnormally, causing a relative fetal hypoxia that is compensated for by preferen-
tial routing blood from one twin to the
hypoxic twin.

2. The incidence of multiple gestations

  a. Decreases with maternal age.

  b. Increases with maternal age.

  c. Is independent of maternal age.

CHAPTER 16:
ISOIMMUNIZATION IN PREGNANCY

1. Which of the following accurately conveys
the relationship between Rh and ABO compati-
bilities?

  a. Rh incompatibility between mother and
fetus occurs only in the presence of concomitant ABO incompatibility.

  b. ABO incompatibility between mother and
fetus increases the chance of Rh isoimmunization.

  c. ABO incompatibility between mother and
fetus decreases the chance of Rh isoimmunization.

  d. ABO and Rh incompatibility have no significant relationship to each other.

2. A G2P0010 female presents at 19 weeks gestation. Routine testing has revealed that she has
Rh antibodies present in her blood. Select the
most accurate statement regarding her continued
management.

  a. Because she is already sensitized, she
should be given Rho-GAM immediately to
prevent isoimmunization during this pregnancy.

  b. Because she is already sensitized, she
should be given prophylactic Rho-GAM at
28 weeks gestation.

  c. She is not a candidate for Rho-GAM because she is already sensitized. Maternal
antibody titer should be determined and

monitored carefully throughout the subsequent weeks.

  d. She is not a candidate for Rho-GAM because she is already sensitized. The fetus is
likely to abort some time during the second
trimester.

3. The Liley curve

  a. Measures maternal Rh antibody titers so as
to assess the risk of transmission of antibodies to the fetus.

  b. Provides a means by which to monitor fetal
hemolysis and thus assess the degree of
fetal compromise secondary to Rh-anti-
body-mediated red blood cell destruction.

  c. Provides a means by which to monitor fetal
hematocrit so as to assess the degree of
hemolysis secondary to Rh-antibody-medi-
ated red blood cell destruction.

  d. Is a means to monitor the degree of fetal
hydropic change and help determine when
delivery is indicated so as to increase the
chances of fetal viability.

CHAPTER 17:
FETAL GROWTH ABNORMALITIES

1. Fetuses failing to grow in utero to their full potential are said to be

  a. Growth-retarded.

  b. Growth-restricted.

  c. Small for gestational age.

  d. Microsomic.

  e. Immature.

2. A 4300 g infant is delivered at 40 weeks gestation to a mother whose pregnancy has been complicated by gestational diabetes. This infant is
probably

  a. Post-term.

  b. Post-mature.

  c. Asymmetrically macrosomic with increased head circumference compared to
abdominal circumference.

  d. Asymmetrically macrosomic with increased abdominal circumference compared to head circumference.

CHAPTER 18:
TERATOLOGY

1. Select the statement regarding birth defects
that is most accurate.

  a. Genetic abnormalities account for approximately 45% of developmental defects.

b. The etiology of birth defects is most often due to fetal exposure to teratogens and other environmental agents.

c. Birth defects are rare in the absence of a family history of genetic anomalies or a maternal history of multiple spontaneous abortions.

d. The etiology of birth defects is frequently multifactorial and often unknown.

Questions 2–6 Match the following drug with the fetal effect with which maternal use during pregnancy has been most commonly associated.

a. Thalidomide

b. Valproic acid

c. Phenytoin

d. Lithium

e. Androgens

f. Diethylstilbestrol

g. Tobacco

h. Marijuana

2. A female infant is born with a T-shaped uterus.

3. An infant is born with rudimentary limb buds.

4. An infant is born premature with low birth weight and head circumference at the fifth percentile.

5. An infant is born with a neural tube defect.

6. An infant exhibits the Ebstein anomaly.

7. The TORCH infections are

a. Toxoplasmosis, rubella, cytomegalovirus (CMV), herpes simplex virus (HSV)

b. Toxoplasmosis, rubella, Chlamydia, HSV

c. Toxoplasmosis, rubella, CMV, human papillomavirus (HPV)

d. Toxoplasmosis, rubella, Chlamydia, HPV

e. Toxoplasmosis, RSV, CMV, HSV

8. An infant is born with microcephaly, micrognathia, cardiac and renal anomalies, and unusually shaped feet. This infant is exhibiting a constellation of features most characteristic of

a. Organic mercury exposure.

b. Organic lead exposure.

c. Exposure to ionizing radiation.

d. Trisomy 13.

e. Trisomy 15.

f. Trisomy 18.

g. Trisomy 21.

CHAPTER 19: PRETERM LABOR

1. Preterm delivery is defined as

a. Delivery of an infant with a lecithin: sphingomyelin ratio of less than 2:1.

b. Delivery of a low-birth-weight infant.

c. Delivery of a very-low-birth-weight infant.

d. Delivery at less than 37 weeks.

e. Delivery at less than 40 weeks.

2. Ritrodine is

a. A beta-antagonist that relaxes uterine smooth muscle and is used as a tocolytic agent to abort preterm labor.

b. A tocolytic agent that may work by competing with calcium in uterine smooth muscle, thus reducing muscle cell excitability.

c. A beta-agonist that relaxes uterine smooth muscle but may be associated with maternal tachycardia and/or pulmonary edema.

d. An alpha-agonist that relaxes uterine smooth muscle and is the preferred agent for tocolysis in most cases.

e. None of the above.

3. A G1P0 patient at 28 weeks gestation presents in preterm labor. If the decision is made to attempt to abort her labor, administration of all of the following might be indicated except:

a. Terbutaline.

b. Magnesium sulfate.

c. Ritodrine.

d. Prostaglandin.

e. Calcium-channel blocker.

4. A G2P1 patient presents in preterm labor at 30 weeks gestation. Results of amniocentesis indicate a lecithin:sphingomyelin ratio of 1.5, consistent with fetal lung immaturity. The decision is made to

a. Administer indomethacin to promote fetal lung maturity.

b. Administer betamethasone to promote fetal lung maturity, as well as ritodrine to abort uterine contractions.

c. Administer ritodrine to promote fetal lung maturity and abort uterine contractions.

d. Administer misoprostol to promote fetal lung maturity, as well as ritodrine to abort uterine contractions.

e. Deliver the infant emergently and prepare for supplemental oxygen and/or intubation if required.

CHAPTER 20:
PREMATURE RUPTURE OF MEMBRANES

1. Which of the following situations most likely represent(s) premature rupture of membranes (PROM) or preterm premature rupture of membranes (PPROM)?

   a. A G1P0 patient at 38 weeks gestation presents in labor with a ruptured amniotic sac, but her infant is not delivered until 60 hours later.

   b. A G2P1 patient at 33 weeks gestation presents with progressive dilation and effacement of the cervix and ruptured membranes. Despite administration of tocolytics, she delivers 48 hours later.

   c. A G6P0 patient at 24 weeks gestation presents in labor with ruptured membranes. After a brief trial of labor, the infant experiences an episode of fetal bradycardia and is delivered by emergent cesarean section 36 hours later.

   d. A G2P1 patient at 36 weeks gestation presents reporting a sudden gush of fluid from her vagina. She is placed on a monitor and no contractions are present. A swab of the vaginal fluid reveals a pH of 6.0 without ferning.

   e. Both a and b.

   f. Both a and c.

   g. Both a and d.

   h. All of the above.

   i. None of the above.

2. A G1P0 patient at 38 weeks gestation presents with a history of her "water breaking." Which of the following features of a vaginal fluid sample taken from the posterior vagina is consistent with the diagnosis of PROM?

   a. Nitrazine paper turns blue

   b. Fluid exhibits ferning

   c. Nitrazine paper turns orange

   d. Fluid exhibits stringing

   e. Both a and b.

   f. Both b and c.

   g. Both a and d.

3. A G2P1 patient at 32 weeks gestation presents with PPROM. Culture of the amniotic fluid reveals group B streptococcus. Which of the following statements regarding her diagnosis and subsequent management is most accurate?

   a. The infant is preterm. Lung maturity should be assessed via phosphotidylglycerol mea-surement and betamethasone administered if the fetal lungs are deemed immature. The patient should be delivered by cesarean section 24 hours after administration of betamethasone.

   b. The patient has chorioamnionitis and the infant is likely to be immature. The mother should receive tocolytics and betamethasone to facilitate fetal lung maturity.

   c. The patient has chorioamnionitis. Delivery should be expedited and intravenous antibiotics begun.

   d. The patient has chorioamnionitis. Intravenous antibiotics should be begun along with administration of tocolytics to attempt to abort labor and premature delivery.

4. All of the following developmental abnormalities have been associated with oligohydramnios except:

   a. Lung hypoplasia.

   b. Compression deformity of the limbs.

   c. Renal hypoplasia.

   d. Facial deformity.

   e. Growth restriction.

   f. Umbilical cord compression.

CHAPTER 21:
THIRD TRIMESTER BLEEDING

1. Placenta previa complicates one in approximately how many births?

   a. 250

   b. 100

   c. 2500

   d. 1000

2. Abdominal pain and third trimester bleeding are classically associated with

   a. Placenta previa.

   b. Abruptio placenta.

   c. Both placenta previa and abruptio placenta.

   d. Neither placenta previa nor abruptio placenta.

3. Which of the following is not considered a direct risk factor for placental abruption?

   a. Gestational diabetes

   b. Maternal hypertension

   c. Polyhydramnios

   d. Antiphospholipid syndrome

4. An appropriate first step in the work-up of third-trimester bleeding includes
   a. Pelvic examination.
   b. Obstetrical ultrasound.
   c. NST and external monitoring of uterine contractions.
   d. Amniocentesis to rule out chorioamnionitis.
   e. None of the above.

5. The Kleihauer-Betke test is used
   a. To detect maternal/fetal Rh isoimmunization.
   b. To test for amniotic fluid.
   c. To detect fetal blood cells in the maternal circulation.
   d. To detect fetal chromosomal anomalies from cells obtained by amniocentesis.

6. An appropriate delivery technique in a woman presenting at 36 weeks gestation with a placenta previa is generally
   a. Cesarean section.
   b. Vaginal delivery.
   c. Most dependent on the patient's Bishop's score of cervical readiness for delivery.

7. Placenta accreta refers to
   a. Trophoblastic invasion into the uterine myometrium and is a complication most commonly associated with abruptio placenta.
   b. Trophoblastic invasion into the uterine submucosa and is a complication most commonly associated with placenta previa.
   c. Trophoblastic invasion into the uterine submucosa and is a complication most commonly associated with abruptio placenta.
   d. Trophoblastic invasion into the uterine myometrium and is a complication most commonly associated with placenta previa.
   e. Stiffening of the uterine myometrium as a result of extravasated blood from an abruptio placenta.

CHAPTER 22:
PRE-ECLAMPSIA AND ECLAMPSIA

1. Which of the following statements most accurately defines the onset of pre-eclampsia?
   a. It classically occurs less than 20 weeks into a patient's first pregnancy.
   b. It classically occurs at more than 20 weeks into a patient's first pregnancy.
   c. It classically occurs in women with a history of essential hypertension.

2. The diagnosis of pre-eclampsia requires the triad of
   a. Hypertension, hematuria, and proteinuria.
   b. Hypertension, glucosuria, and edema.
   c. Hypertension, proteinuria, and edema.
   d. Hypertension, proteinuria, and hypoalbuminemia.
   e. Hypertension, proteinuria, and mental status changes.

3. A 32-year-old G1P0 at 36 weeks gestation presents with right upper quadrant pain. On physical examination, the patient exhibits fluctuating mental status. CBC reveals WBC 9000, Hb 10.3, and platelets 87,000. Of the following choices, which is most likely to assist in the diagnosis?
   a. Fetal ultrasound to rule out ectopic pregnancy
   b. Right upper quadrant ultrasound to rule out the presence of cystic duct obstruction
   c. Liver function tests to rule out viral hepatitis
   d. Liver function tests to evaluate for HELLP syndrome
   e. MRI to rule out an acute hemorrhagic episode secondary to the patient's low platelet count

4. Appropriate treatment for cardiac arrest related to elevated $MgSO_4$ levels includes
   a. Calcium sulfate to stabilize the cardiac cell membrane potential.
   b. Calcium gluconate to stabilize the cardiac cell membrane potential.
   c. Potassium gluconate to stabilize the cardiac cell membrane potential.
   d. Subcutaneous epinephrine to stimulate the heart's electrical activity.
   e. Activated charcoal to block further absorption of magnesium sulfate.

5. The etiology of pre-eclampsia is associated with
   a. Elevated levels of cyclo-oxygenase relative to thromboxane.
   b. Elevated cyclo-oxygenase and thromboxane.
   c. Elevated levels of thromboxane relative to cyclo-oxygenase.

d. Decreased platelet activation.

e. Vascular hypersensitivity to fetal trophoblastic factors.

6. Regarding the seizures associated with eclampsia,

    a. Seizures most commonly occur during delivery.

    b. Seizures occurring immediately postpartum suggests the development of HELLP syndrome.

    c. Seizures occurring after delivery suggest an etiology unrelated to eclampsia.

    d. Preferred seizure prophylaxis is $MgSO_4$.

CHAPTER 23:
MEDICAL AND SURGICAL COMPLICATIONS OF PREGNANCY

1. The most common cause of anemia during pregnancy is

    a. Folate deficiency.

    b. Maternal–fetal transfusion.

    c. Iron deficiency.

    d. Occult bleeding.

2. Of the following statements regarding the etiology of anemia during pregnancy, which is most accurate?

    a. It occurs because a pregnant woman's intestines have a diminished capacity to absorb ingested iron.

    b. It is a dilutional anemia that occurs because a pregnant woman's plasma volume expands while her red cell mass remains constant.

    c. It occurs because a pregnant woman's red blood cell mass falls during pregnancy.

    d. It occurs because a pregnant woman's red blood cell mass rises to a greater extent than her plasma volume.

    e. It occurs because a pregnant woman's plasma volume rises to a greater extent than her red blood cell mass.

3. Which maternal deficiency is most closely associated with fetal neural tube defects?

    a. Folate

    b. Vitamin B_{12}

    c. Thiamine

    d. Iron

    e. AFP

4. An African American couple is referred for genetic counseling. They have two children, one boy and one girl, each of whom has the sickle cell trait. Neither of the parents has sickle cell anemia. The woman is now pregnant with the couple's third child. Without any additional information, you can tell them that the most likely risk of the fetus being born with sickle cell anemia is:

    a. 0% to 25%.

    b. 26% to 50%.

    c. 51% to 75%.

    d. 76% to 100%.

    e. Cannot be determined without further information.

5. The diabetogenic hormone associated with pregnancy is

    a. Prolactin.

    b. Estrogen.

    c. Progesterone.

    d. Human placental lactogen.

6. In patients with no increased risk of gestational diabetes, during what trimester of pregnancy is the glucose tolerance test best performed?

    a. First trimester

    b. Second trimester

    c. Third trimester

    d. During prenatal counseling

7. Which of the following is the most appropriate next step in the management of gestational diabetes refractory to diet therapy alone?

    a. Addition of oral hypoglycemics

    b. Addition of oral insulin

    c. Addition of subcutaneous insulin

    d. Addition of oral hypoglycemics plus subcutaneous insulin as needed

8. Which of the following is (are) appropriate indications for cesarean delivery?

    a. HIV infection or the presence of active herpes simplex vaginal lesions

    b. Gestational diabetes or a history of herpes zoster

    c. The presence of active herpes simplex vaginal lesions or a positive group B streptococcal culture obtained at 26 weeks

    d. The presence of active herpes simplex vaginal lesions

    e. Active or latent herpes simplex infection

9. Which of the following medications has been used as prophylaxis for genital herpes?
   a. Amiodarone
   b. Ganciclovir
   c. Acyclovir
   d. Amantadine

10. A 29-year-old G1P0 schoolteacher has been exposed to a child with rubella. She reports no history of prior rubella immunization. Appropriate management of the patient now includes:
   a. Measurement of serum antibody titers and monitoring of the mother for signs of infection.
   b. Measurement of serum antibody titers and administration of rubella vaccine.
   c. Measurement of serum antibody titers and administration of rubella immune globulin.
   d. Termination of the pregnancy.

11. An infant is born with deafness, cataracts, and a patent ductus arteriorus. Which of the following is most likely to have occurred during the pregnancy?
   a. The mother has a history of herpes simplex infection.
   b. The mother was exposed to varicella zoster during the pregnancy.
   c. During the pregnancy, the mother reported an illness characterized by low-grade fever and lymphadenopathy.
   d. The mother is positive for the hepatitis B surface antigen.
   e. The mother has a history of untreated syphilis.

12. Appropriate management of the infant born to a mother who is positive for hepatitis B surface antigen includes:
   a. Hepatitis immune globulin at delivery.
   b. Hepatitis immunization beginning at delivery.
   c. Hepatitis immune globulin at delivery and hepatitis immunization beginning at birth.
   d. Hepatitis immune globulin at delivery and hepatitis immunization beginning three months after birth.

13. Vertical transmission of hepatitis B is most common when the mother has which of the following antigen profiles?
   a. Hepatitis B surface antigen positive
   b. Hepatitis B surface antigen and e antigen positive
   c. Hepatitis B surface antigen and c antigen positive
   d. Hepatitis B surface antigen and d antigen positive

14. Which of the following statements regarding the management of medical problems during pregnancy is most accurate?
   a. Preferred medical management of hypertension during pregnancy is with thiazide diuretics.
   b. Most adnexal masses discovered routinely are benign.
   c. AZT should be avoided in early pregnancy due to its teratogenic effects.
   d. Inhaled steroids and beta agonists are to be avoided in the treatment of pregnant asthmatics.

CHAPTER 24:
POST-TERM PREGNANCY

1. Select the statement that most accurately describes the post-term pregnancy.
   a. Defined as extension of pregnancy beyond 42 weeks, the causes of post-term pregnancy are often unknown; post-term pregnancy poses a threat mostly for the fetus rather than the mother.
   b. Defined as extension of pregnancy beyond 42 weeks, the causes of post-term pregnancy are often unknown; post-term pregnancy poses a threat mostly for the mother rather than the fetus.
   c. Defined as extension of pregnancy beyond 40 weeks, the causes of post-term pregnancy are often unknown; post-term pregnancy poses a significant threat to both fetus and mother.
   d. Defined as extension of pregnancy beyond 42 weeks, the causes of post-term pregnancy are often unknown; post-term pregnancy poses a significant threat to both fetus and mother.

2. How does perinatal mortality at 42 weeks gestation compare to mortality at term?
   a. 1:1
   b. 2:1
   c. 1:2
   d. 4:1
   e. 1:4

3. Which of the following accurately defines a reactive nonstress test (NST)?

a. Two episodes of fetal heart rate acceleration of ≥15 beats per minute over baseline, lasting ≥15 seconds during a 20-minute observation period

b. Two episodes of fetal heart rate acceleration of ≥ 15 beats per minute over baseline, or two accelerations lasting ≥15 seconds during a 20-minute observation period

c. Two spontaneous decelerations in fetal heart rate of ≤15 beats per minute under baseline, lasting ≤15 seconds in response to two separate uterine contractions during a 20-minute observation period

d. Two episodes of fetal heart rate acceleration of ≥15 beats per minute over baseline, lasting ≤15 seconds during a 20-minute observation period

4. Contraction stress test (CST) results are considered accurate predictors of fetal survival over what time interval?

a. 3 to 4 days

b. 1 week

c. 10 days

d. 2 weeks

5. Which of the following set of test results suggests the most favorable outcome for the fetus?

a. A nonreactive NST and negative CST

b. A reactive NST and positive CST

c. A reactive NST and negative CST

d. A nonreactive NST and positive CST

6. All of the following are used as components of the biophysical profile except:

a. Amniotic fluid volume.

b. Fetal heart rate.

c. Fetal tone.

d. Fetal breathing.

e. Fetal body movement.

f. All of the above are components of the biophysical profile.

CHAPTER 25:
INTRAPARTUM CARE: MANAGEMENT OF LABOR AND DELIVERY

1. Which of the following defines the third stage of normal labor?

a. From the onset of regular contractions until cervical dilation to 10 cm

b. From the onset of regular contractions until full cervical dilation

c. From full cervical dilation until delivery of the fetus and placenta

d. From full cervical dilation until delivery of the fetus

e. From delivery of the fetus until delivery of the placenta

f. From delivery of the placenta through the first one to two hours post-partum

2. Which of the following descriptions is most accurate?

a. Effacement describes the increase in cervical aperture that occurs during normal labor.

b. Dilation refers to the thinning of the cervix that occurs during labor.

c. Dilation is associated with active phase I labor, while effacement occurs during latent phase I labor.

d. Dilation and effacement occur successively during normal labor.

e. None of the above is accurate.

3. Which of the following places the cardinal movements of labor in order from earliest to latest?

a. Flexion, descent, engagement, internal rotation, external rotation, expulsion

b. Engagement, descent, internal rotation, flexion, expulsion, external rotation

c. Flexion, extension, descent, internal rotation, expulsion, external rotation

d. Engagement, descent, flexion, internal rotation, external rotation, extension

e. Engagement, descent, flexion, internal rotation, extension, external rotation

4. Fetal presentation may be determined by performing the

a. Leopold maneuvers.

b. Bishop maneuvers.

c. Cardinal maneuvers.

d. Leonard maneuvers.

e. Ritken maneuvers.

5. The presence of amniotic fluid may be confirmed with which of the following tests?

a. Kleihauer-Betke

b. Nitroblue

c. Bishop

d. Nitrazine

6. Prolonged, latent-phase labor is best treated with

a. Therapeutic rest.

b. Oxytocin.

c. Cesarean section.

d. Magnesium sulfate.

7. Molding is most accurately described as the

a. Overlapping of fetal cranial sutures that occurs during navigation of the fetal head through the birth canal.

b. Encircling of the vulvar ring by the fetal head as it traverses the birth canal.

c. Thinning of the cervix to accommodate the fetal presenting part.

d. Relaxation of the pelvic ligaments to allow passage of the fetal head through the birth canal.

8. Post-partum hemorrhage during a vaginal delivery is defined as loss of

a. >100 cm^3

b. >300 cm^3

c. >500 cm^3

d. >1000 cm^3

CHAPTER 26:
ABNORMAL LABOR AND FETAL DISTRESS

1. Which of the following most accurately characterizes the relative benefits and drawbacks of internal versus external monitoring of fetal heart rate?

a. Internal monitoring provides more accurate data regarding long-term heart rate variability but carries excess risk of infection.

b. External monitoring provides more accurate data regarding long-term heart rate variability, while internal monitoring gives a better record of beat-to-beat variability.

c. Internal monitoring requires rupture of membranes and may introduce infection, but provides a better record of beat-to-beat heart rate variability.

d. Internal monitoring gives better information on beat-to-beat heart rate variability and can also be used to monitor uterine contractions; however, it carries excess risk of infection.

2. Diminished beat-to-beat heart rate variability is often an indicator of

a. Umbilical cord compression.

b. Head compression.

c. Uteroplacental insufficiency.

d. Fetal anoxia or other central nervous system impairment.

e. None of the above.

Questions 3–5 Match the type of deceleration with the cause with which it is most commonly associated. Answers may be used more than once.

a. Late deceleration

b. Delayed deceleration

c. Early deceleration

d. Variable deceleration

e. Invariable deceleration

3. The result of umbilical cord compression

4. A sign of uteroplacental insufficiency

5. The result of head compression

6. A G3P2 patient at 40 weeks gestation is being monitored on the labor and delivery floor. An external fetal heart rate monitor has begun to reveal severe variable decelerations. All of the following may be appropriate in her management except:

a. Change in maternal position.

b. Amnioinfusion.

c. Preparation for possible cesarean delivery.

d. Administration of maternal oxygen.

e. Administration of oxytocin.

7. Components of the Bishop's score include all of the following except:

a. Fetal presentation.

b. Fetal position.

c. Cervical effacement.

d. Cervical dilation.

e. Cervical consistency.

8. A normal fetal lie is defined as

a. Fetal head fully engaged within the pelvis.

b. Fetal spine longitudinal to maternal spine.

c. Flexion of the fetal hips and extension of the fetal legs.

d. Vertex forward occiput position.

Questions 9 and 10 Match the following terms with their appropriate definitions.

a. Frank breech

b. Footling breech

c. Complete breech

d. Incomplete breech

e. Partial breech

f. Transverse breech

9. Flexion of the fetal hips and legs

10. Flexion of the fetal hips and extension of the fetal legs

11. The most common reason for cesarean sections in the United States today is

a. Cephalopelvic disproportion.

b. Fetal distress.

c. Failure of labor to progress.

d. Repeat cesarean section.

12. Contraindications to vaginal birth following a cesarean section include

a. Classical uterine incision.

b. Low vertical incision.

c. Low transverse incision.

d. Two or more previous low transverse cesarean sections.

e. Both a and b.

f. Answers a, b, and d.

CHAPTER 27:
OPERATIVE VAGINAL DELIVERY

1. All of the following criteria are necessary for the use of outlet forceps except:

a. Fetal skull is on the pelvic floor.

b. Fetal head is on the perineum.

c. Rotation > 45°.

d. Fetal scalp visible at the introitus without separating the labia.

e. Sagittal suture in the anterior-posterior or ROA/LOA position.

2. The most common type of female pelvis is

a. Platypelloid.

b. Android.

c. Anthropoid.

d. Gynecoid.

3. The most worrisome complication associated with shoulder dystocia is

a. Shoulder dislocation.

b. Auerbach plexus injury.

c. Radial nerve injury.

d. Brachial plexus injury.

CHAPTER 28:
NEONATAL ASSESSMENT

1. Which of the following accurately outlines the flow of the majority of oxygenated blood carried to the infant from the placenta?

a. Umbilical vein → inferior vena cava → ductus venosus → left atrium → left ventricle

b. Umbilical artery → ductus arteriosus → inferior vena cava → left atrium → left ventricle

c. Umbilical vein → ductus venosus → inferior vena cava → left atrium → left ventricle

d. Umbilical artery → ductus venosus → inferior vena cava → left atrium → left ventricle

e. Umbilical vein → ductus venosus → inferior vena cava → right atrium → right ventricle

2. During fetal life, the direction of blood flow between the ductus arteriosus and the aorta is correctly described by which of the following?

a. From aorta to ductus arteriosus

b. From ductus arteriosus to aorta

3. A patent ductus arteriosus in a three-week-old infant would exhibit blood flow in which direction?

a. From aorta to ductus arteriosus

b. From ductus arteriosus to aorta

4. A preterm infant has a patent ductus arteriosus. To close the ductus, this infant may be treated with

a. Misoprostol.

b. Prostaglandins.

c. Prostaglandin inhibitors.

d. Glucocorticoids.

e. Epinephrine.

Questions 5–7 Match the following component of the fetal circulation with its most accurate description.

a. Shunts blood away from the liver and toward the inferior vena cava

b. Shunts blood away from the liver and toward the umbilical artery

c. Shunts blood away from the fetal lungs and toward the aorta

d. Connects the umbilical artery to the inferior vena cava

e. Connects the right and left ventricles

f. Connects the right and left atria

g. Connects the left atrium and left ventricle

5. Ductus arteriosus

6. Foramen ovale

7. Ductus venosus

8. An infant has just been delivered after a lengthy labor. At one minute, the infant's heart rate is 120 beats per minute and she is gasping for breath. She has good flexion of arms and legs and coughs in response to the insertion of nasal prongs. She is uniformly bluish in color. Based on this information, what is her Apgar score at one minute?

a. 5

b. 6

c. 7

d. 8

9. All of the following are problems commonly associated with prematurity except:

a. Intraventricular hemorrhage.

b. Necrotizing enterocolitis.

c. Shoulder dystocia.

d. Hyaline membrane disease.

10. Vitamin K is administered to infants at delivery so as to

a. Prevent direct hyperbilirubinemia due to immature infant liver conjugating ability.

b. Prevent indirect hyperbilirubinemia and kernicterus in the newborn.

c. Prevent hemorrhagic disease of the newborn.

d. Lessen jaundice and peak bilirubin levels in the newborn.

e. Provide excess nutrition for preterm infants.

11. Peak bilirubin levels in term infants generally occur

a. During the first day of life.

b. During days 3 to 4 of life.

c. During day 7 of life.

d. During days 10 to 14 of life.

CHAPTER 29:
POST-PARTUM CARE

1. Lochia is

a. A term used to describe the period of time immediately after delivery of the newborn.

b. A term used to describe the vaginal dis-

charge that may be present for several weeks following a normal delivery.

c. Suggestive of the presence of retained placental products that should be removed from the uterus.

d. The result of persistent uterine bleeding after delivery and may be stopped with oxytocin or methylergonovine.

2. In women who choose to breast-feed, estrogen-containing oral contraceptives are not recommended primarily because

a. There is increased risk of thromboembolism.

b. Estrogen may decrease milk production.

c. Estrogen may decrease milk nutrient quantity.

d. Estrogen interferes with normal suckling.

e. The estrogen present in the mother's milk affects the sexual development of the infant.

3. Circumcision is

a. A necessary component in the care of the newborn male.

b. May confer some protection from penile cancer and urinary tract infections compared to uncircumcised males.

c. Should be performed under general anesthesia.

d. Protects the male against infection with a variety of sexually transmitted diseases.

CHAPTER 30:
LACTATION

Questions 1–3 Match the following substance(s) with the statement that reflects its function in lactation.

a. Progesterone

b. Estrogen

c. Estrogen and progesterone

d. Oxytocin

e. Luteinizing hormone

f. Prolactin

1. Stimulates milk ejection

2. Its withdrawal permits lactogenesis to occur

3. Required for continued milk production

4. Compared with mature breast milk, colostrum is higher in

a. Fat.

b. Protein.

c. Lactose.

d. Kcal/dL.

e. Both a and d.

f. Both b and d.

5. Which of the following statements regarding breastfed infants compared to formula-fed infants is true?

a. Breastfed infants suffer from fewer upper respiratory and urinary tract infections than formula-fed babies.

b. Breastfed infants appear to have a lower incidence of some diseases that occur after the newborn period.

c. Breast milk has a protective role in the risk of necrotizing enterocolitis.

d. Breastfed infants suffer from less allergies than formula-fed infants.

e. All of the above are true.

6. Progesterone-containing oral contraceptives

a. Are contraindicated in a breast-feeding mother.

b. Confer an added risk of thromboembolic events in breast-feeding women.

c. Have a protective effect against ovarian and endometrial cancer due to their inhibition of ovulation.

d. Have a protective effect against breast and endometrial cancer due to their inhibition of ovulation.

7. Bromocriptine

a. Is an agent that suppresses prolactin secretion and was once recommended to inhibit lactation in women who chose not to breast-feed.

b. Is an agent that suppresses oxytocin secretion and was once recommended to inhibit lactation in women who chose not to breast-feed.

c. Is an agent used to treat mastitis.

d. Is an agent used to stimulate milk formation in women who have limited natural breast milk production.

CHAPTER 31:
POST-PARTUM INFECTION

1. Endomyometritis

a. Is more common after vaginal delivery than cesarean delivery.

b. Is most commonly caused by group B streptococcal infection.

c. Is rarely accompanied by vaginal discharge.

d. Complicates 10% to 20% of vaginal deliveries.

e. Both a and b.

f. Answers a, b, and d.

g. All of the above.

h. None of the above.

2. Risk factors for endomyometritis include

a. Cesarean section.

b. Vaginal delivery.

c. Prolonged rupture of membranes.

d. Preterm delivery.

e. Multiple gestations.

f. Both a and c.

g. Both b and c.

h. Answers a, c, and d.

i. Answers b, c, and d

3. A G1P1 female delivered a full-term infant via spontaneous vaginal delivery six days ago. She developed fevers to 38.6 °C on post-partum day 3. Cultures of the uterus grew multiple organisms, and she was treated empirically with intravenous gentamicin and clindamycin. After failing to improve on antibiotic therapy, a CT of the pelvis was performed, which revealed bilateral thrombi of the pelvic vessels. Her continued management is likely to include

a. Emergent surgical removal of the thrombi.

b. Pelvic revascularization.

c. IV warfarin therapy.

d. IV heparin therapy.

e. Discontinuation of antibiotics with close monitoring and physical therapy to encourage clot dislodgment.

CHAPTER 32:
MANAGING HEMORRHAGING COMPLICATIONS IN OBSTETRICS AND GYNECOLOGY

1. All of the following drugs may be helpful in the management of acute uterine bleeding except:

a. Ergot alkaloids.

b. Progestins.

c. Prostaglandins.

d. Oxytocin.

2. Urgent control of uterine bleeding is often accomplished via ligation of the
   a. Hypogastric artery.
   b. External iliac artery.
   c. Anterior iliac vein.
   d. Cardinal artery.
   e. Uterosacral artery.

3. Ureter injury is not uncommon during the surgical management of a woman hemorrhaging after vaginal delivery because
   a. The uterine artery is the major blood supply of the ureter.
   b. The ureter is frequently compressed by a retroperitoneal hematoma.
   c. The ureter lies in close proximity to the uterine artery and may become injured during uterine artery ligation.
   d. The ureter and uterine artery lie within a common sheath in the pelvis.

4. A 34-year-old woman has just delivered monozygotic twins via a normal vaginal delivery with weights of 5.6 and 6.2 lb. She is now bleeding profusely from the uterus. On the basis of this information alone, which of the following causes is highest on your list of differential diagnoses?
   a. Uterine hyperstimulation
   b. Retained placental fragments
   c. Vaginal laceration
   d. Uterine atony

CHAPTER 33:
FETAL AND MATERNAL DEATH

1. Which of the following places the causes of maternal death in order from most common to least common?
   a. Hypertensive disease, infection, hemorrhage, thromboembolism
   b. Hemorrhage, hypertensive disease, infection, thromboembolism
   c. Thromboembolism, hemorrhage, hypertensive disease, infection
   d. Thromboembolism, hypertensive disease, hemorrhage, infection
   e. Hemorrhage, thromboembolism, hypertensive disease, infection

2. Perinatal death is defined as
   a. The sum of stillbirths and neonatal deaths per 1000 live births.

   b. The sum of intranatal and neonatal deaths per 1000 live births.
   c. The sum of abortions and stillbirths per 1000 live births.
   d. None of the above.

3. According to the National Center for Health Statistics, abortion is defined as
   a. Fetal loss prior to 20 weeks gestation.
   b. Fetal loss after 20 weeks gestation.
   c. Fetal loss after 28 weeks gestation.
   d. Fetal loss during the first or second trimester.
   e. Fetal loss before 28 weeks gestation.

4. The most common cause of fetal loss early in gestation is
   a. Ectopic implantation.
   b. Prematurity.
   c. Chromosomal abnormalities.
   d. Infection.
   e. Poor placental circulation.

5. Fetal death syndrome refers to
   a. Chronic fetal loss early in gestation.
   b. A complication of the retention of a dead fetus in the uterus.
   c. A maternal coagulopathy that adversely affects fetal oxygenation and thus commonly leads to fetal demise.
   d. A coagulopathy caused by fetal–maternal transfusion early in gestation.

6. The maternal mortality ratio refers to the number of maternal deaths from pregnancy-related causes per 100,000 live births.
   a. True
   b. False

CHAPTER 34:
PUBERTY, MENSTRUAL CYCLE, AND REPRODUCTIVE PHYSIOLOGY

1. Which of the following statements is most accurate?
   a. Thelarche is initiated with the production of increased levels of adrenal DHEAS
   b. Adrenarche generally occurs at age 12 to 13 years in females.
   c. Menarche usually occurs at 9 to 10 years of age.
   d. Thelarche refers to breast development and

is a relatively early physical finding of female pubertal development.

e. Just prior to the onset of puberty, serum LH and FSH decrease.

f. Both b and d.

g. Both d and e.

2. Primary amenorrhea in a 16-year-old girl without secondary sexual characteristics and with elevated FSH levels suggests

a. Idiopathic delayed puberty.

b. Pituitary dysfunction.

c. Ovarian insensitivity.

3. A woman has her maximal number of oocytes

a. At birth.

b. During intrauterine life.

c. At puberty.

4. The principal androgens produced by the adrenal gland are

a. Estrogen and progesterone.

b. Testosterone and DHT.

c. LH and FSH.

d. Pregnenolone and androstenedione.

e. DHEA and androstenedione.

f. Androstenedione and testosterone.

g. Spironolactone and DHEA.

5. Anovulatory cycles

a. Are common during the first few years of adolescence.

b. Generally result in a regular pattern of menstrual bleeding.

c. Are uncommon during adolescence but can cause infertility in adult life.

d. Frequently cause painful menses.

6. The average age of menarche in the United States is

a. 7 to 9 years old.

b. 9 to 11 years old.

c. 12 to 13 years old.

d. 13 to 15 years old.

7. A 12-year-old girl with moderate breast buds and Tanner 2 axillary and pubic hair comes to the physician. She is concerned because many of her friends have begun menstruating and she has not. The best advice to offer is to

a. Recommend to the parents a work-up for primary amenorrhea.

b. Recommend to the parents a work-up for secondary amenorrhea.

c. Advise the girl and her parents that her friends have begun menstruating early and she is right on time.

d. Advise the girl and her parents that there is no reason to suspect a pathological cause of the girl's lack of menses.

8. Which of the following set of analogies is most accurate?

a. FSH:granulosa cells as LH:theca cells

b. Estrogen:theca cells as progesterone:granulosa cells

c. LH:granulosa cells as FSH:theca cells

d. Estrogen:granulosa cells as progesterone:theca cells

9. The oocyte completes its first meiotic division

a. During fetal development.

b. Just prior to ovulation.

c. At the time of follicular recruitment.

d. At the time of fertilization.

10. Which of the following hormones support the corpus luteum during pregnancy?

a. Estrogen and progesterone

b. Progesterone

c. Human chorionic gonadotropin

d. Progesterone and human chorionic gonadotropin

11. Human chorionic gonadotropin is produced by the

a. Fetal gonads.

b. Amnion.

c. Chorionic laeve.

d. Placental trophoblast.

12. Fertilization most commonly occurs in the

a. Ampulla of the fallopian tube.

b. Isthmus of the fallopian tube.

c. Cornua of the fallopian tube.

d. Cornua of the uterus.

CHAPTER 35:
EVALUATION OF THE INFERTILE COUPLE

1. Of the following, the one that causes the most infertility is

a. Pelvic inflammatory disease with subsequent fallopian tube scarring.

b. The coital factor.

c. Anovulation.

d. The male factor.

2. Which of the following is most accurate?

    a. Infertility increases with maternal age, but miscarriage decreases.

    b. Infertility and miscarriage increase with maternal age.

    c. Infertility decreases with maternal age, but miscarriage increases.

    d. Infertility and miscarriage decrease with maternal age.

3. Which of the following is not analyzed as part of the routine semen analysis?

    a. Semen volume

    b. Sperm concentration

    c. Semen pH

    d. Sperm antibodies

    e. White blood cells

    f. Motility

4. Of the following, the best test to evaluate for a cervical component of infertility is

    a. Pelvic examination.

    b. Ultrasound.

    c. Basal body temperature analysis.

    d. Measurement of serum progesterone level.

    e. Post-coital analysis.

    f. Hysterosalpingogram.

    g. Pap smear.

5. Abnormal basal body temperature analysis suggests a(n)

    a. Corpus luteum defect.

    b. Endometrial defect.

    c. Ovulatory defect.

    d. Pituitary defect.

6. Fecundability refers to

    a. The percentage of women who become pregnant during one ovulatory cycle.

    b. The percentage of women who become pregnant during 12 ovulatory cycles.

    c. The percentage of women who become pregnant after 12 months of unprotected intercourse.

    d. One hundred minus the percentage of women who become pregnant after 12 months of unprotected intercourse.

CHAPTER 36:
ASSISTED REPRODUCTIVE TECHNIQUES

1. The zona reaction is

    a. The process by which a sperm gains entry into the oocyte.

    b. The process by which a sperm binds to the zona pellucida.

    c. The process by which the fertilized oocyte becomes implanted in the uterine cavity.

    d. A process that prevents fertilization of an oocyte by multiple spermatozoa.

2. Implantation

    a. Generally occurs within the first one to three days of fertilization.

    b. Is marked by the appearance of human chorionic gonadotropin in maternal serum.

    c. Occurs in the ampulla of the uterine cavity.

    d. Occurs just after the zona reaction.

3. Which of the following is true?

    a. Ovarian hyperstimulation is used to induce ovulation in women with premature menopause.

    b. Human menopausal gonadotropins are used to induce ovarian hyperstimulation.

    c. Human menopausal gonadotropins are used to maintain the corpus luteum in a pregnancy achieved by in vitro fertilization.

    d. Ovarian hyperstimulation results in premature menopause due to exhaustion of maternal oocyte stores.

4. Cryopreserved embryos

    a. Rarely lead to successful pregnancies.

    b. Cannot be preserved for more than one month.

    c. Often show an increased rate of chromosomal abnormalities.

    d. None of the above.

    e. Both a and b.

    f. Both a and c.

    g. All of the above.

5. Ovarian hyperstimulation syndrome is characterized by

    a. Excessive uterine bleeding with severe intravascular volume depletion.

    b. Bleeding into the ovaries secondary to excessive ovulatory stimulation.

c. Capillary vasodilatation leading to intravascular volume depletion.

d. Severe abdominal pain due to ovarian rupture.

e. Death or renal failure in more than 50% of patients.

CHAPTER 37:
CONTRACEPTION, STERILIZATION, AND ABORTION

1. For a given form of contraception, the method failure rate refers to the

a. Expected failure rate based on the patient's technique of contraceptive use.

b. Expected failure rate when the contraceptive is used correctly.

c. Expected failure rate when the contraceptive is used by a novice.

d. Expected failure rate based on how often the contraceptive is used.

2. Which of the following most accurately characterizes the benefits and drawbacks of the barrier method of contraception?

a. The barrier methods provide protection against many STDs but their efficacy is highly dependent on proper usage technique.

b. The barrier methods offer an easy-to-use method of contraception but do not afford protection against most STDs.

c. The barrier methods are quite difficult to use and do not provide STD protection.

d. The barrier methods are socially unacceptable to a majority of sexually active people.

3. Regarding intrauterine devices (IUDs),

a. Only the copper-containing type can be kept in place for more than one year.

b. The copper-containing IUD was removed from the market due to the high incidence of infection associated with its use.

c. Progestin-impregnated IUDs can be used for 12 months.

d. They work by eliciting a low-level, benign, infectious inflammatory response.

e. Only IUDs with multifilamented tails are clinically effective at preventing pregnancy.

4. According to WHO data, the overall risk of pelvic inflammatory disease (PID) in women with IUDs in place

a. Is significantly increased relative to that in women using no method of birth control.

b. Is somewhat increased in the first few months after placement.

c. Is significantly increased relative to that in women using other methods of birth control and is the reason why IUDs are rarely used in clinical practice.

d. None of the above are true.

5. Compared to women who use no contraception, the risk of ectopic pregnancy in women using a copper-containing IUD for birth control is

a. Increased.

b. Decreased.

c. About the same.

6. Which of the following contraceptives work by inhibiting the LH surge?

a. Norplant

b. Depo-Provera

c. Oral contraceptive pills

d. Both a and b

e. Both a and c

f. Both b and c

g. All of the above

h. None of the above

7. Regarding the use of oral contraceptive pills (OCPs) and the risk of pelvic inflammatory disease (PID),

a. OCPs have no effect on the rate of PID.

b. OCPs increase PID risk by encouraging increased sexual contact due to decreased fear of pregnancy.

c. OCPs decrease PID risk, probably by their effect on cervical mucus.

d. OCPs increase PID risk by altering the hormonal milieu that normally provides some protection against uterine infection.

8. The most popular method of contraception in the United States is

a. Sterilization.

b. Oral contraceptive pills.

c. Intrauterine devices.

d. Barrier methods (e.g., condoms, diaphragm, sponge).

e. Rhythm method.

9. RU-486 is a(n)

 a. Prostaglandin agent used to induce abortion in early pregnancy.

 b. Estrogen compound used to induce abortion in early pregnancy.

 c. Progesterone antagonist used to induce abortion in early pregnancy.

 d. Muscle stimulant used to induce spontaneous abortion in women for whom pregnancy carries too much health risk.

CHAPTER 38:
ENDOMETRIOSIS

1. Endometriosis

 a. Is a disease of older women in whom multiple menstrual cycles have led to aberrant placement of uterine tissue outside the uterine cavity.

 b. Is most commonly associated with menorrhagia.

 c. Is an infrequent cause of infertility.

 d. None of the above.

2. Elevation of CA-125 levels in a woman with known endometriosis

 a. Suggests underlying ovarian cancer.

 b. Is difficult to interpret because it may be from endometriosis or an underlying pathology.

 c. Suggests an incorrect diagnosis because endometriosis is not associated with elevated levels of CA-125.

3. Pathological findings consistent with endometriosis include the

 a. Presence of endometrial gland within the uterine myometrium.

 b. Presence of normal endometrial glands outside the uterine cavity.

 c. Presence of ovarian tissue outside the ovary.

 d. Presence of malignant endometrial glands outside the uterine cavity.

4. Endometriosis is a diagnosis that

 a. Must be confirmed by direct visualization of tissue, most often by laparoscopy.

 b. Is made based on clinical judgment.

 c. Is always associated with symptoms of menometrorrhagia.

 d. Is generally treated through medical management.

5. Which of the following is not an option for the temporary or sustained treatment of endometriosis?

 a. Danazol

 b. Testosterone

 c. Leuprolide

 d. Oral contraceptive pills

 e. Total abdominal hysterectomy and bilateral salpingo-ophorectomy

 f. Laparoscopic fulguration

CHAPTER 39:
MENOPAUSE

1. Menopause

 a. Occurs when estrogen levels are no longer adequate to sustain ovarian function.

 b. Is suggested by an LH:FSH ratio greater than 2.5.

 c. Represents the point at which ovarian follicles are depleted.

 d. Is marked by decrease in estrogen, LH, and FSH.

2. Which of the following statements is most accurate?

 a. Irregular menses in a 45-year-old woman with previously regular menstrual cycles is highly suggestive of an underlying endometrial pathology.

 b. Irregular menses in a 45-year-old woman with previously regular menstrual cycles may be a sign of perimenopause.

 c. Irregular menses in a 45-year-old woman with previously regular menstrual cycles suggests the onset of menopause.

 d. Irregular menses in a 45-year-old woman with previously regular menstrual cycles suggests the presence of an ectopic pregnancy.

3. In women who have been taking oral contraceptive pills (OCPs) prior to menopause,

 a. Hormone replacement therapy is associated with excess risk of thromboembolic complications.

 b. There is no need to change to another form of hormone replacement because OCPs provide appropriate doses of estrogen and progesterone for the post-menopausal woman.

 c. FSH and LH should be checked occasionally to determine when a patient is entering menopause.

4. Regarding cancer screening in the menopausal woman, which of the following is inaccurate?

   a. The American Cancer Society recommends annual mammograms for women older than 50 years of age.

   b. Fecal occult blood testing is recommended on an annual basis.

   c. Pap smears are not necessary due to decreased estrogen/progesterone stimulation.

   d. Post-menopausal bleeding requires careful work-up.

5. Urinary incontinence in a menopausal woman

   a. May improve with estrogen therapy.

   b. Is generally a sign of underlying disease.

   c. May be secondary to thinning of the urogenital mucosa.

   d. Requires biopsy.

   e. Both a and c.

   f. Both b and d.

6. Osteoporosis is defined as a(n)

   a. Decreased amount of abnormal bone.

   b. Increased amount of abnormal bone.

   c. Decreased amount of normal bone.

   d. Decreased mineralization of a normal amount of bone.

7. Which of the following is true?

   a. Falls in the elderly, though uncommon, are almost always life-threatening.

   b. Although only a small fraction of women older than 75 years experience vertebral fractures secondary to osteoporosis, in those who do, the result is frequently debilitating.

   c. Nearly 25% of women older than 80 years of age experience hip fractures, a significant fraction of which prove fatal.

   d. About 50% of women older than 75 years of age experience hip fractures, a significant fraction of which prove fatal.

8. Regarding hormone replacement therapy and cancer risk, which of the following statements is most accurate?

   a. Although hormone replacement therapy increases the rate of breast cancer, overall mortality in women taking hormone replacement therapy is lower than that in women taking no therapy.

   b. The addition of progesterone is not necessary for women without a uterus.

   c. Progesterone is added to the estrogen replacement regimen because it directly antagonizes the carcinogenic properties of estrogen.

   d. Progesterone therapy increases the risk of uterine cancer slightly, but the effect is not clinically significant except in those patients with a strong family history of uterine cancer.

9. The bisphosphonates

   a. Act by inhibiting osteoclastic bone resorption.

   b. Act by stimulating osteoblastic activity.

   c. Block the growth-stimulating effects of estrogens at the cellular level.

   d. Have mixed estrogen agonist/antagonist properties and thus may have a role in the primary management of post-menopausal females with a history of breast cancer.

CHAPTER 40:
HIRSUTISM AND VIRILIZATION

1. 5-alpha reductase

   a. Converts estrogen to testosterone at the base of the hair shaft to induce terminal hair development.

   b. Converts testosterone to dihydrotestosterone, which acts at the level of the hair shaft to induce terminal hair development.

   c. Converts dihydrotestosterone to its reduced form, which acts at the level of the hair shaft to induce terminal hair development.

   d. Converts estrogen to androstenedione, which acts at the level of the hair shaft to induce terminal hair development.

   e. Is an enzyme found only in males and accounts for the normal male pattern of hair distribution.

2. A 29-year-old woman presents with elevation of testosterone and DHEA-S levels. The most likely source for these hormones is

   a. The pituitary gland.

   b. An arrhenoblastoma.

   c. The adrenal gland.

   d. The ovary.

   e. Occult testicular tissue.

3. All of the following mechanisms contribute to the efficacy of oral contraceptives in the treatment of idiopathic hirsutism except a(n):

   a. Increase in sex-hormone binding globulin.

   b. Decrease in pituitary LH secretion.

c. Decrease in 5-alpha reductase activity.

d. Progestin antagonism of androgen at the receptor level.

e. Decrease in adrenal DHEA-S.

f. All of the above are related to the efficacy of oral contraceptives in the treatment of idiopathic hirsutism.

4. Other drug classes used to treat idiopathic hirsutism include all of the following except:

a. GnRH antagonists.

b. 5-alpha reductase inhibitors.

c. Progestins.

d. Spironolactone.

CHAPTER 41:
AMENORRHEA AND ABNORMAL UTERINE BLEEDING

1. A 13-year-old female presents to her pediatrician for an examination. She is Tanner 3 and has not begun menstruating. She is mildly obese. This girl most likely

a. Has polycystic ovarian syndrome because of her elevated weight and delayed menses.

b. Has primary amenorrhea.

c. Has secondary amenorrhea.

d. Has delayed menarche.

e. Has a pituitary disturbance with obesity and menstrual abnormality suggestive of Cushing's disease.

f. Is normal.

Questions 2–6 Match the following clinical scenario with the most likely diagnosis

a. Turner syndrome

b. Testicular feminization

c. Asherman syndrome

d. Premature ovarian failure

e. Pituitary tumor

f. Sheehan syndrome

g. Pregnancy

h. Anorexia nervosa

i. No abnormality

2. A 39-year-old G2P2 with amenorrhea and elevated FSH

3. A 19-year-old female who presents with primary amenorrhea and palpable inguinal mass

4. A 32-year-old G1P0 who had an abortion two months ago and now presents with secondary amenorrhea

5. A 50-year-old female who presents with amenorrhea, plus elevated FSH and LH levels

6. A 23-year-old female who presents with amenorrhea and an elevated prolactin level

Questions 7–10 Match the following clinical scenario with the appropriate term

a. Menorrhagia

b. Metrorrhagia

c. Polymenorrhea

d. None of the above

7. A 20-year-old female who experiences uterine bleeding unpredictably throughout the month

8. A 50-year-old female who experiences regular uterine bleeding for nine consecutive days each month

9. A 30-year-old female who experiences regular monthly periods plus occasional spotting in between periods

10. A 41-year-old female who experiences regular bleeding every two and a half weeks

11. Dysfunctional uterine bleeding is most common in

a. Women with endometriosis.

b. Women at the extremes of their reproductive years.

c. Multigravidas.

d. Women with uterine myomas.

12. The mechanism by which estrogen is useful in the control of acute uterine bleeding is by

a. Vasoconstriction of uterine vessels.

b. Stabilization of uterine endometrium.

c. Antagonizing the effect of progesterone.

d. Blocking gonadotropin release and consequently stopping uterine endometrial proliferation.

e. Stimulating gonadotropin release and consequently stabilizing the friable endometrial lining.

CHAPTER 42:
CHRONIC PELVIC PAIN

1. Chronic pelvic pain is

a. A diagnosis of exclusion when a woman experiences persistent pelvic pain in the absence of organic pathology.

b. Defined as pelvic pain lasting ≥6 weeks with or without intervals of relief.

c. Defined as pelvic pain lasting ≥6 months with or without intervals of relief.

d. More often than not a psychiatric diagnosis rather than the result of organic pathology.

e. None of the above.

2. The most common cause of chronic pelvic pain of organic etiology is

a. Adenomyosis.

b. Endometriosis.

c. Leiomyoma.

d. Surgical adhesions.

e. Gastrointestinal disorders.

CHAPTER 43:
PELVIC RELAXATION AND URINARY INCONTINENCE

1. Urinary incontinence

a. Is underreported to caregivers but estimated to affect about 5% to 10% of adult American women.

b. Is underreported to caregivers but estimated to affect about 15% to 35% of adult American women.

c. Is underreported to caregivers but estimated to affect about 1.5% to 3.5% of adult American women.

d. Is less common among menopausal women than women of childbearing years.

2. Stress urinary incontinence

a. Commonly occurs during episodes of sneezing, coughing, lifting, or other activities that increase intra-abdominal pressure.

b. May be diagnosed by urodynamic testing.

c. May result from an incompetent bladder outlet.

d. All of the above.

3. Genuine stress incontinence

a. Usually is the result of detrusor muscle instability.

b. Usually results from poor support of the bladder neck.

c. Is suggested by rotation of 30° from normal position on cotton swab examination.

d. Is suggested by rotation of 30° from normal position on cotton swab examination.

e. Both a and c.

f. Both a and d.

g. Both b and c.

h. Both b and d.

4. A female patient complains of intermittently feeling a strange bulge in her vagina along with occasional episodes of urinary incontinence. Which of the following statements about her condition is most accurate?

a. Her symptoms are suggestive of an "overactive bladder" resulting from excess bladder muscle contractile activity.

b. Her symptoms are suggestive of procidentia. She may be a candidate for surgical repair of an incompetent pelvic floor.

c. Her symptoms are suggestive of a cystocele causing bladder prolapse through a defect in the anterior vaginal wall

d. Her symptoms are diagnostic of genuine stress incontinence. Evaluation for urethropexy is probably indicated.

Questions 5–8   Match the following activity related to bladder control with the agent with which it is most closely associated. Answers may be used more than once.

a. Estrogens

b. Progesterones

c. Anticholinergic agents

d. Cholinergic agents

e. Alpha-antagonist agents

f. Alpha-agonist agents

5. A high concentration of receptors for these agents is present in the urethra, and use of these agents may ameliorate urinary urge symptoms.

6. These agents block bladder contractile activity.

7. These agents increase bladder capacity.

8. These agents may improve bladder neck tone.

9. A pessary

a. Is a device placed in the vagina that supports the vaginal walls and may be useful in the treatment of stress incontinence and/or pelvic floor prolapse.

b. Is a device placed in the urethra that maintains bladder neck patency in the setting of uterine prolapse.

c. Is the name of one of the repair procedures used to treat pelvic floor relaxation.

d. None of the above.

CHAPTER 44:
SEXUALLY TRANSMITTED DISEASES

1. The two most common causes of pelvic inflammatory disease are
   a. *Neisseria gonorrhoeae* and *Chlamydia trachomatis.*
   b. Syphilis and *Neisseria gonorrhoeae.*
   c. *Trichomonas* and *Gardnerella.*
   d. Syphilis and *Chlamydia trachomatis.*
   e. *Candida albicans* and gram-negative anaerobes.

2. Pelvic inflammatory disease
   a. Is an infection of the upper genital tract generally resulting from ascent of infection from the lower vaginal canal.
   b. Is usually a blood-borne infection that invades the upper genital tract via the systemic arterial system.
   c. Is a lower genital tract infection the risk of which is increased in women with multiple sexual partners.
   d. Both a and b.
   e. Both a and c.
   f. Both b and c.

3. All of the following antibiotic combinations may form acceptable regimens for the treatment of pelvic inflammatory disease according to CDC guidelines except:
   a. Ceftriaxone + doxycycline.
   b. Clindamycin + gentamicin + doxycycline.
   c. Benzathine penicillin + doxycycline.
   d. Ofloxacin + metronidazole.
   e. All of the following may be acceptable antibiotic combinations when used in the appropriate dosages and routes of administration.

4. Fitz-Hugh-Curtis syndrome
   a. Is the development of a tubo-ovarian abscess due to untreated pelvic inflammatory disease.
   b. Is suggested by the presence of adhesions between the liver and anterior abdominal wall resulting from prior pelvic infection.
   c. Is the name given to infertility resulting from tubal damage secondary to long-standing, untreated pelvic inflammatory disease.
   d. May be diagnosed by VDRL or RPR testing.

5. Syphilis is
   a. A viral infection that may be diagnosed by VDRL or RPR testing.
   b. A bacterial infection with the organism *Treponema pallidum.*
   c. A parasitic infection that can be diagnosed by serology.
   d. A protozoal infection that can be sexually transmitted.

6. Which of the following statements regarding syphilis testing is most accurate?
   a. VDRL and RPR tests measure the presence of nonspecific antibodies associated with *Treponema pallidum* infection.
   b. VDRL and RPR tests measure antibodies specific for the *Treponema* organism.
   c. FTA-ABS testing measures antibodies specific for *Treponema pallidum.*
   d. FTA-ABS testing measures the presence of nonspecific antibodies associated with *Treponema pallidum* infection.
   e. Both a and c.
   f. Both b and d.

Questions 7–15 Match the following description with the stage of syphilis it represents. Answers may be used more than once.
   a. Primary syphilis
   b. Secondary syphilis
   c. Tertiary syphilis
   d. Latent syphilis
   e. None of the above

7. Marked by the presence of a painful genital or oral chancre

8. Marked by the presence of a painless genital or oral chancre

9. Frequently asymptomatic but serological tests are positive

10. Characterized by cardiac or neurological symptoms

11. Marked by the presence of a maculopapular rash classically involving palms and soles

12. Marked by the presence of a papulovesicular rash classically involving palms and soles

13. Marked by the presence of condyloma lata

14. Marked by the presence of condyloma acuminata

15. Painless granulomas may be present

CHAPTER 45:
DYSMENORRHEA AND PREMENSTRUAL SYNDROME

1. Dysmenorrhea
   a. Is synonymous with premenstrual syndrome.
   b. Is pelvic pain that occurs before or during menstruation.
   c. Is usually associated with ovulatory menstrual cycles.
   d. Is usually associated with anovulatory menstrual cycles.
   e. Both b and c.
   f. Both b and d.
   g. Both a and c.
   h. Both a and d.

2. Which of the following are thought to be possible contributors to dysmenorrhea?
   a. Excess uterine contractile activity
   b. Ischemia resulting from reduced blood flow to the pelvis
   c. Excess prostaglandins
   d. Both a and b
   e. Both b and c
   f. Both a and c
   g. All of the above

3. Endometriosis
   a. Is the deposition of endometrial tissue outside the uterine cavity.
   b. Is characterized by hormonally responsive endometrial tissue, regardless of location.
   c. Is thought to be more common in women with cervical stenosis.
   d. Both a and b.
   e. Both b and c.
   f. All of the above.

4. Adenomyosis is
   a. The deposition of endometrial glands in the uterine myometrium.

   b. The deposition of endometrial tissue outside the uterine cavity.
   c. The deposition of endometrial glands on the uterine serosa.
   d. Abnormal hypertrophy of normally placed endometrial glands.

5. The pain associated with premenstrual syndrome usually occurs
   a. During the luteal phase of the menstrual cycle.
   b. During the follicular phase of the menstrual cycle.
   c. During ovulation.
   d. During menses.

6. All of the following therapies are routinely used in the treatment of PMS except:
   a. Fluoxetine.
   b. GnRH agonists.
   c. Surgical removal of the ovaries.
   d. Exercise therapy.

CHAPTER 46:
VULVOVAGINITIS

1. Select the features associated with *Candida albicans* overgrowth in the vagina.
   a. pH < 4.7
   b. pH > 5.0
   c. "Cheesy" discharge
   d. "Fishy" odor
   e. Hyphae on potassium hydroxide wet-mount slide
   f. Flagellated organisms on wet-mount slide
   g. Answers a, c, and e
   h. Answers b, c, and e
   i. Answers a, d, and f

2. A sexually active female patient presents with diffuse inguinal lymphadenopathy, malaise, and painful genital ulcers. A swab of the vesicular fluid is obtained. Which of the following findings is most consistent with the suspected diagnosis based on clinical presentation?
   a. The presence of multinucleated giant cells on Tzanck smear
   b. The presence of hyphae on potassium hydroxide wet-mount preparation
   c. The presence of Donovan inclusion bodies
   d. The presence of spirochetes on dark-field microscopic examination

3. Medical therapy for herpes simplex infection may include

a. Acyclovir.
b. Amantadine.
c. Clotrimazole.
d. Metronidazole.
e. Benzathine penicillin.

4. Condyloma acuminata are the result of infection with

a. HSV-1.
b. HSV-2.
c. HPV.
d. Syphilis.
e. Gonorrhea.

Questions 5–7 Match the following disease with its characteristic feature.

a. Donovan bodies
b. Chanchroid
c. Condyloma lata
d. Lymphogranuloma venereum

5. Syphilis

6. *Haemophilus ducreyi*

7. Granuloma inguinale

8. Lichen sclerosis

a. Is a condition of hyperplasia of the vulvar epithelium that may be treated with corticosteroids.
b. Is a condition of vulvar atrophy associated with loss of normal rete pegs.
c. Is a precancerous condition that requires biopsy.
d. May respond to topical corticosteroids and/or topical progesterone or testosterone agents.
e. Both a and d.
f. Answers a, c, and d.
g. Both b and d.
h. None of the above.

9. Behçet's syndrome is

a. A condition causing hyperplasia of the vulvar epithelium.
b. A condition marked by atrophy of the vulvar epithelium.
c. A condition characterized by herpetiform

lesions of the genital region, oral cavity, and other areas of the body.
d. An uncommon complication of Crohn's disease.

Chapter 47:
Ectopic Pregnancy

1. A patient presents to her physician complaining of abdominal pain and nausea. She states that a home pregnancy test taken one week ago was positive. A transvaginal ultrasound examination fails to reveal the presence of an intrauterine pregnancy. Her serum beta hCG level returns at 1500 mIU/mL. Four days later, the beta hCG level is 1800 mIU/mL. This woman's clinical and laboratory picture is most consistent with the diagnosis of

a. Ectopic pregnancy.
b. Spontaneous abortion.
c. Multiple gestation.
d. Incomplete abortion.

2. Methotrexate halts the growth of trophoblastic tissue by

a. Blocking implantation.
b. Inducing uterine contractions that dislodge the newly implanted embryo.
c. Blocking thymidylate synthetase enzymatic activity, thereby inhibiting DNA synthesis.
d. Blocking the dihydrofolate reductase enzyme, thereby inhibiting DNA synthesis.

Chapter 48:
Disorders of the Breast

1. Routine mammographic examination should commence at

a. 30 years.
b. 35 years.
c. 40 years.
d. 45 years.
e. 50 years.
f. Menopause.

2. Which of the following is not considered a risk factor for breast cancer?

a. Obesity
b. Multiparity
c. Early menarche
d. All of the above are risk factors for breast cancer.

3. Select the statement that most accurately characterizes fibroadenomas of the breast.

   a. They are thought to be premalignant and should therefore be excised if discovered.

   b. They frequently increase in size at menopause.

   c. They may exhibit "popcorn" calcification on mammogram.

   d. None of the above are accurate.

4. Which of the following statements regarding breast cysts is most accurate?

   a. They may be notable on palpation but can be confirmed by ultrasound examination.

   b. Cytological analysis of the fluid from a simple cyst is routinely performed to rule out pathology.

   c. They may vary in size during different stages of the menstrual cycle.

   d. Both a and b.

   e. Both b and c.

   f. Both a and c.

   g. All of the above.

Questions 5–7   Indicate whether the following features are characteristic of fibroadenomas or simple breast cysts.

   a. Fibroadenoma

   b. Simple breast cyst

   c. Both

   d. Neither

5. Often contain "spiculated" calcifications on mammogram

6. Frequently associated with visible changes of the breast skin

7. Are generally immobile breast masses

8. Mastalgia

   a. Is more common in the menopausal period.

   b. Is usually due to enhanced responsiveness of the breast tissue to hormonal fluctuations that occur during the menstrual cycle.

   c. Is uncommon in the absence of a dominant breast mass.

   d. Both a and b.

   e. Both b and c.

   f. All of the above.

9. Spontaneous nipple discharge

   a. Is a rare but significant symptom that may indicate breast pathology, notably intraductal papilloma.

   b. Is a relatively common symptom of breast pathology, notably intraductal papilloma.

   c. Is serious only when the discharge is grossly bloody.

10. Periductal mastitis

   a. Is the result of bacterial infection and can be managed with antibiotic therapy in most cases.

   b. Is more common in women of perimenopausal age.

   c. Is marked by a serosanguineous nipple discharge.

   d. All of the above.

   e. None of the above.

CHAPTER 49:
VULVAR AND VAGINAL NEOPLASMS

Questions 1–3   Match the following characteristic with the neoplasm with which it is most commonly associated.

   a. Paget's disease

   b. Bowen's disease

   c. Bowenoid papulosis

1. Associated with human papillomavirus infection

2. Patients often present with vulvar pruritus and eczematoid lesions

3. Approximately 20% of the patients have an underlying adenocarcinoma

4. Select the statement that most accurately characterizes vulvar malignancies.

   a. They are most frequently squamous cell in origin and often spread by local extension.

   b. They are most frequently adenocarcinomas and often spread by local extension.

   c. They are most frequently endometrioid and often spread hematogenously.

   d. They occur most commonly on the labia minora.

Questions 5–7   Match the following characteristic with the neoplasm with which it is most commonly associated. Answers may be used more than once.

    a. Endodermal sinus tumor

    b. Squamous cell carcinoma of the vagina

    c. Adenocarcinoma of the vagina

    d. Sarcoma botryoides

    e. Leiomyosarcoma

5. The most common vaginal tumor of adolescents

6. The most common vaginal tumor cell type

7. Females born to mothers treated with diethylstilbestrol during pregnancy are at increased risk for this type of vaginal neoplasm

8. A woman with a 2 cm vulvar cancer with one groin lymph node on the same side as the lesion containing metastatic disease has what stage of vulvar cancer?

    a. I

    b. II

    c. III

    d. IV

9. Women with in utero exposure to DES are at risk for which of the following problems?

    a. Cervical dysplasia

    b. Clear cell carcinoma of the vagina

    c. Uterine structural anomalies

    d. Adenosis of the vagina

    e. All of the above

10. The most common vaginal cancer is

    a. Sarcoma botryoides

    b. Clear cell adenocarcinoma

    c. Squamous cell carcinoma

    d. Metastatic from the cervix or vulva

    e. Endodermal sinus tumor

11. Which of the following is not considered a benign vulvar neoplasm?

    a. Bowenoid papulosis

    b. Bowen's disease

    c. Endometriosis

    d. Leiomyoma

    e. All of the above are benign vulvar neoplasms.

Questions 12–15 Match the following description with the stage of vaginal carcinoma that it represents. Answers may be used more than once.

    a. Stage 0

    b. Stage I

    c. Stage II

    d. Stage III

    e. Stage IV

    f. Stage V

12. Vaginal carcinoma with extension to the pelvic wall.

13. Vaginal carcinoma with extension beyond the true pelvis.

14. Vaginal carcinoma limited to the vaginal wall.

15. Vaginal carcinoma with involvement of the rectal mucosa.

CHAPTER 50:
DISORDERS OF THE CERVIX

1. Which of the following statements regarding the Pap smear is (are) correct?

    a. Samples of the endocervix are obtained.

    b. Samples of the ectocervix are obtained.

    c. Routine examinations should begin at coitarche or age 18 years.

    d. Both a and c.

    e. Both b and c.

    f. Answers a, b, and c.

2. Which of the following statements is most accurate?

    a. The Pap smear is one method of diagnosing cervical dysplasia that may be clinically silent.

    b. The Pap smear screens for cervical dysplasia and abnormal findings should be further evaluated with colposcopy and biopsy.

    c. The Pap smear does not detect non-dysplastic cervical changes such as those caused by human papillomavirus infection.

    d. The Pap smear is used to stage cervical neoplasms.

3. All of the following statements regarding the colposcopic examination are correct except:

    a. The exam is considered inadequate unless the entire transformation zone is visualized.

    b. Application of acetic acid is a method to highlight dysplastic cervical cells.

c. The examination is used to identify the location(s) appropriate for biopsy.

d. Normal cervical tissue reveals a mosaic-like vascular pattern as opposed to the punctate vessels that typically surround dysplastic tissue.

4. Cervical carcinoma

   a. Is the leading cause of gynecologic malignancy in the United States.

   b. Is the leading cause of death due to gynecologic malignancy in the United States.

   c. Is the third leading cause of gynecologic malignancy in the United States.

   d. Is the third leading cause of death due to gynecologic malignancy in the United States.

5. All of the following are risk factors for cervical dysplasia except:

   a. Cigarette smoking.

   b. Human papillomavirus infection.

   c. Nulliparity.

   d. Multiple sexual partners.

   e. Early age at coitarche.

6. Which of the following places the histological types of cervical cancer in correct order of frequency from most common to least common?

   a. Adenocarcinoma > adenosquamous cancer > squamous cancer

   b. Squamous cancer > adenosquamous cancer > adenocarcinoma

   c. Adenosquamous cancer > squamous cancer > adenocarcinoma

   d. Squamous cancer > adenocarcinoma > adenosquamous cancer

7. Cervical cancer is staged

   a. Surgically.

   b. Clinically.

8. A woman has a 5 cm lesion of the cervix with right parametrial involvement. A CT scan reveals right hydroureter and hydronephrosis. Her stage is

   a. Ib2.

   b. IIa.

   c. IIb.

   d. IIIa.

   e. IIIb.

9. Based on the stage of cervical cancer present in the woman in Question 8, her management is most likely to include

a. Surgical resection of the transformation zone.

b. Surgical resection of the transformation zone with pelvic lymph node dissection.

c. Radical hysterectomy with lymph node dissection.

d. Radiation and possibly chemotherapy.

10. The best predictor of survival in cervical cancer is based on

   a. The HPV serotype identified in the dysplastic cells.

   b. The stage of the carcinoma.

   c. The grade of dysplasia.

   d. The size of the cervical lesion.

11. Which of the following HPV serotypes is most strongly associated with cervical cancer?

   a. HPV 6

   b. HPV 11

   c. HPV 16

   d. HPV 35

Questions 12–15 Match the following description with the stage of cervical cancer it describes.

   a. Stage Ia

   b. Stage Ib

   c. Stage IIa

   d. Stage IIb

   e. Stage IIIa

   f. Stage IIIb

   g. Stage IVa

   h. Stage IVb

12. Tumor has spread to adjacent organs

13. Tumor involves the lower one-third of the vagina

14. Clinically apparent lesion involving only the cervix

15. Tumor has spread to the upper two-thirds of the vagina and does not involve the parametria

CHAPTER 51:
UTERINE LEIOMYOMA

1. Which of the following statements regarding uterine leiomyomata is (are) correct?

   a. They are composed of benign fibrous tissue.

b. They are more common in African American women.

c. They are sometimes referred to as "fibroids."

d. They are most common among women in their reproductive years.

e. Both a and d.

f. Answers a, c, and d.

g. Both b and d.

h. Answers b, c, and d.

i. All of the above.

2. A 43-year-old, G3P3, African American female has suffered from menorrhagia and dysmenorrhea from uterine leiomyomata for several years. She presents to her physician today complaining of an increased feeling of pelvic pressure escalating over the last three months. She says that she cannot button her pants and feels like she is pregnant. Her uterine size is equivalent to a gravid uterus of approximately 14 weeks gestation. Her only medication is an oral contraceptive pill for birth control that she has been taking for several years. Which of the following statements regarding her condition and continued management is most accurate?

a. The apparent rapid growth of her leiomyomata is worrisome and she should be evaluated with MRI or CT scan of the pelvis to rule out leiomyosarcoma or other malignancy.

b. She should stop her oral contraceptive pill, as the estrogen is likely to be causing the excess growth in her leiomyomata.

c. She should be reassured that uterine leiomyomata are benign neoplasms and may actually regress as she approaches menopause.

d. She may benefit from hysteroscopic removal of her leiomyomata.

3. Which of the following statements regarding the use of GnRH agonists in the treatment of uterine leiomyomata is most accurate?

a. They may be used as long-term therapy to manage the symptoms and size of the leiomyomata.

b. They are often used preoperatively to shrink the leiomyomata to a size more easily managed by surgical removal and to reduce preoperative bleeding caused by the leiomyomata.

c. They are known to induce permanent reduction in size and amount of bleeding

from uterine leiomyomata even when therapy is discontinued.

d. They no longer have a role in the management of uterine leiomyomata.

e. None of the above.

CHAPTER 52:
MALIGNANT DISORDERS OF THE UTERUS

1. Endometrial cancer

a. Arises from the uterine myometrium.

b. Is the fourth leading cause of gynecologic malignancy.

c. Is most commonly sarcomatous in origin.

d. None of the above.

2. Which of the following ranks the frequency of gynecologic malignancies in the United States from most common to least common?

a. Ovarian > cervical > vaginal > endometrial

b. Endometrial > ovarian > cervical > vaginal

c. Cervical > endometrial > ovarian

d. Ovarian > endometrial > cervical

3. A 53-year-old, G3P3, female comes to the physician's office with the complaint of vaginal bleeding. She entered menopause at 48 years of age and has never taken hormone replacement therapy. Which of the following statements regarding her continued management is most accurate?

a. She should be evaluated with a Pap smear.

b. She should be evaluated with a colposcopic exam.

c. She should be evaluated with an endometrial biopsy.

d. She is likely experiencing perimenopausal menstrual irregularity that is not pathological.

e. She should be given a trial of hormone replacement therapy to stabilize her uterine lining.

4. A 55-year-old, G0P0, female comes to her gynecologist for a routine evaluation. Her gynecologic history is unremarkable except that she reports she and her husband chose to adopt their two children because she was unable to conceive. She continues to menstruate normally. She is obese and has suffered from diabetes mellitus since age 38 years. Factors in this woman's his-

tory that place her at increased risk for endometrial cancer include

    a. Nulliparity and obesity.

    b. Nulliparity, obesity, and late-onset meno-
pause.

    c. Nulliparity, obesity, late-onset menopause,
and diabetes mellitus.

5. Which of the following statements accurately
characterizes the role of the Pap smear in the
work-up of endometrial cancer?

    a. The Pap smear is frequently abnormal in
women with endometrial cancer and can
be used as an efficient screening test for the
disease.

    b. The Pap smear is frequently abnormal in
women with endometrial cancer but is not
routinely used to evaluate possible endometrial cancer.

    c. The Pap smear infrequently reveals abnor-
mal endometrial cells in women with endometrial cancer.

    d. The Pap smear is a specific but not sensi-
tive test for endometrial cancer.

6. An endometrial stripe of 5 mm found on pelvic ultrasound examination is

    a. Reassuring of the likely absence of endo-
metrial carcinoma.

    b. Worrisome for possible endometrial malig-
nancy.

    c. Suggestive of endometrial hyperplasia of
either a benign or malignant etiology.

    d. Suggestive of endometrial atrophy possibly
consistent with menopause.

7. Endometrial cancer is staged

    a. Clinically.

    b. Surgically.

8. The most common cell type of endometrial
carcinoma is

    a. Squamous.

    b. Papillary serous.

    c. Mucinous.

    d. Myometrial.

    e. Adenosquamous.

    f. Endometrioid.

9. Uterine sarcomas

    a. Are noted for hematogenous spread.

    b. Are especially responsive to chemothera-
peutics.

    c. All of the above.

    d. None of the above.

10. The majority of women diagnosed with endometrial cancer in the United States are found
to have what stage of disease?

    a. I

    b. II

    c. III

    d. IV

11. A woman is found to have a deeply invasive
endometrial cancer with implants on the uterine
serosa. No other disease is found. Her stage is

    a. Ic.

    b. IIb.

    c. IIIa.

    d. IVb.

CHAPTER 53:
EVALUATION OF THE PELVIC MASS

1. The median age of patients diagnosed with
ovarian cancer is

    a. 32 years.

    b. 42 years.

    c. 52 years.

    d. 62 years.

    e. 72 years.

2. A woman presents with a history of infertility
and menorrhagia. On examination, she is obese
and somewhat hirsute. A pelvic ultrasound reveals bilateral cystic irregularities of the ovaries.
Based on this evaluation, her symptoms may be
caused by

    a. Mature ovarian teratoma.

    b. Polycystic ovarian syndrome.

    c. The presence of bilateral follicular cysts.

    d. The presence of bilateral luteal cysts.

    e. Ovarian carcinoma.

3. All of the following statements regarding ovarian teratomas are true except:

    a. They are also called dermoid cysts.

    b. They most commonly affect women in their
reproductive years.

    c. They have not been known to undergo ma-
lignant degeneration.

    d. They are bilateral in 10% to 15% of cases.

    e. All of the above statements are true.

Questions 4–6 Match the following marker with the ovarian tumor type with which it is most commonly associated.

    a. Endodermal sinus tumor

    b. Epithelial cell ovarian tumor

    c. Dysgerminoma

    d. Mature teratoma

4. CA-125

5. Lactate dehydrogenase

6. Alpha-fetoprotein

7. Which of the following ultrasound features of an ovarian mass is more worrisome for malignancy?

    a. Cystic components

    b. Solid components

8. Which of the following conditions may be associated with an elevated CA-125 level?

    a. Endometriosis

    b. Leiomyomata

    c. Breast cancer

    d. Cirrhosis

    e. All of the above

    f. None of the above

CHAPTER 54:
OVARIAN CANCER

1. Complete the following statement: Ovarian cancer ranks _____ in causes of cancer mortality in women in the United States.

    a. first

    b. second

    c. third

    d. fourth

2. Nulliparity, early menarche, and late menopause are all considered risk factors for ovarian cancer presumably because of

    a. The gonadotropin suppression associated with these states.

    b. The anovulatory cycles associated with these states.

    c. The elevated progesterones associated with these states.

    d. The increased number of ovulations associated with these states.

3. Which of the following statements regarding familial ovarian cancer syndromes is (are) true?

    a. They account for about 30% of cases of ovarian cancer.

    b. They include the Lynch II, breast–ovary, and site-specific ovarian cancer syndromes.

    c. They appear to be transmitted in an autosomal recessive pattern with variable penetration.

    d. They appear to be transmitted in an autosomal dominant pattern with variable penetration.

    e. Answers a, b, and c.

    f. Answers a, b, and d.

    g. Both b and c.

    h. Both b and d.

4. The Lynch II syndrome poses an increased risk for all of the following cancers except:

    a. Ovarian.

    b. Breast.

    c. Endometrial.

    d. Colorectal.

5. Epithelial cell ovarian tumors are

    a. The most common cell type associated with ovarian cancers.

    b. Frequently bilateral.

    c. Spread via peritoneal seeding.

    d. All of the above.

    e. None of the above.

6. Select the statement that most accurately reflects the relationship between endometrial carcinoma and granulosa cell ovarian tumors.

    a. Granulosa cell ovarian tumors frequently spread to the uterus via the lymphatics.

    b. Granulosa cell ovarian tumors frequently spread to the uterus via hematogenous spread.

    c. Granulosa cell ovarian tumors may secrete estrogen that can "feed" endometrial hyperplasia and dysplastic changes.

    d. There is no relationship between the two cancers.

7. A 34-year-old, G1P1, female presents to her physician with the complaint of excess hair growth on her abdomen and face. Meanwhile, she thinks her scalp hair is thinning. She also reports that her skin has been "breaking out" lately.

She is most concerned because these problems are new and seem to be getting worse rapidly. Which of the following statements is most accurate?

   a. Her history is worrisome for an androgen-secreting Sertoli-Leydig tumor, and she should undergo further evaluation.

   b. Her symptoms are suggestive of polycystic ovarian syndrome, and she may benefit from a trial of oral contraceptives to regulate her hormone levels.

   c. Her history is worrisome for a granulosa cell tumor, and she should undergo further evaluation.

   d. Her symptoms are not uncommon in women of their reproductive years, and she might benefit from the use of hair removal or hair bleaching systems.

8. A 54-year-old female has undergone a staging work-up for serous ovarian cancer. Her examination reveals extension of the neoplasm from the ovary to the pelvis. Based on this information, her stage is

   a. Ib.

   b. Ic.

   c. II.

   d. IIIa.

   e. IIIb.

CHAPTER 55:
GESTATIONAL TROPHOBLASTIC DISEASE

1. Choriocarcinomas are

2. Usually extremely responsive to chemotherapy.

3. Usually extremely responsive to radiation.

4. Known to spread via the lymphatics

5. Observed to frequently secrete alpha-fetoprotein.

6. Gestational trophoblastic disease may occur concomitant with a(n)

   a. Ectopic pregnancy.

   b. Normal pregnancy.

   c. Spontaneous abortion.

   d. Both a and b.

   e. Both a and c.

   f. Both b and c.

   g. All of the above.

7. During work-up of an incomplete molar gestation, bilateral cystic lesions of the ovaries are noted. Which of the following statements regarding these lesions is most accurate?

   a. They are suspicious for carcinomatous spread and should be sampled by frozen section before the operation is completed and removed if found to be malignant.

   b. They are likely to be theca lutein cysts that have developed as a result of stimulation by beta human gonadotropin produced by the molar gestation and should be removed during the operation.

   c. They are likely to be theca lutein cysts that should regress with removal of the molar gestation and therefore should not be surgically removed.

   d. They are probably benign follicular cysts unrelated to the molar gestation and need not be further evaluated at this time.

8. The most common site for metastatic gestational trophoblastic disease is the

   a. Ovary.

   b. Lungs.

   c. Bone.

   d. Brain.

   e. Breast.

Questions 5–7 Match the following characteristics with the type of molar gestation with which it is most commonly associated. Answers may be used more than once.

   a. Complete mole

   b. Incomplete mole

5. 46, XX chromosomal pattern

6. 69, XXY chromosomal pattern

7. Villi are markedly edematous

8. Patients recovering from the evacuation of a molar gestation are advised not to become pregnant for at least one year mainly because

   a. Serum beta-hCG is used to monitor disease recurrence and pregnancy would interfere with the interpretation of beta-hCG levels.

   b. There is an increased risk of a second molar gestation in the year following treatment.

   c. The chemotherapeutic agents used to induce uterine evacuation may have deleterious effects on the fetus.

   d. None of the above.

9. All of the following are features of good-prognosis metastatic gestational trophoblastic disease except:

   a. Serum beta-hCG of less than 40,000 mIU/mL.

   b. Disease duration of less than four months.

   c. Gestational trophoblastic disease following a normal term pregnancy.

   d. No metastases to the brain or liver.

   e. All of the above are features of good-prognosis gestational trophoblastic disease.

CHAPTER 56:
LEGAL ISSUES IN OBSTETRICS AND GYNECOLOGY

1. An "informed refusal" most commonly refers to

   a. The record of a physician's desire to terminate a physician–patient relationship.

   b. The record of a patient's unwillingness to accept responsibility for his or her medical conditions and the acknowledgment of the desire to have a guardian appointed on his or her behalf.

   c. The record of a patient's refusal to receive a recommended medical or surgical procedure.

   d. The record of a patient's refusal to participate in an experimental procedure.

2. A durable power of attorney

   a. Is generally the preferred surrogate decision maker when an individual becomes unable to make decisions on his or her own, because this individual has been appointed by the patient prior to becoming incapacitated.

   b. Is an individual appointed by the court to execute medical decision-making authority for an individual who is no longer able to make these decisions on his or her own.

   c. Is a set of written instructions that express a patient's wishes in the event of loss of ability to communicate or give consent for medical interventions.

3. A general medical records release

   a. May or may not include the release of HIV test results.

   b. Must include all medical information, including the diagnosis of AIDS.

   c. Is in most cases performed only with a patient's prior written authorization.

   d. Both a and c.

   e. Both b and c.

4. Which of the following most accurately characterizes the rights and responsibilities implicit in the physician–patient relationship?

   a. Physicians are obliged to treat all patients that come for care, regardless of their compliance with medical recommendations.

   b. Patients, but not physicians, may formally terminate a doctor–patient relationship.

   c. A physician may terminate a therapeutic relationship with the proper advanced written notice of his or her intent to do so.

   d. None of the above.

5. A physician is seeing a female patient for a routine prenatal examination. She is escorted by her husband and five-year-old daughter. The daughter has a large bruise on her forearm. It is wintertime and she has come with no coat. While her daughter and husband are out of the room, the patient starts crying. The patient states that her husband hit her daughter as punishment for a bad grade she received in school. Which of the following statements regarding the physician's responsibilities in this situation is most accurate?

   a. She should make a telephone report of the child abuse immediately and encourage her patient to report any domestic violence to the authorities.

   b. She should make a written report of the child abuse within 36 hours and encourage her patient to report any domestic violence to the authorities.

   c. She should make a written report of the child abuse and domestic violence within 36 hours of the visit.

   d. She should make a telephone report of the child abuse and domestic violence within 36 hours of the visit.

CHAPTER 57:
ETHICS IN OBSTETRICS AND GYNECOLOGY

1. A patient tells her gynecologist that she is depressed and wants "to kill myself with my shotgun." Her physician orders her held in a locked psychiatric ward against her will. This case is an example of

   a. Abandonment.

   b. Autonomy.

c. Paternalism.

d. Abuse.

2. According to the American College of Obstetricians and Gynecologists, sexual contact concurrent with a doctor–patient relationship is

a. Unethical.

b. Immoral.

c. Illegal.

d. Sometimes acceptable.

3. A chaperone should be present during a pelvic examination

a. If the patient is a minor.

b. Only if the patient and physician are of the opposite sex.

c. In all situations.

d. Unless the clinic is extremely busy.

CHAPTER 58:
DOMESTIC VIOLENCE

1. Typically, a battered woman is

a. Poor.

b. Poorly educated.

c. Abusing alcohol or drugs.

d. From any ethnic, religious, or socioeconomic group.

2. It is estimated that domestic violence is present at one time or another in what percentage of marriages and ongoing relationships?

a. 10%

b. 20%

c. 30%

d. 40%

e. 50%

3. A past history of abuse or rape

a. Is more common in battered women.

b. Is less common in battered women.

c. Has no significant relationship to a woman's vulnerability to future domestic violence.

4. Screening for domestic violence

a. Should include direct questions about potential emotional and physical abuse.

b. Should include a careful physical examination with attention to signs of healed injuries, bruises, and cuts.

c. Should be part of the routine medical care of all women.

d. Both a and b.

e. Both b and c.

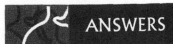 ANSWERS

Chapter 1
History of Obstetrics and Gynecology
1. c
2. a
3. b
4. d
5. b
6. a
7. c
8. e
9. a
10. b

Chapter 2
Clinical Anatomy of the Pelvis
1. d
2. a
3. c
4. b
5. a
6. d
7. c
8. a

Chapter 3
History and Physical Examination
1. d
2. e
3. a

Chapter 4
Gynecologic Procedures
1. d
2. g
3. f
4. d
5. c

Chapter 5
Anesthesia in Obstetrics and Gynecology
1. d
2. f
3. i
4. g
5. a
6. b
7. c
8. e
9. e
10. d

Chapter 6
Obstetric and Gynecologic Sonography
1. a
2. c
3. b

Chapter 7
Psychosocial Aspects of Women's Care
1. e
2. c
3. b
4. a
5. c

Chapter 8
Preventive Screening Guidelines
1. c
2. d
3. b

Chapter 9
Human Sexuality
1. c
2. b
3. h

Chapter 10
HIV in Obstetrics and Gynecology
1. c
2. d
3. b

Chapter 11
Maternal/Fetal Physiology
1. f
2. a
3. b
4. g
5. i
6. b
7. a
8. b
9. a
10. a
11. c
12. g

Chapter 12
Preconception and Antepartum Care
1. a
2. g
3. e
4. i
5. g

Chapter 13
Genetic Counseling
1. i
2. c
3. e
4. b

Chapter 14
First Trimester Bleeding
1. c
2. c
3. a
4. e
5. c
6. c

Chapter 15
Multiple Gestations
1. a
2. b

Chapter 16
Isoimmunization in Pregnancy
1. c
2. c
3. b

Chapter 17
Fetal Growth Abnormalities
1. b
2. d

Chapter 18
Teratology
1. d
2. f
3. a
4. g
5. b
6. d
7. a
8. f

ANSWERS

Chapter 19
Preterm Labor
1. d
2. c
3. d
4. b

Chapter 20
Premature Rupture of Membranes
1. a
2. e
3. c
4. c

Chapter 21
Third Trimester Bleeding
1. a
2. b
3. a
4. b
5. c
6. a
7. d

Chapter 22
Pre-eclampsia and Eclampsia
1. b
2. c
3. d
4. b
5. c
6. d

Chapter 23
Medical and Surgical Complications of Pregnancy
1. c
2. e
3. a
4. a
5. d
6. b
7. c
8. d
9. c
10. a
11. c
12. c
13. b
14. b

Chapter 24
Post-term Pregnancy
1. d
2. b
3. a
4. b
5. c
6. b

Chapter 25
Intrapartum Care: Management of Labor and Delivery
1. e
2. e
3. e
4. a
5. d
6. a
7. a
8. c

Chapter 26
Abnormal Labor and Fetal Distress
1. c
2. d
3. d
4. a
5. c
6. e
7. a
8. b
9. c
10. a
11. d
12. a

Chapter 27
Operative Vaginal Delivery
1. c
2. d
3. d

Chapter 28
Neonatal Assessment
1. c
2. b
3. a
4. c
5. c
6. f
7. a
8. c
9. c
10. c
11. b

Chapter 29
Post-partum Care
1. b
2. b
3. b

Chapter 30
Lactation
1. d
2. c
3. f
4. b
5. e
6. c
7. a

Chapter 31
Post-partum Infection
1. h
2. f
3. d

Chapter 32
Managing Hemorrhaging Complications in Obstetrics and Gynecology
1. b
2. a
3. c
4. d

Chapter 33
Fetal and Maternal Death
1. e
2. a
3. a
4. c
5. b
6. a

Chapter 34
Puberty, Menstrual Cycle, and Reproductive Physiology
1. d
2. c
3. b
4. e
5. a
6. c
7. d
8. a
9. b
10. d
11. d
12. a

Chapter 35
Evaluation of the Infertile Couple
1. d
2. b
3. d
4. e
5. c
6. a

Chapter 36
Assisted Reproductive Techniques
1. d
2. b
3. c
4. d
5. c

Chapter 37
Contraception, Sterilization, and Abortion
1. b
2. a
3. c
4. b
5. b
6. g
7. c
8. a
9. c

Chapter 38
Endometriosis
1. d
2. b
3. b
4. a
5. b

Chapter 39
Menopause
1. c
2. b
3. c
4. c
5. e
6. c
7. c
8. b
9. a

Chapter 40
Hirsutism and Virilization
1. b
2. c
3. c
4. a

Chapter 41
Amenorrhea and Abnormal Uterine Bleeding
1. f
2. d
3. b
4. c
5. i
6. e
7. b
8. a
9. d
10. c
11. b
12. b

Chapter 42
Chronic Pelvic Pain
1. c
2. b

Chapter 43
Pelvic Relaxation and Urinary Incontinence
1. b
2. d
3. h
4. c
5. a
6. c
7. c
8. f
9. a

Chapter 44
Sexually Transmitted Diseases
1. a
2. a
3. c
4. b
5. b
6. e
7. e
8. a
9. d
10. c
11. b
12. e
13. b
14. e
15. c

Chapter 45
Dysmenorrhea and Premenstrual Syndrome
1. e
2. g
3. f
4. a
5. a
6. c

Chapter 46
Vulvovaginitis
1. g
2. a
3. a
4. c
5. c
6. b
7. a
8. g
9. c

Chapter 47
Ectopic Pregnancy
1. a
2. d

Chapter 48
Disorders of the Breast
1. c
2. b
3. c
4. f
5. d
6. d
7. d
8. b
9. a
10. b

Chapter 49
Vulvar and Vaginal Neoplasms
1. b
2. a
3. a
4. a
5. d
6. b
7. c
8. c
9. e
10. d
11. e
12. d
13. e
14. b
15. e

ANSWERS

Chapter 50
Disorders of the Cervix
1. f
2. b
3. d
4. c
5. c
6. d
7. b
8. e
9. d
10. b
11. c
12. g
13. e
14. b
15. c

Chapter 51
Uterine Leiomyoma
1. h
2. a
3. b

Chapter 52
Malignant Disorders of the Uterus
1. d
2. b
3. c
4. c
5. c
6. a
7. b
8. f
9. a
10. a
11. c

Chapter 53
Evaluation of the Pelvic Mass
1. c
2. b
3. c
4. b
5. c
6. a
7. b
8. e

Chapter 54
Ovarian Cancer
1. d
2. d
3. h
4. b
5. d
6. c
7. a
8. c

Chapter 55
Gestational Trophoblastic Disease
1. a
2. g
3. c
4. b
5. a
6. b
7. a
8. a
9. c

Chapter 56
Legal Issues in Obstetrics and Gynecology
1. c
2. a
3. d
4. c
5. a

Chapter 57
Ethics in Obstetrics and Gynecology
1. c
2. a
3. c

Chapter 58
Domestic Violence
1. d
2. e
3. a
4. f

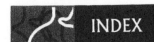

INDEX

Note: Page numbers with an *f* indicate figures; those with a *t* indicate tables.

Printed and bound by CPI Group (UK) Ltd, Croydon, CR0 4YY